PRINCIPLES AND PRACTICE

Springer
Berlin
Heidelberg
New York
Barcelona
Budapest
Hong Kong
London
Milan
Paris
Singapore
Tokyo

E. Raz (Ed.)

Gene Vaccination: THEORY AND PRACTICE

With 44 Figures and 12 Tables

Springer

Eyal Raz, M.D., Associate Professor
Department of Medicine
University of California, San Diego
9500 Gilman Drive
La Jolla, CA 92093-0663
USA

ISBN-13: 978-3-642-46869-8

Library of Congress Cataloging-in-Publication Data applied for

Die Deutsche Bibliothek – CIP-Einheitsaufnahme

Gene vaccination : theory and practice ; with 12 tables / E. Raz (ed.). - Berlin ; Heidelberg ; New York ; Springer, 1998
(principles and practice)
ISBN-13: 978-3-642-46869-8 e-ISBN-13: 978-3-642-46867-4
DOI: 10.1007/978-3-642-46867-4

Softcover reprint of the hardcover 1st edition 1998

Production: PRO EDIT GmbH, 69126 Heidelberg, Germany
Cover Design: Frido Steinen-Pro, Estudio Calamar, Spain
Typesetting: Mitterweger Werksatz GmbH, 68723 Plankstadt, Germany
SPIN: 10673570 27/3136-5 4 3 2 1 0 - Printed on acid-free paper

Contents

List of Contributors

BLAZCYK-THURIN, M.A.
The Wistar Institute, 3601 Spruce Street, Philadelphia, PA 19104, USA

BRAZOLOT MILLAN, CYNTHIA L.
Loeb Research Institute,
Ottawa Civic Hospital,
1053 Carling Avenue, Ottawa,
Canada K1Y 4E9

BROIDE, DAVID
Department of Medicine,
University of California San Diego,
9500 Gilman Drive, La Jolla,
CA 92093-0663, USA

CARSON, DENNIS A.
Department of Medicine and the Sam and Rose Stein Institute for Research on Aging, University of California, San Diego, 9500 Gilman Drive, La Jolla, CA 92093-0663, USA

CHAROENVIT, YUPIN
Malaria Program, Naval Medical
Research Institute Annex,
12300 Washington Avenue, Rockville,
MD 20852 USA

CONOVER, JACQUELINE
Section of Retroviral Immunology, Division of Viral Products, Center for Biologics Research and Evaluation, Food and Drug Administration, Bldg. 29A Rm 3D 10HFM 454, Bethesda, MD 20892, USA

CORR, MARIPAT
Department of Medicine and The Sam and Rose Stein Institute for Research on Aging, University of California, San Diego, 9500 Gilman Drive, La Jolla, CA 92093-0663, USA

DAVIS, HEATHER L.
Loeb Research Institute,
Ottawa Civic Hospital,
1053 Carling Avenue, Ottawa,
Canada K1Y 4E9
and Faculties of Health Sciences & Medicine, University of Ottawa, Ottawa, Canada

DENG, H.
The Wistar Institute, 3601 Spruce Street, Philadelphia, PA 19104, USA

DOOLAN, DENISE L.
Malaria Program, Naval Medical
Research Institute Annex,
12300 Washington Avenue, Rockville,
MD 20852 USA

ERTL, H.C.J.
The Wistar Institute, 3601 Spruce Street, Philadelphia, PA 19104, USA

GARDNER, MALCOLM J.
Malaria Program, Naval Medical
Research Institute Annex,
12300 Washington Avenue, Rockville,
MD 20852 USA

GERLONI, MARA
The Department of Medicine
and Cancer Center,
University of California,
San Diego, 9500 Gilman Drive, La Jolla,
CA 92093-0063, USA

GRAMZINSKI, ROBERT A.
Malaria Program, Naval Medical
Research Institute Annex,
12300 Washington Avenue, Rockville,
MD 20852 USA

GU, MILLI
Section of Retroviral Immunology,
Division of Viral Products, Center for
Biologics Research and Evaluation,
Food and Drug Administration,
Bldg. 29A Rm 3D 10HFM 454, Bethesda,
MD 20892, USA

HE, Z.
The Wistar Institute, 3601 Spruce Street,
Philadelphia, PA 19104, USA

HEDSTROM, RICHARD C
Malaria Program, Naval Medical
Research Institute Annex,
12300 Washington Avenue, Rockville,
MD 20852 USA

HOBART, PETER
Vical Incorporated, San Diego, CA, USA

HOFFMAN, STEPHEN L.
Malaria Program, Naval Medical
Research Institute Annex,
12300 Washington Avenue, Rockville,
MD 20852 USA

ICHINO, MOTOHIDE
Section of Retroviral Immunology,
Division of Viral Products,
Center for Biologics Research
and Evaluation,
Food and Drug Administration,
Bldg. 29A Rm 3D 10HFM 454, Bethesda,
MD 20892, USA

INCHAUSPÉ, GENEVIÈVE
INSERM U 271, 151 Cours Albert-Thomas,
69003 Lyon, France

KIM, JONG J.
Department of Chemical Engineering
and Department of Pathology
and Laboratory Medicine,
University of Pennsylvania,
505 Stellar-Chance, 422 Curie Blvd.,
Philadelphia, PA 19104, USA

KIPPS, THOMAS J.
UCSD Human Gene Therapy Program,
Division of Hematology/Oncology,
Department of Medicine,
UCSD School of Medicine, La Jolla,
CA 92093-0663, USA

KLINMAN, DENNIS M.
Section of Retroviral Immunology,
Division of Viral Products,
Center for Biologics Research
and Evaluation,
Food and Drug Administration,
Bldg. 29A Rm 3D 10HFM 454, Bethesda,
MD 20892, USA

KUMAR, ANITA
Malaria Program, Naval Medical
Research Institute Annex,
12300 Washington Avenue, Rockville,
MD 20852 USA

LAMBERT, PAUL-HENRI
WHO Collaboration Center for Neonatal
Vaccinology, Departments of Pathology
and Pediatrics, University of Geneva,
1 rue Michel Servet, 1211 Geneva 4,
Switzerland

LEE, DELPHINE J.
Department of Medicine and the Sam
and Rose Stein Institute for Research
on Aging, University of California,
San Diego, 9500 Gilman Drive, La Jolla,
CA 92093-0663, USA

Lowrie, Douglas B.
National Institute for Medical Research,
The Ridgeway, Mill Hill,
London NW7 1AA, UK

Margalith, Michal
Vical Incorporated, San Diego, CA, USA

Mendoza, Robert B.
UCSD Human Gene Therapy Program,
Division of Hematology/Oncology,
Department of Medicine,
UCSD School of Medicine, La Jolla,
CA 92093-0663, USA

Mor, Gil
Section of Retroviral Immunology,
Division of Viral Products, Center for
Biologics Research and Evaluation,
Food and Drug Administration,
Bldg. 29A Rm 3D 10HFM 454, Bethesda,
MD 20892, USA

Norman, Jon A.
Vical Incorporated, San Diego, CA, USA

Pasquini, S.
The Wistar Institute, 3601 Spruce Street,
Philadelphia, PA 19104, USA

Raz, Eyal
Department of Medicine,
University of California San Diego,
9500 Gilman Drive, La Jolla,
CA 92093-0663, USA

Roman, Mark
Dynavax Technologies Coporation,
3099 Science Park Road, San Diego,
CA 92121, USA

Sacci Jr., John B.
Malaria Program, Naval Medical
Research Institute Annex,
12300 Washington Avenue, Rockville,
MD 20852
and Department of Microbiology and
Immunology, University of Maryland
School of Medicine, Baltimore, MD, USA

Sedegah, Martha
Malaria Program, Naval Medical
Research Institute Annex,
12300 Washington Avenue, Rockville,
MD 20852
and Department of Microbiology and
Immunology, University of Maryland
School of Medicine, Baltimore, MD, USA

Siegrist, Claire-Anne
WHO Collaboration Center for Neonatal
Vaccinology, Departments of Pathology
and Pediatrics, University of Geneva,
1 rue Michel Servet, 1211 Geneva 4,
Switzerland

Silva, Celio L.
University of Sao Paulo, Sao Paulo,
Brazil

Spiegelberg, Hans L.
Department of Pediatrics,
University of California San Diego,
School of Medicine, La Jolla,
CA 92093, USA

Takeno, Mitsuhiro
Section of Retroviral Immunology,
Division of Viral Products, Center for
Biologics Research and Evaluation,
Food and Drug Administration,
Bldg. 29A Rm 3D 10HFM 454, Bethesda,
MD 20892, USA

Tascon, Ricardo E.
National Institute for Medical Research,
The Ridgeway, Mill Hill,
London NW7 1AA, UK

Tighe, Helen
Department of Medicine and The Sam
and Rose Stein Institute for Research
on Aging, University of California,
San Diego, Clinical Sciences Building,
Room 126, 9500 Gilman Drive, La Jolla,
CA 92093-0663, USA

Wang, Ruobing
Malaria Program, Naval Medical Research Institute Annex, 12300 Washington Avenue, Rockville, MD 20852 USA

Wang, Y.
The Wistar Institute, 3601 Spruce Street, Philadelphia, PA 19104, USA

Weiner, David B.
Department of Pathology and Laboratory Medicine, University of Pennsylvania, 505 Stellar-Chance, 422 Curie Blvd., Philadelphia, PA 19104, USA

Weiss, Walter R.
Malaria Program, Naval Medical Research Institute Annex, 12300 Washington Avenue, Rockville, MD 20852 USA

Wu, Yunqi
UCSD Human Gene Therapy Program, Division of Hematology/Oncology, Department of Medicine, UCSD School of Medicine, La Jolla, CA 92093-0663, USA

Xiang, Z.Q.
The Wistar Institute, 3601 Spruce Street, Philadelphia, PA 19104, USA

Xiong, Sidong
The Department of Medicine and Cancer Center, University of California, San Diego, 9500 Gilman Drive, La Jolla CA 92093-0063, USA

Yamshchikov, Galina
Section of Retroviral Immunology, Division of Viral Products, Center for Biologics Research and Evaluation, Food and Drug Administration, Bldg. 29A Rm 3D 10HFM 454, Bethesda, MD 20892, USA

Zanetti, Maurizio
The Department of Medicine and Cancer Center, University of California, San Diego, 9500 Gilman Drive, La Jolla CA 92093-0063, USA

Introduction:
gene vaccination, current concepts and future directions

Eyal Raz

Department of Medicine, University of California San Diego, 9500 Gilman Drive,
La Jolla, CA 92093-0663, USA

Gene vaccination: the phenomenon

Intramuscular (i.m.) inoculation with plasmid (p) DNA encoding a specific antigen (gene vaccination) has been shown to induce both antibodies and cytotoxic T lymphocyte (CTL) responses [12, 23, 37, 40, 41]. In different models of viral diseases, in which challenge of immunized animals with virulent virus is possible, these responses have been found to be protective [28, 37]. Antibodies have been raised in various species (e.g., chickens, mice, ferrets, cattle and non-human primates) by the injection of pDNA that encode various antigens such as: hemagglutinin [37], matrix protein and nucleoprotein from the influenza virus [9], glycoprotein (gp) 120 and pg160 from the HIV-1 ([40, 41] and Kim et al. in this issue), gIV from bovine herpes virus [7], surface gp from rabies virus [43], hepatitis B virus (HBV) surface antigen ([8, 14] and Davis et al. in this issue), the malaria sporozoite protein ([16] and Hedstorm et al. in this issue), the heat-shock protein (hsp) 65 antigen from mycobacteria tuberculosis ([36] and Lowrie et al. in this issue), and hepatitis C virus (HCV) core antigen ([15] and Inchauspe in this issue). The immune response induced by injection of pDNA-encoded viral antigens persisted more than 12 months in Rhesus monkeys [9, 40, 41].

Gene vaccination has also been successfully utilized to elicit anti-tumor [4], anti-idiotype [35, 42], and alloimmune responses [13], to suppress an autoimmune disease such as experimental allergic encephalitis [39] as well as to inhibit IgE formation and allergic responses ([17, 29, 30] and Roman et al. in this issue).

However, muscle is not considered the best site for antigen presentation because it contains few, if any, dendritic cells (DC), macrophages and lymphocytes [28]. The skin and mucous membranes are the anatomical sites where most exogenous antigens are normally encountered [33]. The skin-associated lymphoid tissue contains specialized cells which enhance immune responses [34]. The keratinocytes produce interleukin-1 (IL-1), tumor necrosis factor-α (TNF-α) and IL-12 [1], which can activate macrophages, lymphocytes and DC. The Langerhans' cells (LC) of the skin carry the antigen from the skin to the draining lymph nodes. Antigen-loaded antigen-presenting cells (APC) such as LC or DC are potent activators of naive T lymphocytes. Furthermore, it has recently been shown that in gene-vaccinated animals, bone marrow-derived cells (e.g., APC) and not somatic cells (e.g., myocytes) dictate the nature of the subsequent immune response to the gene product ([15] and Corr et al. in this issue). Therefore, the in vivo transfection of dermal and epidermal cells, and especially APC, would be expected to provide an efficient route for gene immunization that mimics the physiological response to viral infections of the skin, as has recently been demonstrated [4, 28]. Indeed, intradermal (i.d.) injection of pDNA encoding influenza nucleoprotein (NP) or *Escherichia coli* β-galactosidase (β-gal) in a human cytomegalovirus-based expression vector led to prolonged intracellular antigen expression by keratinocytes, fibroblasts and cells with the morphology of macrophages and DC in the dermis [5, 28]. The i.d. gene vaccination induced both antibodies and CTLs specific for the gene product which persisted for at least 17 months post-inoculation [28], and protected the gene vaccinated mice from lethal challenge by the influenza virus [28]. Thus, i.d. or i.m. gene vaccination are both effective routes for the induction of antigen-specific humoral and cellular immune responses.

Analysis of the T cell response to the gene product induced by the i.m. and the i.d. routes has shown that gene vaccination elicits an antigen-specific Th1 response to the encoded antigen [22, 29], whereas gene gun immunization generates Th0/Th2 immune response [10]. The induction of a Th1 response to protein antigens, such as allergens, has been used to down-regulate IgE and allergic responses (see Roman et al. in this issue).

The adjuvanticity of DNA: the role of the immunostimulatory DNA sequences

One of the most intriguing questions that is frequently asked is "Why does gene vaccination which generates only picograms or nanograms of gene product (antigen) induces a strong immune response that is usually a Th1 response, whereas immunization of animals with the same dose of antigen (picograms or a few nanograms) does not elicit any respone at all"!?

In animals models potent adjuvants magnify the immune response to low concentrations of the injected antigen. However, since gene vaccination is usually employed without any adjuvant, as "naked" pDNA (dissolved in normal saline), it was difficult to understand why it is such an effective vaccine. It was then discovered that certain DNA sequences in the pDNA backbone act as adjuvants and may control the nature of the subsequent immune response to the gene product [20, 31].

Several types of polynucleotides are mitogenic for lymphocytes. For example, polymers composed of guanosine and cytosine (poly G:C), or inosine and cytosine (poly I:C), are potent inducers of interferon-α (IFN-α) and activate the lytic potential of macrophages and natural killer (NK) cells [46]. By synthesizing oligodeoxynucleotides (ODN) from different regions of the mycobacterial genome, single-stranded 45mer ODN were identified which also activate macrophages and NK cells. This cell activation was attributed to DNA sequences containing a CpG motif within a palindromic hexamer that follow the formula: 5′-purine-purine-CG-pyrimidine-pyrimidine-3′ (e.g., 5′-GACGTC-3′, 5′-AGCGCT-3′ and 5′-AACGTT-3′) in the ODN [45]. Bacterial DNA (but not vertebrate) was also shown to induce B cell proliferation and immunoglobulin secretion [24]. The mechanism of this B cell stimulation has been unclear. Structural differences between bacterial and vertebrate DNA such as the presence of adenosine or cytosine methylation in the vertebrate genome, and/or the absence of CpG suppression in bacteria, were claimed to be responsible for the observed phenomenon [26]. Indeed, Krieg et al. [21] showed that the elimination of the CpG in a particular ODN invariably abolished immune stimulation, but changes in the ODN sequences that did not affect the CpG or the flanking bases did not alter the immunostimulatory (IS) effect. Furthermore, they extended the initial observations of the IS effects to non-palindromic CpG-enriched ODN [21]. Subsequent studies showed that CpG-enriched ODN also induce the secretion of IL-6 and IL-12 [19] and IFN-α [6, 27].

By adding or deleting various IS sequences (ISS)-ODN to or from different pDNAs, it was demonstrated that the ISS have a pivotal role in the induction of the subsequent immune response to the gene product in gene-vaccinated animals. The enhanced Th1 immune response induced by gene vaccination is the consequence of the activation of the innate immune response by the ISS in the pDNA backbone [30, 31], rather than the low dose of intracellularly produced antigen. The cell activation products induced by the ISS, i.e., IFN-α [3], IFN-β [43], IL-12 [37], and IL-18 [25], are established inducers of IFN-γ synthesis and promote the differentiation of naive T helper cells to Th1 lymphocytes. Thus, the ISS activate the precise innate cytokine network required to promote Th1 differentiation (see Fig. 1). In a recent study it was demonstrated that this approach is also applicable to a protein antigen. Protein antigen(s) co-administered with ISS-enriched, non-coding pDNA or with ISS-ODN, elicited a Th1 response, while proteins co-administered with ISS-deficient pDNA induced a Th2 response [30]. Thus, this particular property of ISS-induced cell activation can be used to evoke a Th1 response to co-administered protein antigens (see Fig. 1).

Based on empirical results, Freund et al. [11] utilized mycobacterial as a major constituent in their adjuvant formula [11]. This finding led to the discovery of immunomodulatory DNA sequences (in the mycobacterial genome) that selectively enhanced NK cell activity [18]. Preliminary data suggest that the potent IS effects of Freund's adjuvant may depend upon these ISS in the mycobacterial genome [18] in addition to the cell wall ingredients such as lipids and protein, to which the adjuvant properties have been previously attributed [11]. It is of interest that the in vivo administration of ISS-enriched pDNA (i.e., pUC19), in contrast to complete Freund's adjuvant, does not induce inflammatory reactions at the injected site [28]. Thus, the ISS-pDNA adjuvant can provide, in part, the IS effects of the Freund's adjuvant without the severe inflammatory and toxic side effects attributed to the paraffin oil and the mycobacterial cell wall products.

Transfection of fresh human macrophages with ISS-enriched pDNA or with ISS-ODN, but not with ISS-deficient pDNA or mutated ODN (where the CG are replaced with GG), increased IFN-α, IFN-β, IL-12, and IL-18 mRNA levels [30, 31]. These cytokines of the innate immune system are established inducers of IFN-γ synthesis. Incubation of human macrophages with IFN-α raised IL-12 and IL-18 mRNA in a dose-dependent manner, suggesting an amplifying role for the former cytokine in ISS-induced stimulation [30] and possibly in the induction of a Th1 response in this system. Furthermore, transfection of human peripheral blood mononuclear cells with ISS-ODN but not with mutated ODN resulted in the production of IFN-γ by NK cells, as previously described [18], in addition to the production of IFN-α, IFN-β and IL-12 by macrophages [30].

Thus, pDNA vaccines contain two conceptually distinct units: (i) a transcription unit that directs antigen synthesis, and (ii) an adjuvant unit (ISS) in the pDNA backbone which elicits the production of IFN-α, IFN-β, IL-12 and IL-18 from the transfected APC (macrophages) and IFN-γ from NK cells. These cytokines synergisticly

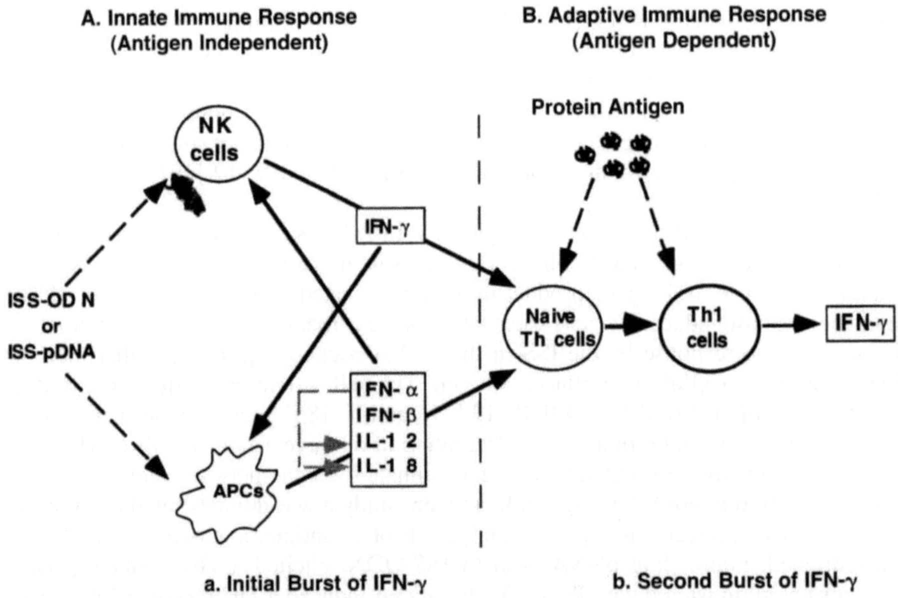

Fig. 1 A, B. A postulated mechanism for the induction of a Th1 response by gene vaccination or protein/pDNA co-immunization (**A**) immunostimulatory sequence (ISS)-pDNA trigger the release of interferon-γ (*IFN*-γ and IFN-γ inducers by natural killer (*NK*) cells and antigen-presenting cells (*APC*) e.g., macrophages), respectively. These responses result in the initial burst of IFN-γ in an antigen-independent fashion (in tissue culture, the level of the initial IFN-γ burst is in the pg/ml range). IFN-α has an amplification role on IL-12 and IL-18 synthesis. The release of IL-12 from APC results in further IFN-γ production by T cells [2]. **B** In the presence of an antigen, the secreted innate cytokines prime naive T helper cells to differentiate toward Th1 cells that produce additional IFN-γ in an antigen-dependent fashion (Th1 response). The level of the second IFN-γ burst is in the ng/ml range. Vectors for gene vaccination provide both the adjuvant (ISS) and the genetic information for the encoded antigen

promote Th1 differentiation of naive T cells and Th1 response to the encoded antigen. Therefore pDNA for gene vaccination should be designed to include ISS to enhance the subsequent immune response to the encoded gene as shown in Fig. 1.

Future directions

The mechanism by which naked pDNA transfects somatic cells in vivo is still unclear. Transfection of mycocytes can be amplified by pretreatment with local anesthetics [40, 41] or with cardiotoxin [39], which induce local tissue damage and consequently activate myoblast regeneration. Understanding the mechanism of naked pDNA uptake in vivo and its import into the nucleus may lead to improved applications for gene therapy in general and for gene vaccination in particular.

In general, the antibody response induced by gene vaccination is usually significantly lower than that induced by protein vaccination. The reason for this may be the minute amount of gene product (pg/ml to a few ng/ml) produced in vivo which is inadequate to stimulate sufficient number of B cells. Improved gene expression combined with a better DNA adjuvant (ISS) engineered into the pDNA backbone in *cis* or delivered as an adjuvant in *trans*, may enhance the antibody responses to the gene products and expand the applications of gene vaccinations as an important preventive modality for infectious diseases where high levels of neutralizing antibody titers are required.

The use of gene vaccination to modify an on-going immune response (therapeutic vaccine) should be further explored. In theory, gene vaccination may provide an important tool for eliciting an immune response in patients with chronic viral infections such as HIV, HBV or HCV. Due to the continuous expression of the gene product, e.g., the microbial antigen, in a immunologically privileged milieu containing many APC such as the skin (which provide the necessary cellular interactions for enhanced immune response), gene vaccination may promote a successful therapeutic immune response which is not obtained by the current protein vaccines.

Finally, the relevance of the data obtained in various animal models to human diseases has to be evaluated. Application of gene vaccination for infectious, allergic and malignant diseases relies mainly on the usefulness of this new method to elicit a unique and protective immune response in humans. Also, various important safety considerations have not yet been fully addressed (discussed by Klinman et al. and Siegrist et al. in this issue). Once toxicity, safety and the related regulatory issues have been approved, the way for appropriate clinical trials will be paved.

Acknowledgement. This work was supported by grant from the National Institute of Health – AI37305, and AI40682, and Nature Medicine for the permission to reproduce Fig. 1.

References

1. Aragane Y, Riemann H, Bhardway RS, Schwarz A, Sawada Y, Yamada H, Luger TA, Kubin M, Trinchieri G, Schwarz T (1994) IL-12 is expressed and released by human keratinocytes and epidermoid carcinoma cell lines. J Immunol 153 : 5366
2. Bradley LM, Dalton DK, Croft MA (1996) Direct role for IFN-gamma in regulation of Th1 cell development. J Immunol 157 : 1350
3. Brinkmann V, Geiger T, Alkan S, Heusser CH (1993) Interferon alpha increases the frequency of interferon gamma-producing human CD4+ T cells. J Exp Med 178 : 1655
4. Condon C, Watkins SC, Celluzi CM, Thompson K, Falo LD Jr (1996) DNA based immunization by in vivo transfection of dendritic cells. Nature Med 2 : 1122
5. Corr M, Lee DJ, Carson DA, Tighe H (1996) Gene vaccination with naked plasmid DNA: mechanism of CTL priming. J Exp Med 184 : 1555
6. Cowdery JS, Chace JH, Yi AK, Krieg AM (1996) Bacterial DNA induces NK cells to produce IFN-gamma in vivo and increases the toxicity of lipopolysaccharides. J Immunol 156 : 4570
7. Cox GJ, Zamb T, Babiuk LA (1993) Bovine herpesvirus 1: immune response in mice and in cattle injected with plasmid DNA. J Virl 67 : 5664
8. Davis HL, McCluskie MJ, Gerin JL, Purcell RH (1996) DNA vaccine for hepatitis B: evidence for immunogenicity in chimpanzees and comparison with other vaccines. Proc Natl Acad Sci USA 93 : 7213
9. Donnelly JJ, Ulmer JB, Liu MA (1994) Immunization with DNA. J Immunol Methods 176 : 145
10. Feltquate DM, Heany S, Webster RG, Robinson HL (1997) Different T helper cell types and antibody isotypes generated by saline and gene gun DNA immunization. J Immunol 158 : 2278
11. Freund J, Casals J, Hosmer EP (1937) Sensitization and antibody formation after injection of tubercle bacilli and parafin oil. Proc Soc Exp Biol Med 37 : 509
12. Fynan EF, Webster RG, Fuller DH, Haynes JR, Santoro JC, Robinson HL (1993) DNA vaccines: protective immunizations by parenteral, mucosal, and gene-gun inoculations. Proc Natl Acad Sci USA 90 : 11478
13. Geissler EK, Wang J, Fechner JH Jr, Burlingham WJ, Knechtle SJ (1994) Immunity to MHC class I antigen after direct DNA transfer into skeletal muscle. J Immunol 152 : 413

14. Geissler M, Tokushige K, Chante CC, Zurawski VR Jr, Wands JR (1997) Cellular and humoral immune response to hepatitis B virus structural proteins in mice after DNA-based immunization. Gastroenterology 112 : 1307
15. Geissler M, Geisen A, Tokushige K, Wands JR (1997) Enhancement of cellular and humoral immune response to hepatitis C virus protein using DNA based vaccines augmented with cytokine expressing plasmids. J Immunol 158 : 1231
16. Hoffman SL, Doolan DL, Sedegah M, Gramzinski R, Wang H, Gowda K, Hobart P, Margalith M, Norman J, Hedstrom RC (1995) Nucleic acid malaria vaccines. Current status and potential. Ann N Y Acad Sci 772 : 88
17. Hsu CH, Chua KY, Tao MH, Lai YL, Wu HD, Huang SK, Hsieh KH (1996) Immunoprophylaxis of allergen induced immunoglobulin E synthesis and airway hyperresponsiveness in vivo by genetic immunization. Nature Med 2 : 540
18. Kimura Y, Sonehara K, Kuramoto E, Makino T, Yamamoto S, Yamamoto T, Kataoka T, Tokunaga T (1994) Binding of oligoguanylate to scavenger receptors is required for oligonucleotides to augment NK cell activity and induce IFN. J Biochem 116 : 991
19. Klinman DM, Yi AK, Beaucage SL, Conove J, Krieg AM (1996) CpG motifs present in bacteria DNA rapidly induce lymphocytes to secrete interleukin 6, interleukin 12, and interferon gamma. Proc Natl Acad Sci USA 93 : 2879
20. Klinman DM, Yamschikov G, Ishigatsubo Y (1997) Contribution of CpG motifs to the immunogencity of DNA vaccine. J Immunol 158 : 3635
21. Krieg AM, Yi AK, Matson S, Waldschmidt TJ, Bishop GA, Teasdale R, Koretzky GA, Klinman DM (1995) CpG motifs in bacterial DNA trigger direct B-cell activation. Nature 374 : 546
22. Manickan E, Rouse RJ, Yu Z, Wire WS, Rouse BT (1995) Genetic immunization against herpes simplex virus. Protection is mediated by $CD4^+$ T lymphocytes. J Immunol 155 : 259
23. McDonnell WM, Squires HR Jr (1996) DNA vaccines. N Engl J Med 334 : 42
24. Messina JP, Gilkeson GS, Pisetsky DS (1991) Stimulation of in vitro murine lymphocyte proliferation by bacterial DNA. J Immunol 147 : 1759
25. Okamura H, Tsutsi H, Komatsu T et al. (1995) Cloning of a new cytokine that induces IFN-gamma production by T cells. Nature 378 : 88
26. Pisetsky SD (1996) The immunologic properties of DNA. J Immunol 156 : 421
27. Pisetsky SD (1997) DNA and the immune system. Ann Intern Med 126 : 169
28. Raz E, Carson DA, Parker SE et al. (1994) Intradermal gene immunization: the possible role of DNA uptake in the induction of cellular immunity to viruses. Proc Natl Acad Sci USA 91 : 9519
29. Raz E, Tighe H, Sato Y, Roman M, Corr MP, Swain SL, Spiegelberg HL, Carson DA (1996) Preferential induction of Th1 response by intradermal gene vaccination. Proc Natl Acad Sci USA 93 : 5141
30. Raz E, Roman M, Orozco EM, Carson EM (1997) Immunostimulatory (ISS) sequences are a Th1 promoting adjuvant (Abstract). J Allergy Clin Immunol 99 : S365
31. Sato Y, Roman M, Tighe H, Lee D, Corr M, Nguyen M-D, Silverman GJ, Lotz M, Carson DA, Raz E (1996) Immunostimulatory DNA sequences necessary for effective intradermal gene immunization. Science 273 : 352
32. Slater JE, Zhang YJ, Arthur-Smith A (1997) A DNA vaccine inhibits IgE response to the latex allergen Hev b 5 in mice (Abstract). J Allergy Clin Immunol 99 : S504
33. Steinman RM (1991). The dendritic cell system and its role in immunogenicity. Annu Rev Immunol 9 : 271
34. Streilein JW (1993) Dermal cells: underappreciated components of skin associated lymphoid tissues. In: Nickoloff BJ (ed) The dermal immune system. CRC Press, Boca Raton, pp 25–38
35. Syrengelas AD, Chen TT, Levy R (1996) DNA immunization induces protective immunity against B-cell lymphoma. Nature Med 2 : 1038
36. Tascon RE, Colston MJ, Ragno S, Stavropoulos E, Gregory D, Lowrie DB (1996) Vaccination against tuberculosis by DNA injection. Nature Med 2 : 888
37. Trinchieri G (1995) Interleukin-12: a proinflammatory cytokine with immunoregulatory functions that bridge innate resistance and antigen-specific adaptive immunity. Annu Rev Immunol 13 : 251
38. Ulmer JB, Donnelly JJ, Parker SE, et al (1993) Heterologous protection against influenza by injection of DNA encoding a viral protein. Science 259 : 1745
39. Waisman A, Ruiz PJ, Hirschberg DL, Gelman A, Oksenberg JR, Brocke S, Mor F, Cohen IR, Steinman L (1996) Suppressive vaccination with DNA encoding a variable region gene of the T-cell receptor prevents autoimmune encephalomyelitis and activates Th2 immunity. Nature Med 2 : 899

40. Wang B, Ugen KE, Srikantan V, Agadjanyan MG, Dang K, Refaeli Y, Sato AI, Boyer J, Williams WV, Weiner DB (1993) Gene inoculation generates immune responses against human immunodeficiency virus type 1. Proc Natl Acad Sci USA 90 : 4156
41. Wang B, Boyer J, Srikantan V, et al (1993) DNA inoculation induces neutralizing immune responses against human immunodeficiency virus type 1 in mice and nonhuman primates. DNA Cell Biol 9 : 799
42. Watanabc A, Raz E, Kohsaka H, Tighe H, Baird SM, Kipps TJ, Carson DA (1993) Induction of antibodies to a kappa V region by gene immunization. J Immunol 151 : 2871
43. Xiang Z, Ertl HC (1995) Manipulation of the immune response to a plasmid-encoded viral antigen by coinoculation with plasmids expressing cytokines. Immunity 2 : 129
44. Yaegashi Y, Nielsen P, Sing A, Galanos C, Freudenberg MA (1995) Interferon beta, a cofactor in the interferon gamma production induced by gram-negative bacteria in mice. J Exp Med 181 : 953
45. Yamamoto S, Yamamoto T, Shimada S, Kuramoto E, Yano O, Kataoka T, Tokunaga T (1992) DNA from bacteria, but not from vertebrates, induces interferons, activates natural killer cells and inhibits tumor growth. Microbiol Immunol 36 : 983
46. Yamamoto T, Yamamoto S, Kataoka T, Komuro K, Kohase M, Tokunaga T (1994) Synthetic oligonucleotides with certain palindromes stimulate interferon production of human peripheral blood lymphocytes in vitro. Jpn J Cancer Res 85 : 775

Plasmid DNA vaccination: mechanism of antigen presentation

Maripat Corr, Helen Tighe

Department of Medicine and The Sam and Rose Stein Institute for Research on Aging, University of California, San Diego, Clinical Sciences Building, Room 126, 9500 Gilman Drive, La Jolla, CA 92093-0663, USA

Introduction

Direct injection of naked plasmid DNA either intramuscularly or intradermally induces strong, long-lived immune responses to the antigen encoded by the gene vaccine. While the intradermal route of administration appears to be the most efficient, there is evidence that either route leads to production of antibody and the activation of major histocompatibility complex (MHC) class I-restricted, antigen-specific cytotoxic T lymphocytes (CTL) and MHC class II-restricted CD4+ T cells secreting Th1-type cytokines such as interferon-γ (IFN-γ) [1–9]. Plasmid DNA immunization has potential advantages compared to traditional protein vaccination due to the strong CTL and Th1 responses induced, the prolonged antigen expression, and the resistance of the antigen source to antibody-mediated clearance. As a consequence, gene vaccination has potential applications in the fields of infectious diseases, allergy and cancer.

Gene vaccination induces both MHC class I- and class II-restricted responses. The majority of CD4+ T cells recognize peptides derived from exogenous proteins endocytosed by antigen-presenting cells (APC), degraded to peptide fragments and loaded onto MHC class II molecules [10]. The expression of MHC-encoded class II molecules is generally limited to cells of bone marrow origin and, hence, it is likely that these bone marrow-derived cells are responsible for antigen presentation. The ability of such cells to process exogenous antigens and present their peptides in the context of MHC class II for CD4+ T cell stimulation means that the cell initially transfected by the gene vaccination need only produce the protein which is later taken up by the professional APC.

In contrast, CD8+ T cells generally recognize peptides derived from endogenous proteins presented in the context of MHC class I molecules. By this pathway, peptides derived from proteosome processing of intracellular proteins are transported into the lumen of the endoplasmic reticulum by membrane-associated transporters of antigenic peptides (TAP-1 and TAP-2). These peptides then bind nascent MHC class I complexes [11–14]. In contrast to MHC class II, MHC class I molecules are widely ex-

---

Correspondence to: H. Tighe

pressed by almost all cell types, consequently there is the potential of presentation of gene-encoded antigen to T cells by cells other than professional APC. This endogenous route of peptide loading onto MHC class I molecules would be most efficiently used following gene vaccination if the protein were expressed by the APC. To utilize this peptide-loading mechanism the APC would need to be itself transfected by plasmid DNA. Alternatively, both MHC class I and MHC class II molecules of an APC could be loaded with peptides from exogenously produced protein. In this case transfected somatic cells would express protein that could then be extracellularly transferred to the APC. Several investigators have done a series of experiments to explore these different potential pathways.

Plasmid DNA is expressed by resident APC in the dermis

Within the dermis of the skin, there are a variety of "professional" APC such as Langerhans cells, dendritic cells and tissue macrophages which could be transfected by the injected plasmid DNA [12]. Indeed, intradermal gene vaccination has been shown to induce expression of the gene product in cells with macrophage-like morphology as well as keratinocytes and dermal fibroblasts [4]. Furthermore, delivery of plasmid DNA into the skin by gold particle bombardment has been demonstrated to directly transfect dendritic cells that can be later detected in the draining lymph nodes [15]. These transfected dendritic cells should be capable of priming both MHC class I-restricted and MHC class II-restricted responses as they bear the presenting molecules on their cell surface as well as co-stimulatory ligands.

Plasmid DNA remains primarily in muscle tissue

Within muscle tissue, "professional" APC are sparse, although they may be recruited to muscle by the local irritation that follows injection [11, 14, 16]. Surveys of different tissues for the presence of plasmid DNA following intramuscular plasmid injection show little or no plasmid in non-muscle tissues using a sensitive polymerase chain reaction (PCR) technique [17]. Therefore, it is unlikely that circulating cells recruited to the site of injection internalize the plasmids and transport them to a remote site for protein expression. These data suggest that the transfected muscle cells are the major source of expressed protein following intramuscular plasmid DNA injection.

Plasmid DNA immunizes not tolerizes

Following intramuscular DNA immunization, muscle cells are directly transfected by plasmid DNA, produce a protein product [13] and can confer CTL-mediated immune protection from influenza vira challenge [7, 18]. However, priming a naïve $CD8^+$ T cell requires both recognition of an appropriate MHC class I/peptide complex on the APC and a second nonspecific co-stimulatory signal usually provided by the interaction of CD28 on the T cell with CD86 on the APC [19, 20]. Numerous experimental systems have shown that presentation of antigen by non-professional APC which lack appropriate co-stimulatory molecules is more likely to tolerize than stimulate T cells [21–24]. Myocytes form the overwhelming majority of cells which express transgene-encoded protein following intramuscular injection. This poses the question of how priming rather than tolerization could actually occur. A number of experiments have provided a theoretical basis for answering this question. It has been shown that non-professional APC such as transfected fibroblasts are able to induce an antigen-specific MHC class I-restricted response if they are physically relocated to secondary lymphoid tissue [25]. This implies that antigen presentation and co-stimulation do not need to be provided by the same cell but must be in the same local environment. Thus, it is possible that CTL could receive a first signal from peptide/MHC class I complexes expressed by the muscle tissue and a second signal from hemopoietic cells recruited by a local inflammatory response to the site of injection. Alternatively, a number of investigators have shown that contrary to conventional dogma, exogenous antigens can be presented in the context of MHC class I molecules, particularly if encountered in particulate or denatured form [26–28]. Consequently, determination of whether the MHC class I-restricting element is provided by transfected myocytes or professional APC provides valuable information regarding the mechanism of antigen presentation.

Bone marrow-derived cells facilitate CTL induction

A series of experiments using chimeric animals has been performed by different investigators to evaluate the role of antigen presentation by transfected myocytes following naked DNA inoculation. Mice with severe combined immunodeficiency (SCID) lack functional B and T cells which permits the engraftment of allogeneic lymphocytes from immunocompetent mice [29, 30]. H-2^d SCID mice were infused with splenocytes from CB6F1 (H-2^{bxd}) mice and immunized intramuscularly with plasmid DNA [31]. The resulting CTL response was H-2^d restricted, suggesting that antigen presentation was restricted to the recipient's myocytes or possibly macrophages. However, if the H-2^d SCID mice were infused with a mixture of bone marrow cells and splenocytes from CB6F1 mice then both the H-2^d- and the H-2^b-restricted CTL responses could be elicited. These data suggested that cells of hematopoetic origin facilitated the priming of a CTL response to the donor haplotype following naked DNA injection into the muscle. However, in these experiments the role of antigen presentation by the muscle cells was still not clearly defined, as the CTL response restricted to the recipient's MHC haplotype may have been induced by either the recipient's or the donor's hematopoetic cells or the injected muscle tissue.

A separate series of experiments using chimeric mice were performed to evaluate whether somatic cells at the site of plasmid DNA injection can prime a specific CTL response by presenting antigen in the context of their endogenous MHC complexes or whether presentation was restricted to professional APC of hemopoietic origin [32]. To resolve which cell type provided the specific restricting element for intramuscular plasmid DNA vaccination parent → F1 bone marrow chimeras were generated in which H-2^{bxd} recipient mice received bone marrow that expressed only H-2^b or H-2^d MHC molecules. These mice were injected intramuscularly with naked plasmid DNA that encoded the nucleoprotein (NP) from the A/PR/8/34 influenza strain, which as a single antigen had epitopes for both H-$2D^b$ and H-$2K^d$. The resulting CTL responses were restricted to the MHC haplotype of the bone marrow alone and not to the second haplotype expressed by the recipient's myocytes.

These data indicate that muscle cells at the site of plasmid DNA injection do not themselves present gene-encoded antigen to the immune system. Instead, presentation occurs at the surface of a professional bone marrow-derived APC. Such APC may be directly transfected by plasmid DNA at the site of injection, resulting in endogenous expression of NP. Loading of NP-derived cytoplasmic peptides onto MHC class I molecules can then occur through the "endogenous" pathway involving proteosomes and TAP complexes [33–36]. However, the paucity of professional bone marrow-derived APC at the site of injection, favors the hypothesis that gene-transfected muscle cells produce NP protein which is then transferred to conventional APC.

Protein expressed by myoblasts is transferred to APC

Under certain circumstances exogenous antigens can be presented in the context of MHC class I [28, 37–39]. Consequently, presentation may occur by protein transfer from transfected muscle cells to a professional APC. This potential mechanism is supported by a report that H-2^{k} transfected myoblasts when injected intraperitoneally into a F1 hybrid (H-2^{kxd}) were able to elicit a H-2^{d}-restricted CTL response [40]. As the myoblasts did not express the H-2^{d} haplotype this response was presumably induced by the recipient's cells which were not endogenously expressing the transfected protein product. This potential mechanism of protein transfer is consistent with the original cross-priming experiments of Bevan et al. [41] in which bystander cells were shown to present MHC class I-restricted minor histocompatibility antigens in vivo. In addition, it is supported by more recent experiments in which a test antigen expressed by tumors of one haplotype can cross-prime CTL restricted to another MHC haplotype when transferred to F1 hybrid recipient mice, presumably through protein/peptide transfer [42].

It has now been shown by a number of groups that exogenous protein molecules can prime MHC class I-restricted CTL responses when administered as either particulate or denatured protein [38, 39]. Alternatively, peptide fragments or denatured proteins can be transferred intercellularly by heat shock protein chaperones [43]. Presentation involves endocytosis/phagocytosis of the protein by either macrophages or dendritic cells [38, 39, 43]. Loading of MHC class I molecules may occur externally by peptides regurgitated from phagosomes of the same or neighboring cells [39, 44] or internally, either through leakage of digested proteins into the cytosol due to phagocytic overload [28], or through a phagosome to cytoplasm shuttle [27], which then feeds peptides into the conventional TAP-dependent pathway for MHC class I loading. Recent experiments analyzing presentation of tumor-associated antigens by bone marrow-derived APC support this latter mechanism by demonstrating an absolute requirement for functional TAP expression by the bone marrow-derived APC [45].

Conclusions

The injection of naked plasmid DNA directly into the muscle cells of mice is a novel method of vaccination which has been shown to induce potent antibody responses and highly effective MHC class I-restricted CTL and MHC class II-restricted Th1 cells which secrete IFN-γ. The expression of MHC-encoded class II molecules is generally limited to cells of bone marrow origin and, hence, it is likely that these bone marrow-derived cells are responsible for initiating MHC class II-restricted responses. In contrast, MHC class I molecules are widely expressed by almost all cell types. To prime a

MHC class I-restricted CTL response a naïve T cell must receive a cognate signal from MHC class I complexes and a second nonspecific signal through co-stimulatory ligands. The potential mechanisms of priming a CTL response after an intramuscular plasmid DNA injection could include the cognate signal from the MHC class I molecules expressed by the transfected myocytes or by hematopoetic cells that are considered to be "professional" APC. Although the introduction of plasmid DNA into the dermis of mice by gold particle bombardment has been demonstrated to directly transfect professional APC, injection of plasmid DNA into the muscle tissue results in expression relatively limited to myocytes. These transfected myocytes, however, do not directly prime T cells, as chimeric animal experiments have indicated that antigen presentation for inducing CTL responses is restricted to cells of hematopoetic origin. The role of somatic tissues that express protein from injected plasmids may be to serve as a reservoir for antigen which is then transferred to these APC. This could occur by transfer of whole protein or peptide fragments which may be accompanied by chaperonins. However, the exact mechanism of antigen transfer from transfected somatic cells to hematopoetic cells has yet to be elucidated. The data do suggest that the mechanism of priming in this novel method for vaccination utilizes the MHC from bone marrow-derived APC, which are efficient at providing all of the necessary signals for priming the T cell.

Acknowledgements. This work was supported in part by an award from CaPCURE Foundation and grant AR25443 from the National Institutes of Health. H.T. and M.C. are recipients of Arthritis Foundation Investigators Awards.

References

1. Fynan EF, Webster RG, Fuller DH, Haynes JR, Santoro JC, Robinson HL (1993) DNA vaccines: protective immunizations by parenteral, mucosal, and gene-gun inoculations. Proc Natl Acad Sci USA 90:11478
2. Davis HL, Schirmbeck R, Reimann J, Whalen RG (1995) DNA-mediated immunization in mice induces a potent MHC class I-restricted cytotoxic T lymphocyte response to the hepatitis B envelope protein. Hum Gene Ther 6:1447
3. Manickan E, Rouse RJ, Yu Z, Wire WS, Rouse BT (1995) Genetic immunization against herpes simplex virus. Protection is mediated by CD4+ T lymphocytes. J Immunol 155:259
4. Raz E, Carson DA, Parker SE, et al (1994) Intradermal gene immunization: the possible role of DNA uptake in the induction of cellular immunity to viruses. Proc Natl Acad Sci USA 91:9519
5. Whalen RG, Leclerc C, Deriaud E, Schirmbeck R, Reimann J, Davis HL (1995) DNA-mediated immunization to the hepatitis B surface antigen. Activation and entrainment of the immune response. Ann N Y Acad Sci 772:64
6. Xiang Z, Ertl HC (1995) Manipulation of the immune response to a plasmid-encoded viral antigen by coinoculation with plasmids expressing cytokines. Immunity 2:129
7. Ulmer JB, Donnelly JJ, Parker SE, et al (1993) Heterologous protection against influenza by injection of DNA encoding a viral protein [see comments]. Science 259:1745
8. Raz E, Tighe H, Sato Y, Corr M, Dudler JA, Roman M, Swain SL, Spiegelberg HL, Carson DA (1996) Preferential induction of a Th1 immune response and inhibition of specific IgE antibody formation by plasmid DNA immunization. Proc Natl Acad Sci USA 93:5141
9. Watanabe A, Raz E, Kohsaka H, Tighe H, Baird SM, Kipps TJ, Carson DA (1993) Induction of antibodies to a kappa V region by gene immunization. J Immunol 151:2871
10. Neefjes JJ, Ploegh HL (1992) Intracellular transport of MHC class II molecules. Immunol Today 13:179
11. Hohlfeld R, Engel AG (1994) The Immunobiology of muscle. Immunol Today 15:269
12. Nickloff BM (1993) Dermal immune system. CRC Press, Boca Raton
13. Wolff JA, Malone RW, Williams P, Chong W, Acsadi G, Jani A, Felgner PL (1990) Direct gene transfer into mouse muscle in vivo. Science 247:1465

14. Austyn JM, Hankins DF, Larsen CP, Morris PJ, Rao AS, Roake JA (1994) Isolation and characterization of dendritic cells from mouse heart and kidney. J Immunol 152:2401
15. Condon C, Watkins SC, Celluzzi CM, Thompson K, Falo LD Jr (1996) DNA-based immunization by in vivo transfection of dendritic cells. Nature Med 2:1122
16. Pardoll DM, Beckerleg AM (1995) Exposing the immunology of naked DNA vaccines. Immunity 3:165
17. Nichols WW, Ledwith BJ, Manam SV, Troilo PJ (1995) Potential DNA vaccine integration into host cell genome. Ann N Y Acad Sci 772:30
18. Ulmer JB, Donnelly JJ, Deck RR, DeWitt CM, Liu MA (1995) Immunization against viral proteins with naked DNA. Ann N Y Acad Sci 772:117
19. Schwartz RH (1992) Costimulation of T lymphocytes: the role of CD28, CTLA-4, and B7/BB1 in interleukin-2 production and immunotherapy. Cell 71:1065
20. Schwartz RH (1996) Models of T cell anergy: is there a common molecular mechanism? [comment]. J Exp Med 184:1
21. Lamb JR, Skidmore BJ, Green N, Chiller JM, Feldmann M (1983) Induction of tolerance in influenza virus-immune T lymphocyte clones with synthetic peptides of influenza hemagglutinin. J Exp Med 157:1434
22. Jenkins MK, Schwartz RH (1987) Antigen presentation by chemically modified splenocytes induces antigen-specific T cell unresponsiveness in vitro and in vivo. J Exp Med 165:302
23. Quill H, Schwartz RH (1987) Stimulation of normal inducer T cell clones with antigen presented by purified Ia molecules in planar lipid membranes: specific induction of a long-lived state of proliferative nonresponsiveness. J Immunol 138:3704
24. Mueller DL, Jenkins MK, Schwartz RH (1989) Clonal expansion versus functional clonal inactivation: a costimulatory signalling pathway determines the outcome of T cell antigen receptor occupancy. Annu Rev Immunol 7:445
25. Kundig TM, Bachmann MF, DiPaolo C, et al (1995) Fibroblasts as efficient antigen-presenting cells in lymphoid organs. Science 268:1343
26. Kovacsovics-Bankowski M, Rock KL (1994) Presentation of exogenous antigens by macrophages: analysis of major histocompatibility complex class I and II presentation and regulation by cytokines. Eur J Immunol 24:2421
27. Kovacsovics-Bankowski M, Rock KL (1995) A phagosome-to-cytosol pathway for exogenous antigens presented on MHC class I molecules. Science 267:243
28. Reis e Sousa C, Germain RN (1995) Major histocompatibility complex class I presentation of peptides derived from soluble exogenous antigen by a subset of cells engaged in phagocytosis. J Exp Med 182:841
29. Rudolphi A, Spiess S, Conradt P, Claesson MH, Reimann J (1991) $CD3^+$ T cells in severe combined immunodeficiency (scid) mice. II. Transplantation of dm2 lymphoid cells into semi-allogeneic scid mice. Eur J Immunol 21:1591
30. Claesson MH, Rudolphi A, Tscherning T, Reimann J (1991) $CD3^+$ T cells in severe combined immunodeficiency (scid) mice. IV. Graft-vs.-host resistance of H-2d scid mice to intravenous injection of allogeneic H-2b (C57BL/6) spleen cells. Eur J Immunol 21:2057
31. Doe B, Selby M, Barnett S, Baenziger J, Walker CM (1996) Induction of cytotoxic T lymphocytes by intramuscular immunization with plasmid DNA is facilitated by bone marrow-derived cells. Proc Natl Acad Sci USA 93:8578
32. Corr M, Lee DJ, Carson DA, Tighe H (1996) Gene vaccination with naked plasmid DNA: mechanism of CTL priming. J Exp Med 184:1555
33. Monaco JJ, Cho S, Attaya M (1990) Transport protein genes in the murine MHC: possible implications for antigen processing. Science 250:1723
34. Townsend A, Trowsdale J (1993) The transporters associated with antigen presentation. Semin Cell Biol 4:53
35. Yewdell JW, Bennink JR (1992) Cell biology of antigen processing and presentation to major histocompatibility complex class I molecule-restricted T lymphocytes. Adv Immunol 52:1
36. Dick LR, Aldrich C, Jameson SC, Moomaw CR, Pramanik BC, Doyle CK, DeMartino GN, Bevan MJ, Forman JM, Slaughter CA(1994) Proteolytic processing of ovalbumin and beta-galactosidase by the proteasome to a yield antigenic peptides. J Immunol 152:3884
37. Schirmbeck R, Melber K, Reimann J (1995) Hepatitis B virus small surface antigen particles are processed in a novel endosomal pathway for major histocompatibility complex class I-restricted epitope presentation. Eur J Immunol 25:1063

38. Bohm W, Schirmbeck R, Elbe A, Melber K, Diminky D, Kraal G, Rooijen N van, Barenholz Y, Reimann J (1995) Exogenous hepatitis B surface antigen particles processed by dendritic cells or macrophages prime murine MHC class I-restricted cytotoxic T lymphocytes in vivo. J Immunol 155:3313
39. Martinez-Kinader B, Lipford GB, Wagner H, Heeg K (1995) Sensitization of MHC class I-restricted T cells to exogenous proteins: evidence for an alternative class I-restricted antigen presentation pathway. Immunology 86:287
40. Ulmer JB, Deck RR, Dewitt CM, Donnhly JI, Liu MA (1996) Generation of MHC class I-restricted cytotoxic T lymphocytes by expression of a viral protein in muscle cells: antigen presentation by non-muscle cells. Immunology 89:59
41. Bevan MJ (1976) Cross-priming for a secondary cytotoxic response to minor H antigens with H-2 congenic cells which do not cross-react in the cytotoxic assay. J Exp Med 143:1283
42. Huang AY, Golumbek P, Ahmadzadeh M, Jaffee E, Pardoll D, Levitsky H (1994) Role of bone marrow-derived cells in presenting MHC class I-restricted tumor antigens. Science 264:961
43. Suto R, Srivastava PK (1995) A mechanism for the specific immunogenicity of heat shock protein-chaperoned peptides. Science 269:1585
44. Harding CV, Song R (1994) Phagocytic processing of exogenous particulate antigens by macrophages for presentation by class I MHC molecules. J Immunol 153:4925
45. Huang AY, Bruce AT, Pardoll DM, Levitsky HI (1996) In vivo cross-priming of MHC class I-restricted antigens requires the TAP transporter. Immunity 4:349

The development of a multivalent DNA vaccine for malaria

Richard C. Hedstrom[1], Denise L. Doolan[1], Ruobing Wang[1], Malcolm J. Gardner[1,*], Anita Kumar[1], Martha Sedegah[1,2], Robert A. Gramzinski[1], John B. Sacci Jr.[1,2], Yupin Charoenvit[1], Walter R. Weiss[1], Michal Margalith[3], Jon A. Norman[3], Peter Hobart[3], Stephen L. Hoffman[1]

[1] Malaria Program, Naval Medical Research Institute Annex, 12300 Washington Avenue, Rockville, MD 20852, USA
[2] Department of Microbiology and Immunology, University of Maryland School of Medicine, Baltimore, Maryland, USA
[3] Vical Incorporated, San Diego, California, USA

The problem of malaria

According to the latest report from the World Health Organization (December 1996), malaria is still a public health problem in more than 90 countries, inhabited by a total of some 2.4 billion people or 40% of the world's population. Worldwide incidence of the disease is estimated to be 300–500 million clinical cases each year. Mortality due to malaria is estimated to be in the range of 1.5–2.7 million deaths annually. The vast majority of deaths occur among young children in Africa, especially in remote rural areas with poor access to health services. Immunity to malaria seems to occur among residents of malarious areas with increasing age which prevents an even greater number of deaths. However, this type of protection is short-lived and requires frequent exposure to the malaria parasite.

The magnitude of the malaria problem is of increasing concern to a broad range of people who do not reside in the endemic areas. During the twentieth century, United States military forces have lost more person days to malaria than to bullets in every operation conducted in a malarious region [4]. The number of civilian travelers to malarious areas continues to grow as more people throughout the world become increasingly mobile. Why does malaria remain such a problem? Some of the main reasons are these: the parasite has become increasingly resistant to antimalarial drugs; the mosquito vectors that transmit the parasites have developed resistance to the commonly used insecticides; infrastructures required to deliver mosquito control and treatment of patients in many developing countries have been inadequate; and, nonimmune populations have migrated to malarious areas as sometimes occurs in refugee situations. The

Correspondence to: R. C. Hedstrom
* *Present address:* The Institute for Genomic Research, Gaithersburg, Maryland

development of new drugs against malaria is an ongoing effort but this race to stay ahead may one day be lost. The continuing search for tools to combt this disease includes efforts to develop a vaccine.

The life-cycle of the parasite

To understand vaccination strategies it is important to know something about the complex life cycle of the malaria parasite. These are protozoan parasites that belong to the genus *Plasmodium*. The *Plasmodium* life cycle consists of distinct morphological stages broadly categorized as pre-erythrocytic stage (sporozoite and liver), erythrocytic stage (asexual and sexual) and mosquito stage. The host becomes infected when bitten by a female anopheline mosquito carrying the infective sporozoite stage of the malaria parasite which is transmitted during the act of taking a bloodmeal. Sporozoites inoculated into the peripheral circulation then invade hepatocytes. In the hepatocyte, the uninucleated sporozoite undergoes development by entering into a 2- to 10-day cycle of asexual multiplication, called schizogony. This period of schizogony differs among parasite species (at least 5 days for human *Plasmodium* species). A single liver-stage schizont gives rise to as many as 30,000 uninucleate parasites of the next developmental stage of the parasite, the merozoite. During this period of the host infection, the disease is symptomatically silent. The parasite exists in a parasitophorous vacuole bounded by an elaborate protective structure derived from both host and parasite membranes. Eventually, the infected hepatocyte ruptures, releasing thousands of mature merozoites into the bloodstream. Freed merozoites rapidly invade red blood cells initiating the erythrocytic stage of the life cycle of the parasite. Within the red blood cell the parasite undergoes another round of asexual reproduction lasting for 48–72 h, resulting in the release of up to 36 new merozoites from each parasitized erythrocyte. Most of these merozoites quickly invade more erythrocytes. This repeated amplification cycle of asexual reproduction in erythrocytes is the stage of the infection associated with the characteristic manifestations of malaria. During this period, a few parasites differentiate into male and female forms called gametocytes. While taking a bloodmeal, a feeding mosquito ingests male and female gametocytes that undergo gametogenesis. The resultant male and female gametes pair to form zygotes that develop into ookinetes. This sexual reproduction occurs in the mosquito midgut. The ookinete penetrates the midgut wall and develops into an oocyst within which thousands of new sporozoites develop and mature. Following their release from the oocyst, these sporozoites migrate to the salivary gland of the mosquito from which they are injected into the next host during a bloodmeal.

A vaccine against malaria

Vaccination strategies are aimed at inducing immunological responses to attack and disrupt the replicative amplification of the malaria parasite. The development of a vaccine against malaria is an active area of research that has been enormously challenging. As the parasite proceeds from a sporozoite through the liver stage to the replicative cycling of the blood stage, it changes morphological forms and surface antigens, some of which display antigenic variation. These features endow the parasite with the ability to evade protective immune responses. As a result, the acquisition of long-term sterilizing immunity, typically associated with recovery from many other infectious diseases, does not occur with malaria. For example, 85% of adults who had lived their entire lives in the same village in Kenya and been exposed thousands of times to the bites of *Plasmodium*-infected mosquitos, became reinfected within 4 months after being cured of malaria with antimalarial drugs [27]. Nevertheless, the development of a vaccine against malaria is thought to be feasible. This optimism is based on a number of studies. In one, immunization of Rhesus monkeys with asexual-stage parasites in Freund's complete adjuvant induced a level of immunity that rapidly cleared the infection [38]. In addition, field studies have shown that the density of parasitemia and the severity of the clinical manifestations that occur with malaria decrease with age: survival beyond the age of 5 years for an individual in an area of intense malaria transmission indicates that repeated infections induces immune responses that reduce parasite burden ([4] and reviewed in [2]). In other studies it was shown that the transfer of immunoglobulin from life-long adult residents of West Africa into naive recipients provided passive immunity against *P. falciparum* [11] and that immunoglobulin from adults in West Africa, administered to children in Thailand who were suffering from multidrug-resistant *P. falciparum* infection, reduced peripheral parasitemia by 99% [48]. However, perhaps the most compelling evidence that vaccination against malaria is feasible has come from laboratory studies in which sporozoites attenuated by irradiation induce sterile protective immunity in rodents, monkeys, and human subjects (reviewed in [30]).

A vaccine directed against the liver stage

The primary focus of our laboratory is to develop a pre-erythrocytic vaccine designed to induce protective T cell effector mechanisms able to destroy or inactivate parasites during maturation in the liver. An effective pre-erythrocytic stage vaccine would thus eliminate all infection before the appearance of clinical malaria since during the liver stage there are no symptoms, signs or pathology. A vaccine to prevent the release of infective parasites from the liver would block parasite invasion of erythrocytes and thereby prevent the development of symptomatic disease.

Furthermore, this vaccine would stop transmission since no sexual-stage parasites could develop. Thus, the liver stage, due to its duration and lack of association with any manifestations of disease, provides the ideal target for vaccine development. Even an incompletely effective liver-stage vaccine could provide some benefit by reducing the numbers of parasites released from the liver into the bloodstream. This attenuation of the parasite burden could lessen morbidity and mortality. Indeed, indirect evidence supports this argument. Widespread use of insecticide impregnated bednets has been shown to reduce mortality in sub-Saharan Africa [1, 3] by decreasing the exposure to infected mosquitoes. Furthermore, in an area of Western Kenya where virtually all children aged 6 months – 1 year have *P. falciparum* parasitemia every day of the year, the blood-stage parasite density is directly correlated with the numbers of infective mosquitoes to which the children have been exposed during the preceding month [4, 37]. This suggests that reduced exposure to infective mosquitoes corresponds to decreased frequency of exposure to sporozoites which results in lower blood-stage parasitemia, fewer clinical symptoms and reduced mortality. A partially effective sporozoite or liver-stage vaccine might have the same effect as a bednet.

Radiation-attenuated sporozoites have been used as an effective pre-erythrocytic vaccine in human experiments since the early 1970s (reviewed in [26]). However, the usefulness of this vaccine continues to be as an experimental tool limited to small studies as it is impractical for large-scale human use. Although encouraging protection results were reported in a recent clinical trial with a recombinant pre-erythrocytic protein vaccine in adjuvant [56], a malaria vaccine capable of inducing solid immunity, comparable to that obtained by immunization with irradiated sporozoites, is not yet available. During the past decade, there has been significant progress towards identifying the protective immune mechanisms, identifying the antigenic targets of these immune mechanisms, and developing vaccine delivery systems that induce the desired immune response against these targets (reviewed in [30]). It is now known that $CD8^+$ T cells are critical for sporozoite immunity. This dependence was first demonstrated with experimental models of malaria in rodent hosts [50, 58] in which $CD8^+$ T cells alone, without any other parasite immune responses, were shown to be sufficient for protection [33, 44, 47, 61]. The mechanism of the immunity is thought to be due to the activation of $CD8^+$ T cells that recognize and engage infected hepatocytes via genetically restricted major histocompatibility complex (MHC) class I molecules presenting parasite-derived peptides on the cell surface. Thus, $CD8^+$ T cells recognize parasite-derived peptides presented within MHC class I molecules on the surface of infected hepatocytes and destroy the infected host cell or mediate inactivation of the parasite within. It was shown that $CD8^+$ cytotoxic T lymphocytes (CTL) can recognize an epitope from the *Plasmodium yoelii* circumsporozoite protein (PyCSP) expressed on *P. yoelii*-infected hepatocytes [60] and that MHC-restricted immune elimination of infected hepatocytes expressing parasite antigens can protect against malaria following sporozoite challenge [28, 29]. Therefore, our initial goal is to produce a pre-erythrocytic vaccine that will induce protective $CD8^+$ T cells. Hepatocytes that harbor *Plasmodium spp.* parasites are the only target of such $CD8^+$ T cells since sporozoites and merozoites in circulation are extracellular and MHC class I molecules are not present on the surface of mature erythrocytes.

A DNA vaccine against malaria

Vaccine delivery systems designed to induce protective $CD8^+$ T cell responses against *Plasmodium*-infected hepatocytes have been studied extensively and have been judged as being suboptimal for inducing protective immunity against malaria. Such systems include synthetic peptides, purified recombinant proteins and live recombinant organisms. This assessment is based primarily on model studies in the highly rigorous *P. yoelii* rodent malaria system, in which the ID_{50} has been determined to be one to two sporozoites [32, 33], utilizing the PyCSP, which is one of the principal target antigens of protective $CD8^+$ T cells (reviewed in [30]). There has been no demonstration of protection after immunization with several different live recombinant vaccines engineered to express PyCSP. These included vaccinia virus [51], recombinant *Salmonella typhimurium* [20], and recombinant pseudorabies virus [52, 53]. These vaccines failed to provide protection even though high levels of PyCSP-specific CTL activity were induced, as shown in two of the studies [20, 53]. On the other hand, protection that was $CD8^+$ T cell dependent was achieved by immunization with recombinant murine mastocytoma cells (P815) that stably expressed PyCSP [32] and with a PyCSP recombinant influenza/vaccinia combination [35, 43]. However, the practical application of such vaccines is limited. It is doubtful that mastocytoma cells would ever be approved for human use and there are many disadvantages to consider regarding the use of live-attenuated vaccines (summarized in [24]).

The emerging technology of DNA vaccines offers many of the features desired in a malaria vaccine. Plasmid DNA introduced directly into the cells of the vaccinee encodes antigen expression which stimulates a specific immunological response. This technique provides a practical and relatively simple approach toward designing a multivalent vaccine capable of delivering those antigens necessary to induce a protective immune response. This capability is especially relevant for a malaria vaccine since it is well established that there are only a few target epitopes for T cells, that these sequences vary from one strain of parasite to another, and that the specific variants do not often induce immunologically cross-reactive responses. Indeed, an effective DNA vaccine against malaria is expected to be a multi-gene vaccine (reviewed in [16]).

Our strategy is to develop a *P. falciparum* DNA vaccine for human use by first demonstrating in the *P. yoelii* mouse model protective efficacy and biological activity of the induced immune responses with *P. yoelii* genes encoding protective antigens, the analogous genes of which have been identified in the *P. falciparum* parasite. Our major focus is on pre-erythrocytic antigens. The resultant candidate DNA vaccine against *P. falciparum* will be comprised of genes able to induce T cell responses against pre-erythrocytic-stage antigens expressed in the infected hepatocyte. This does not preclude the addition of one or more plasmids encoding antigen genes designed to induce protective antibodies, and $CD4^+$ T cell helper responses, against erythrocytic-stage antigens [16].

DNA vaccine studies in the *P. yoelii* rodent malaria model

It is well established that both MHC and non-MHC genes exert control over protection against *P. yoelii* malaria in mice [59] and that immune responses to many *P. falciparum*, *P. vivax*, *P. yoelii*, and *P. berghei* $CD8^+$ and $CD4^+$ T cell epitopes and B cell epitopes are also genetically restricted. Therefore, our DNA vaccine studies utilized five inbred strains of mice that differed in both genetic background and H-2 haplotype: BALB/cByJ (H-2^d); A/J (H-2^a); B10.BR/SgSnJ (H-2^k); B10.Q/SgJ (H-2^q); and C57BL/6J (H-2^b). Studies with outbred CD-1 mice were included as a model for an outbred human population. The standard immunization regime was three doses of 100 µg DNA encoding the protective antigen at 3-week intervals either intramuscularly (tibialis anterior muscle) or intradermally (base of the tail). Mice were challenged 2 weeks following the final immunization by tail-vein injection with 100 *P. yoelii* sporozoites or with 200 parasitized erythrocytes. Protection was defined as the complete absence of blood-stage parasitemia, as determined by Giemsa-stained blood smears, for at least 2 weeks after challenge. Plasmids expressing the following candidate antigens were tested in this *P. yoelii* model system.

P. yoelii circumsporozoite protein

The major surface coat protein of sporozoites PyCSP [34] is also expressed on the parasitophorous vacuole membrane of developing exoerythrocytic parasites in the infected hepatocyte and it is a target antigen for inducing protective immune responses. Adoptive transfer of protection has been demonstrated in vivo with PyCSP-specific cytotoxic T cell clones of both $CD8^+$ [44, 47, 61] and $CD4^+$ [41] phenotypes. Furthermore, infected hepatocytes can be eliminated from in vitro culture by MHC-restricted

$CD8^+$ cytotoxic T cells specific for PyCSP [60]. The first published report of a DNA vaccine against malaria utilized cytomegalovirus (CMV) promoter-driven plasmids (pDIP and nkCMVintPL) to express the PyCSP gene in mice [54]. Protection against challenge initially was 56% (9/16) in BALB/c mice immunized with pDIP/PyCSP [54]. Shortly after these initial trials, protection as high as 83% was achieved in BALB/c mice immunized with nkCMVint/PyCSP DNA (unpublished). The nkCMVint plasmid vector was shown to express substantially greater levels of PyCSP in vitro as compared with the pDIP construction (unpublished). Immunizations with either of these plasmids induced high levels of CSP-specific antibody production as determined both by indirect fluorescence antibody test (IFAT) against *P. yoelii* sporozoites and by ELISA against recombinant protein [54]. Antibody titers were 10–15 times higher than titers induced by immunization with irradiated sporozoites. These DNA induced antibodies had little biological activity, however, as assessed by the in vitro inhibition of sporozoite invasion and development assay [54]. However, and more importantly, immunization with a plasmid DNA encoding PyCSP induced antigen-specific, MHC-restricted $CD8^+$ CTL directed against a previously identified nonamer CTL epitope from PyCSP [54]. As with the antibody titers, the levels of CTL induced by PyCSP DNA vaccine immunization (70–80% specific lysis) were greater than those induced by immunization with irradiated sporozoites (20–30% specific lysis). Furthermore, the number of liver-stage schizonts were reduced by 86% in BALB/c mice immunized with PyCSP DNA vaccine compared to controls immunized with empty (without the PyCSP gene) plasmid [54]. Finally, the PyCSP DNA vaccine-induced protective immunity was found to be genetically restricted [18]: BALB/c mice ($H\text{-}2^d$) were highly protected against sporozoite challenge but four other inbred strains were not. Restriction of the immunological response to this vaccine was also observed in antibody production as three strains of mice were judged to be high responders and two strains were low responders [18]. Together these results suggest that a DNA vaccine based solely on the CSP gene will not protect outbred human populations against malaria; a multigene DNA vaccine will be required to approach the efficacy of an irradiation-attenuated sporozoite vaccine [16].

P. yoelii hepatocyte erythrocyte protein 17

The *P. yoelii* hepatocyte erythrocyte protein 17 (PyHEP17) antigen is a 17-kDa protein found on the parasitophorous vacuole membrane of infected hepatocytes and erythrocytes [9]. The role played by PyHEP17 as a target of protective immunity was first demonstrated with the anti-PyHEP17 monoclonal antibody, NYLS3. NYLS3 eliminated liver-stage parasites from culture in vitro; and, in vivo, this antibody reduced the density and delayed the onset of blood-stage parasitemia in mice experimentally infected with *P. yoelii* sporozoites [9]. The PyHEP17 antigen is encoded by two exons [17]. A partial-length cDNA of PyHEP17 (designated PyHEP17Ex1.2) that consisted of the complete exon 1 and a truncated exon 2 (lacking the NYLS3 epitope encoding sequence) was used to construct a DNA vaccine in the nkCMVint plasmid. Immunization with nkCMVint/PyHEP17Ex1.2 DNA protected three of five inbred strains of mice (A/J, BALB/c and B10.BR) against sporozoite but not blood-stage challenge [18]. A full-length cDNA vaccine showed similar protection against sporozoite challenge in three strains of mice [17]. Immunization with PyHEP17 DNA vaccine induced a MHC-restricted $CD8^+$ CTL response in mice but, in contrast to immunizations with the PyCSP DNA vaccine, this response did not correlate with the induced level of antibody (Doolan, manuscript in preparation). Indeed, PyHEP17 DNA immunization induced little to no antibody response in all five strains of mice tested. Those weakly positive sera did not recognize *P. yoelii* liver-stage parasites but did react with blood-stage parasites [18]. No correlation between antibody titer and protection was found: protected mice had the lowest levels of anti-PyHEP17 antibody, whereas the highest levels of antibody were found in C57BL/6 mice which were not protected against challenge with sporozoites [18].

Combined DNA vaccine

Although protective immunity induced by either a PyHEP17 DNA vaccine or a PyCSP DNA vaccine given alone was genetically restricted, simultaneous DNA immunization with both plasmids circumvented this restriction [18]. The combination of PyHEP17 and PyCSP DNA vaccines protected 80–90% of higher responder strains (A/J and BALB/c) as well as a moderate responder strain (B10.BR). In two non-responder strains (B10.Q and C57BL/6), a delay in the onset of parasitemia was noted in most mice with the combination relative to either vaccine alone, consistent with the effect being due to protection at the level of the liver stage (Doolan, unpublished). Thus, bivalent DNA immunization broadened the immunity and argues strongly that a combination vaccine will protect mice of diverse genetic backgrounds and H-2 haplotypes.

P. yoelii sporozoite surface protein 2

The *P. yoelii* sporozoite surface protein 2 (PySSP2) antigen is a 140-kDa protein expressed on the surface of sporozoites [8, 23, 46] and is present throughout the liver stage in *P. yoelii*-infected hepatocytes (J. Sacci, unpublished). PySSP2 is the target of protective immune responses against sporozoite challenge based on experiments using both active immunization with recombinant murine mastocytoma cells that expressed PySSP2 [32] and passive immunization by transfer of PySSP2-specific $CD8^+$ T cells [33]. Preliminary studies with DNA vaccines encoding PySSP2 have demonstrated immunogenicity by the production of antigen-specific antibodies and partial protection against sporozoite challenge (unpublished).

P. yoelii merozoite surface protein-1

The *P. yoelii* merozoite surface protein-1 (PyMSP-1) antigen is a 230-kDa protein expressed on the surface of late stage schizonts and merozoites (reviewed in [15]). Since MSP-1 is expressed by liver-stage parasites, cellular immune responses directed against MSP-1 might confer protection by inhibition or destruction of infected hepatocytes. Thus MSP-1, like the antigens discussed above, is also considered a pre-erythrocytic vaccine candidate. Studies show that MSP-1 generates a protective antibody response in both rodent and primate malaria models. Passive transfer of a monoclonal antibody that recognizes a conformational epitope in the C terminus of PyMSP-1 protected mice against a lethal blood stage challenge [6] and antibodies to the *P. falciparum* MSP-1 inhibited the invasion of merozoites into erythrocytes in vitro [5]. Active immunization with *P. falciparum* MSP-1 protected *Aotus* [55] and *Saimiri* [19, 40] monkeys against blood-stage challenge. Immunization with PyMSP-1 [21, 31] or with recombinant fusion proteins of the C terminus [12, 13, 36] protected mice. Protection in these studies appeared to be due to the production of antibodies that recognized a conformational epitope the structure of which could be abolished by reduction and alkylation of the protein [36]. Recent data using *P. yoelii* in mice indicate that, whereas antibodies to MSP-1 are required to reduce parasitemia during the first 12 days after challenge, $CD4^+$ T cells are required to achieve complete protection [13]. Recently, the DNA sequence encoding the C terminus of PyMSP-1 was used to construct several plasmid vaccines. Some of these plasmid constructs incorporated fusing MSP-1 sequences to promiscuous T helper epitopes from tetanus toxin [39, 57]. BALB/c mice immunized with these DNA vaccines produced specific anti-PyMSP-1 antibodies that recognized blood-stage parasites. However, antibody titers were significantly lower than those obtained by immunization with recombinant protein in adjuvant. Nevertheless, these mice demonstrated partial protection from challenge with infected erythrocytes as reflected by a delay in patency, a slower rise to peak parasitemia, and extended survival as compared to controls (M. Gardner et al., manuscript in preparation). Current efforts with experimental PyMSP-1 DNA vaccines in mice include plasmids that encode the N terminus of the molecule and others that utilize the full-length gene. Recently, studies have shown that, compared to the vaccine that encoded the full-length molecule, the C terminus and N terminus encoding vaccines given separately induced a greater level of protection (S. Becker, M, Gardner et al., manuscript in preparation).

A PyCSP DNA vaccine study in the *Aotus* non-human primate malaria model

To optimize an immunization regime in a primate and begin the transition of DNA vaccines from rodents to human subjects, a study was performed to assess the immunogenicity of a PyCSP DNA vaccine in *Aotus* monkeys. Briefly, intradermal but not intramuscular immunization of *Aotus* monkeys induced antibodies directed against PyCSP as determined by IFAT on *P. yoelii* sporozoites and by ELISA with recombinant PyCSP protein [22]. The titer of antibody induced was equivalent to that obtained by immunization with PyCSP multiple antigenic peptide in adjuvant which was used as a control immunogen.

DNA vaccines against pre-erythrocytic *P. falciparum* malaria

The *P. yoelii* DNA vaccine studies discussed here provided the basis for choosing the *P. falciparum* antigen genes that are analogous to PyCSP, PyHEP17 and PySSP2 for inclusion in a *P. falciparum* DNA vaccine. The *P. falciparum* DNA vaccine will probably include plasmids encoding the following analogous *P. falciparum* antigens: circumsporozoite protein (PfCSP) [7], sporozoite surface protein 2 [45], also described as thrombospondin-related anonymous protein or TRAP (PfSSP2/TRAP) [42]; exported protein 1, the *P. falciparum* analogue of PyHEP17 [49] and, *P. falciparum* liver-stage antigen 1 (PfLSA-1) [62]. Although no *P. yoelii* counterpart for PfLSA-1 was available for efficacy testing in mice, the inclusion of this antigen is based on the following: the pattern of PfLSA-1 expression on infected hepatocytes; the detection of PfLSA-1 specific CTL in irradiated sporozoite immunized volunteers and naturally exposed individuals from Kenya; the presence of an invariant HLA-Bw53-restricted CTL PfLSA-1 epitope in naturally exposed Gambians, in whom this haplotype has been associated with resistance to severe malaria [25]; and, the high level of immunogenicity of the PfLSA-1 DNA vaccine in the rodent model (unpublished).

P. falciparum DNA vaccine expression and immunogenicity in mice

The four *P. falciparum* pre-erythrocytic antigen genes discussed above were cloned into DNA vaccine plasmids, examined for expression by transfection of cells in vitro and finally tested for immunogenicity in mice by injection of plasmid DNA (R. Hedstrom et al., manuscript in preparation). Mammalian cell expression of each malarial antigen was optimized by constructing plasmids that encoded the leader peptide sequence (first 23 amino acid residues) of human tissue plasminogen activator protein (TPA) fused to the N terminus of the *P. falciparum* antigen protein [14]. In addition, a portion of the upstream 5′-untranslated region of the human TPA gene was included in these plasmid constructs in an effort to enhance translational efficiency in eukaryotic cells. In each case, *P. falciparum* antigen expression was increased by the use of these TPA sequences as determined by immunoblot analysis of transiently transfected tissue culture cells. Plasmids that expressed well in transiently transfected cells, in every case, induced an immunological response in mice as measured by the induction of specific antibody and CTL. This study demonstrated, however, that the magnitude of expression in vitro may not always be an accurate reflection of murine immunogenicity in vivo. The results of this study provided the basis for further testing of these plasmids in primates.

P. falciparum DNA vaccine immunogenicity in Rhesus monkeys

The next step was to determine if the *P. falciparum* DNA vaccines were immunogenic in non-human primates by intramuscular immunization and, if so, would mixing the plasmids have any stimulatory or suppressive effects on the induction of cellular immune responses to the vaccine antigens. Rhesus monkeys were immunized intramuscularly three times with 500 μg of an individual plasmid, with two plasmids given at different sites, or with combinations of the four plasmids. Antigen-specific, MHC-restricted and $CD8^+$ T cell-dependent CTL activity was induced in all vaccinated monkeys. The level of interferon-γ mRNA in peripheral blood mononuclear cells isolated from vaccinated monkeys was found to be significantly elevated following in vitro stimulation, as compared with control monkeys that were immunized with empty plasmid. Significant antigen-specific lymphoproliferation was also observed for all antigens. Most importantly, no significant negative effects on CTL and antibody responses to the individual antigens were observed in monkeys immunized with plasmid mixtures (R. Wang et al., manuscript in preparation). These data provided the foundation for trials of multi-component pre-erythrocytic DNA vaccines in human volunteers.

Future studies

The next goal will be to begin clinical trials. Initially, a single plasmid expressing PfCSP will be tested for safety and immunogenicity at varying doses. If the single plasmid is safe and immunogenic, a mixture of four to six plasmids will be tested for safety, immunogenicity and efficacy to prevent experimentally induced malaria [10]. Different doses and immunization intervals will be assessed in the initial clinical trials. However, questions concerning the optimization of other vaccine parameters, for instance multivalent mixture(s) versus individual vaccines, will be difficult to assess in human subjects given the preclinical safety requirements for investigational new drug applications. Careful preclinical studies in experimental animals may be the only practical, although imperfect, method of studying these important variables. It may be necessary to increase the number of antigen encoding genes in the vaccine to reach an acceptable level of protective efficacy. Other *P. falciparum* antigens do exist that are expressed within infected hepatocytes, but will not be included in our studies (reviewed in [30]). These could be used in future trials if necessary. Never before has a method of vaccine preparation been so ideally suited to the rapid formulation and testing of multiple antigens both individually and in combinations.

Conclusion

The development of a vaccine to protect human subjects against malaria is a feasible goal; sterile protective immunity can be induced by experimentally infecting human subjects with live sporozoites that have been attenuated by radiation. This multi-antigen exposure has been problematic to replicate with a practical vaccine. The emergence of DNA vaccine technology offers a simple approach to formulating such a multivalent vaccine. The first DNA vaccine studied encoded a single antigen, the major surface antigen of the sporozoite of *P. yoelii*, (PyCSP [54]). Preclinical studies in experimental animals showed that this vaccine induced antigen-specific CTL, antibody responses and protection against sporozoite challenge in some strains of mice, and antigen-specific antibody in *Aotus* monkeys. The genetic restriction of protection observed in the rodent model was circumvented by a bivalent (PyCSP and PyHEP17) vaccine that broadened the protective response and induced protection in other strains of mice. Since then promising results have been obtained using DNA vaccines encoding other *P. yoelii* antigens (PySSP2 and PyMSP1). These studies in mice provided the rationale for development of *P. falciparum* DNA vaccines destined for clinical evaluation as a multivalent malaria vaccine in human volunteers. DNA vaccines were constructed with the *P. falciparum* analogs of those *P. yoelii* genes under investigation. Each candidate *P. falciparum* antigen-encoding plasmid was designed for optimal expression in mammalian cells and tested for immunogenicity in the rodent model and in a nonhuman primate, the Rhesus monkey. Clinical trials in human subjects of a multivalent *P. falciparum* DNA vaccine are planned for the near future.

Acknowledgement. The work was supported by the Naval Medical Research and Development Command Work Units nos. 62787A00101EFX and 63002AA0101HFX. The opinions and assertions contained herein are the private ones of the authors and do not reflect the official policy of the Department of the Navy, Department of Defense, or the U.S. Government. The experiments reported herein, were conducted according to the principles set forth in the "Guide for the Care and Use of Laboratory Animals," Institute of Laboratory Animal Resources, National Research Council, National Academy Press, 1996.

References

1. Alonso PL, Lindsay SW. Armstrong Schellenberg JRM, Keita K, Gomez P, Shenton FC, Hill AG, David PH, Fegan G, Cham K, Greenwood BM (1993) A malaria control trial using insecticide-treated bed nets and targeted chemoprophylaxis in a rural area of The Gambia, West Africa. Trans R Soc Trop Med Hyg 87 : 37
2. Baird J (1995) Host age as a determinant of naturally acquired immunity to *Plasmodium falciparum*. Parasitol Today 11 : 105
3. Beach RF, Ruebush TK, Sexton JD, Bright PL, Hightower AW, Breman JG, Mount DL, Oloo AJ (1993) Effectiveness of permethrin-impregnated bed nets and curtains for malaria control in holoendemic area of western Kenya. Am J Trop Med Hyg 49 : 290
4. Beadle C, McElroy PD, Oster CN, Beier JC, Oloo AJ, Onyango FK, Chumo DK, Bales JD, Sherwood JA, Hoffman SL (1995) Impact of transmission intensity and age on *Plasmodium falciparum* density and associated fever: implications for malaria vaccine design. J Infect Dis 172 : 1047
5. Blackman MJ, Heidrich HG, Donachie S, McBride JS, Holder AA (1990) A single fragment of a malaria merozoite surface protein remains on the parasite during red cell invasion and is the target of invasion–inhibiting antibodies. J Exp Med 172 : 379
6. Burns JM, Majarian WR, Young JF, Daly TM, Long CA (1989) A protective monoclonal antibody recognizes an epitope in the carboxyl-terminal cysteine-rich domain in the precursor of the major merozoite surface antigen of the rodent malarial parasite, *Plasmodium yoelii*. J Immunol Methods 143 : 2670
7. Campbell JR (1989) DNA sequence of the gene encoding a *Plasmodium falciparum* malaria candidate vaccine antigen. Nucleic Acids Res 17 : 5854
8. Charoenvit Y, Leef ML, Yuan LF, Sedegah M, Beaudoin RL (1987) Characterization of *Plasmodium yoelii* monoclonal antibodies directed against stage-specific sporozoite antigens. Infect Immun 55 : 604
9. Charoenvit Y, Mellouk S, Sedegah M, Toyoshima T, Leef MF, De la Vega P, Beaudoin RL, Aikawa M, Fallarme V, Hoffman SL (1995) *Plasmodium yoelii*: 17-kDa hepatic and erythrocytic stage protein is the target of an inhibitory monoclonal antibody. Exp Parasitol 80 : 419
10. Church LWP, Le TP, Bryan JP, Gordon DM, Edelman R, Fries L, Davis JR, Herrington DA, Clyde DF, Shmuklarsky MJ, Schneider I, McGovern TW, Chulay JD, Ballou WR, Hoffman SL (1997) Clinical manifestations of *Plasmodium falciparum* malaria experimentally induced by mosquito challenge. J Infect Dis 175 : 915
11. Cohen S, McGregor IA, Carrington S (1961) Gamma-globulin and acquired immunity to human malaria. Nature 192 : 733
12. Daly TM, Long CA (1993) A recombinant 15-kilodalton carboxyl-terminal fragment of *Plasmodium yoelii* yoelli 17XL merozoite surface protein 1 induces a protective immune response in mice. Infect Immun 61 : 2462
13. Daly TM, Long CA (1995) Humoral response to a carboxyl-terminal region of the merozoite surface protein-1 plays a predominant role in controlling blood-stage infection in rodent malaria. J Immunol 155 : 236
14. Degen SJ, Rajput B, Reich E (1986) The human tissue plasminogen activator gene. J Biol Chem 261 : 6972
15. Diggs CL, Ballou WR, Miller LH (1993) The major merozoite surface protein as a malaria vaccine target. Parasitol Today 9 : 300
16. Doolan DL, Hoffman SL (1997) Multi-gene vaccination against malaria: a multi-stage, multi-immune response approach. Parasitol Today 13 : 171
17. Doolan DL, Hedstrom RC, Rogers WO, Charoenvit Y, Rogers M, de la Vega P, Hoffman SL (1996) Characterization of the protective hepatocyte erythrocyte protein 17-kDa gene of *Plasmodium yoelii*: homolog of *P. falciparum* exported protein-1. J Biol Chem 271 : 17861
18. Doolan DL, Sedegah M, Hedstrom RC, Hobart P, Charoenvit Y, Hoffman SL (1996) Circumventing genetic restriction of protection against malaria with multi-gene DNA immunization: $CD8^+$ T cell, interferon-γ, nitric oxide-dependent immunity. J Exp Med 183 : 1739
19. Etlinger HM, Caspers P, Matile H, Schoenfeld HJ, Stueber D, Takacs B (1991) Ability of recombinant or native proteins to protect monkeys against heterologous challenge with *Plasmodium falicparium*. Infect Immun 59 : 3498
20. Flynn JL, Weiss WR, Norris KA, Seifert HS, Kumar S, So M (1990) Generation of a cytotoxic T-lymphocyte response using a Salmonella antigen-delivery system. Mol Microbiol 4 : 2111
21. Freeman RR, Holder AA (1983) Characteristics of the protective response of BALB/c mice immunized with a purified *Plasmodium yoelii* schizont antigen. Clin Exp Immunol 54 : 609

22. Gramzinski RA, Maris DC, Obaldia N, Rossan R, Sedegah M, Wang R, Hobart P, Margalith M, Hoffman S (1996) Optimization of antibody responses of a malaria DNA vaccine in *Aotus* monkeys. Vaccine Res 5 : 173
23. Hedstrom RC, Campbell JR, Leef ML, Charoenvit Y, Carter M, Sedegah M, Beaudoin RL, Hoffman SL (1990) A malaria sporozoite surface antigen distinct from the circumsporozoite protein. Bull World Health Org 68 : 152
24. Hedstrom RC, Sedegah M, Hoffman SL (1994) Prospects and strategies for development of DNA vaccines against malaria. Res Immunol 145 : 476
25. Hill AVS, Allsopp CEM, Kwiatkowki D, Anstey NM, Twumasi P, Rowe PA, Bennett S, Brewster D, McMichael A, Greenwood BM (1991) Common West African HLA antigens are associated with protection from severe malaria. Nature 352 : 595
26. Hoffman SL (1997) Experimental challenge of volunteers with malaria. Ann Int Med 127 : 233
27. Hoffman SL, Oster CN, Plowe CV, Woollett GR, Beier JC, Chulay JD, Wirtz RA, Hollingdale MR, Mugambi M (1987) Naturally acquired antibodies to sporozoites do not prevent malaria: vaccine development implications. Science 237 : 639
28. Hoffman SL, Isenbarger D, Long GW, Sedegah M, Szarfman A, Waters L, Hollingdale MR, Miede PH van der, Finbloom DS, Ballou WR (1989) Sporozoite vaccine induces genetically restricted T cell elimination of malaria from hepatocytes. Science 244 : 1078
29. Hoffman SL, Weiss W, Mellouk S, Sedegah M (1990) Irradiated sporozoite vaccine induces cytotoxic T lymphocytes that recognize malaria antigens on the surface of infected hepatocytes. Immunol Lett 25 : 33
30. Hoffman SL, Franke ED, Hollingdale MR, Druilhe P (1996) Attacking the infected hepatocyte. In: Hoffman SL (ed) Malaria vaccine development. ASM Press, Washington DC, pp 35–75
31. Holder AA, Freeman RR (1981) Immunization against blood-stage rodent malaria using purified parasite antigens. Nature 294 : 361
32. Khusmith S, Charoenvit Y, Kumar S, Sedegah M, Beaudoin RL, Hoffman SL (1991) Protection against malaria by vaccination with sporozoite surface protein 2 plus CS protein. Science 252 : 715
33. Khusmith S, Sedegah M, Hoffman SL (1994) Complete protection against *Plasmodium yoelii* by adoptive transfer of a $CD8^+$ cytotoxic T cell clone recognizing sporozoite surface protein 2. Infect Immun 62 : 2979
34. Lal AA, De la Cruz VF, Welsh JA, Charoenvit Y, Maloy WL, McCutchan TF (1987) Structure of the gene encoding the circumsporozoite protein of *Plasmodium yoelii*. J Biol Chem 262 : 2937
35. Li S, Rodrigues M, Rodriguez D, Rodriguez JR, Esteban M, Palese P, Nussenzweig RS, Zavala F (1993) Priming with recombinant influenza virus followed by administration of recombinant vaccinia virus induces $CD8^+$ T-cell-mediated protective immunity against malaria. Proc Natl Acad Sci USA 90 : 5214
36. Ling IT, Ogun SA, Holder AA (1994) Immunization against malaria with a recombinant protein. Parasite Immunol 16 : 63
37. McElroy PD, Beier JC, Oster CN, Beadle C, Sherwood JA, Oloo AJ, Hoffman SL (1994) Predicting outcome in malaria: correlation between rate of exposure to infected mosquitoes and level of *Plasmodium falciparum* parasitemia. Am J Trop Med Hyg 51 : 523
38. Mitchell GH, Butcher GA, Cohen S (1975) Merozoite vaccination against *Plasmodium knowlesi* malaria. Immunology 29 : 397
39. Panina Bordignon P, Tan A, Termijtelen A, Demotz S, Corradin G, Lanzavecchia A (1989) Universally immunogenic T cell epitopes: promiscuous binding to human MHC class II and promiscuous recognition by T cells. Eur J Immunol 19 : 2237
40. Perrin LH, Merkli B, Loche M, Chizzolini C, Smart J, Richle R (1984) Antimalarial immunity in Saimiri monkeys. Immunization with surface components of asexual blood stages. J Exp Med 160 : 441
41. Renia L, Grillot D, Marussig M, Corradin G, Miltgen F, Lambert PH, Mazier D, Del Giudice G (1993) Effector functions of circumsporozoite peptide primed $CD4^+$ T cell clones against *Plasmodium yoelii* liver stages. J Immunol 150 : 1471
42. Robson KJ, Hall JR, Jennings MW, Harris TJ, Marsh K, Newbold CI, Tate VE, Weatherall DJ (1988) A highly conserved amino acid sequence in thrombospondin, properdin and in proteins from sporozoites and blood stages of a human malaria parasite. Nature 335 : 79
43. Rodrigues M, Li S, Murata K, Rodriguez D, Rodriguez JR, Bacik I, Bennink JR, Yewdell JW, Garcia Sastre A, Nussenzweig RS, Esteban M, Palese P, Zavala F (1994) Influenza and vaccinia viruses expressing malaria $CD8^+$ T and B cell epitopes. Comaprison of their immunogenicity and capacity to induce protective immunity. J Immunol 153 : 4636

44. Rodrigues MM, Cordey A-S, Arreaza G, Corradin G, Romero P, Maryanski JL, Nussenzweig RS, Zavala F (1991) CD8+ cytolytic T cell clones derived against the *Plasmodium yoelii* circumsporozoite protein protect against malaria. Int Immunol 3 : 579
45. Rogers WO, Malik A, Mellouk S, Nakamura K, Rogers MD, Szarfman A, Gordon DM, Nussler AK, Aikawa M, Hoffman SL (1992) Characterization of *Plasmodium falciparum* sporozoite surface protein 2. Proc Natl Acad Sci USA 89 : 9176
46. Rogers WO, Rogers MD, Hedstrom RC, Hoffman SL (1992) Characterization of the gene encoding sporozoite surface protein 2, a protective *Plasmodium yoelii* sprozoite antigen. Mol Biochem Parasitol 53 : 45
47. Romero P, Maryanski JL, Corradin G, Nussenzweig RS, Nussenzweig V, Zavala F (1989) Cloned cytotoxic T cells recognize an epitope in the circumsporozoite protein and protect against malaria. Nature 341 : 323
48. Sabchareon A, Burnouf T, Quattara D, Attanath P, Bouharoun Tayoun H, Chantavanich P, Foucault C, Chongsuphajaisiddhi T, Druilhe P (1991) Parasitologic and clinical human response to immunoglobulin administration in falciparum malaria. Am J Trop Med Hyg 45 : 297
49. Sanchez GI, Rogers WO, Mellouk S, Hoffman SL (1994) *Plasmodium falciparum*: exported protein-1, a blood stage antigen, is expressed in liver stage parasites. Exp Parasitol 79 : 59
50. Schofield L, Villaquiran J, Ferreira A, Schellekens H, Nussenzweig RS, Nussenzweig V (1987) Gamma-interferon, CD8+ T cells and antibodies required for immunity to malaria sporozoites. Nature 330 : 664
51. Sedegah M, Beaudoin RL, De la Vega P, Leef MF, Ozcel MA, Jones E, Charoenvit Y, Yuan LF, Gross M, Majarian WR, Robey FA, Weiss W, Hoffman SL (1988) Use of a vaccinia construct expressing the circumsporozoite protein in the analysis of protective immunity to *Plasmodium yoelii*. In: Lasky L (ed) Technological advances in vaccine development. Liss, New York, pp 295–309
52. Sedegah M, Beaudoin RL, Majarian WR, Cochran MD, Chiang CH, Sadoff J, Aggarwal A, Charoenvit Y, Hoffman SL (1990) Evaluation of vaccines designed to induce protective cellular immunity against the *Plasmodium yoelii* circumsporozoite protein: vaccinia, pseudorabies, and salmonella transformed with circumsporozoite gene. Bull World Health Org 68 : 109
53. Sedegah M, Chiang CH, Weiss WR, Mellouk S, Cochran MD, Houghton RA, Beaudoin RL, Smith D, Hoffman SL (1992) Recombinant pseudorabies virus carrying a plasmodium gene: herpes virus as a new live viral vector for inducing T- and B-cell immunity. Vaccine 10 : 578
54. Sedegah M, Hedstrom RC, Hobart P, Hoffman SL (1994) Protection against malaria by immunization with plasmid DNA encoding circumsporozoite protein. Proc Natl Acad Sci USA 91 : 9866
55. Siddiqui WA, Tam LQ, Kramer KJ, Hui GS, Case SE, Yamaga KM, Chang SP, Chan EB, Kan SC (1987) Merozoite surface coat precursor protein completely protects Aotus monkeys against *Plasmodium falciparum* malaria. Proc Natl Acad Sci USA 84 : 3014
56. Stoute JA, Slaoui M, Heppner DG, Monin P, Kester K, Desmons P, Wellde BT, Garcon N, Krzych U, Marchand M, Ballou WR, Cohen JD, for the RTS,S Malaria Vaccine Evaluation Group (1997) A preliminary evaluation of a recombinant circumsporozoite vaccine against *Plasmodium falciparum* malaria. N Engl J Med 336 : 86
57. Valmori D, Pessi A, Bianchi E, Corradin G (1992) Use of human universally antigenic tetanus toxin T cell epitopes as carriers for human vaccination. J Immunol Methods 149 : 717
58. Weiss WR, Sedegah M, Beaudoin RL, Miller LH, Good MF (1988) CD8+ T cells (cytotoxic/suppressors) are required for protection in mice immunized with malaria sporozoites. Proc Natl Acad Sci USA 85 : 573
59. Weiss WR, Good MF, Hollingdale MR, Miller LH, Berzofsky JA (1989) Genetic control of immunity to *Plasmodium yoelii* sporozoites. J Immunol 143 : 4263
60. Weiss WR, Mellouk S, Houghten RA, Sedegah M, Kumar S, Good MF, Berzofsky JA, Miller LH, Hoffman SL (1990) Cytotoxic T cells recognize a peptide from the circumsporozoite protein on malaria-infected hepatocytes. J Exp Med 171 : 763
61. Weiss WR, Berzovsky JA, Houghten R, Sedegah M, Hollingdale M, Hoffman SL (1992) A T cell clone directed at the circumsporozoite protein which protects mice against both *P. yoelii* and *P. berghei*. J Immunol 149 : 2103
62. Zhu J, Hollingdale MR (1991) Structure of *Plasmodium falciparum* liver stage antigen-1. Mol Biochem Parasitol 48 : 223

Genetic adjuvants for DNA immunization

Robert B. Mendoza, Thomas J. Kipps

UCSD Human Gene Therapy Program, Division of Hematology/Oncology, Department of Medicine, UCSD School of Medicine, La Jolla, CA 92093-0663, USA

Introduction

The injection of naked plasmid DNA expression vectors into animal muscle or skin has been shown to be an effective means to stimulate cellular and humoral immunity against the expressed protein [36]. However, even though such DNA vaccines in some cases may be more effective than inactivated virus or subvirion vaccines in inducing anti-viral immunity [8, 12], the immune response that they elicit is often too weak or too late in developing to provide protective immunity [10, 23]. For this reason, investigators have attempted to enhance the efficacy of DNA vaccines by co-injecting plasmids encoding immune stimulatory cytokines, such as IL-2 and GM-CSF, along with plasmid encoding the antigen [17, 29, 35, 37].

Recently, two groups reported that the delayed-type hypersensitivity response or CTL activity against a transgene antigen could be enhanced by co-injecting skeletal muscle with the DNA vaccine together with plasmid expressing CD86 (B7-2) [15, 33]. Conceivably, co-expression of antigen and CD86 allowed the transfected muscle cell to present the transgene antigen more efficiently to T helper cells. However, recent studies suggest that bone marrow-derived APCs present the transgene antigen to T cells being transfected at the site of injection or after taking up antigen expressed by transfected connective tissue cells [7]. In either case, co-injection of DNA vaccines with plasmids expressing accessory molecules that can activate such APCs for T cell antigen presentation should enhance the immune response to a trangene antigen.

Our strategy to enhance the efficacy of nucleic acid vaccines has been to evaluate the murine CD40-ligand (CD154) as a type of genetic adjuvant within a DNA immunization protocol. The CD40-ligand is a 39 kDa type II membrane glycoprotein [3] that has homology to TNF-α [2, 25] and is primarily expressed on activated CD4+ T cells [19, 20]. The engagement of CD154 with its counter-receptor (CD40) on B cells [6, 27] induces activities that are critical for humoral immunity, such as B cell proliferation [2], Ig class switching [32], and germinal center formation [11, 16] (Fig. 1). The significance of CD40-ligand expression *in vivo* is noted in patients that lack expression of functional CD154 and develop the X-linked hyper-IgM syndrome (HIGM). This disease is characterizaed by elevated levels of serum IgM and absent or negligible levels of IgA, IgE and IgG isotypes [26]. HIGM patients also have a high degree of susceptibility to opportunistic infections that are typically eliminated by the cellular immune response. Utilizing expression vectors encoding CD154 and a target antigen, we hypothesized that co-immunization with these vectors may augment CD154/CD40 cross-linking events thereby enhancing the proliferation of B cells and inducing an immune response against the target antigen.

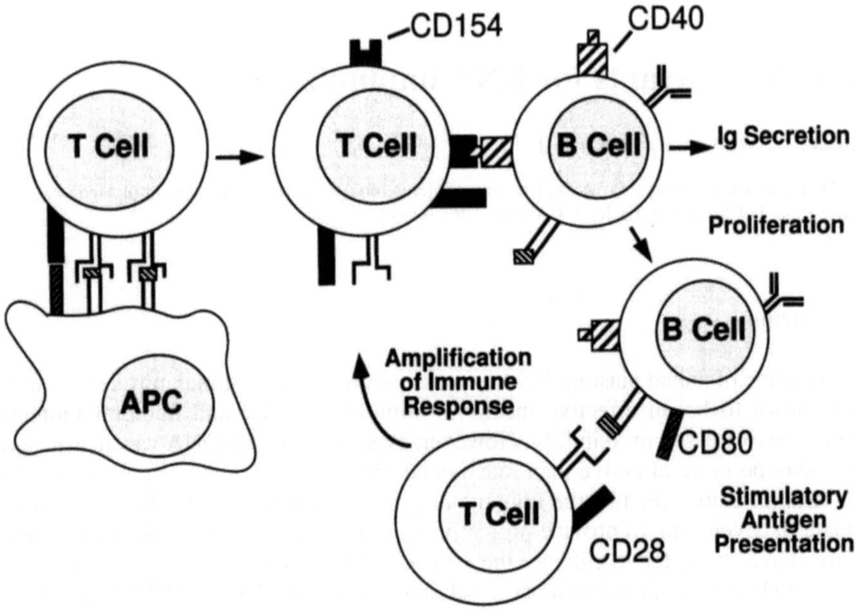

Fig. 1. Interaction between T and B cells through CD154:CD40 cross-linking induces the proliferation, differentiation, and immunoglobulin class switching of B cells. T cells that do not express functional CD154 are unable to promote the amplification and maturation of B cells thereby leading to hyper-IgM syndrome.

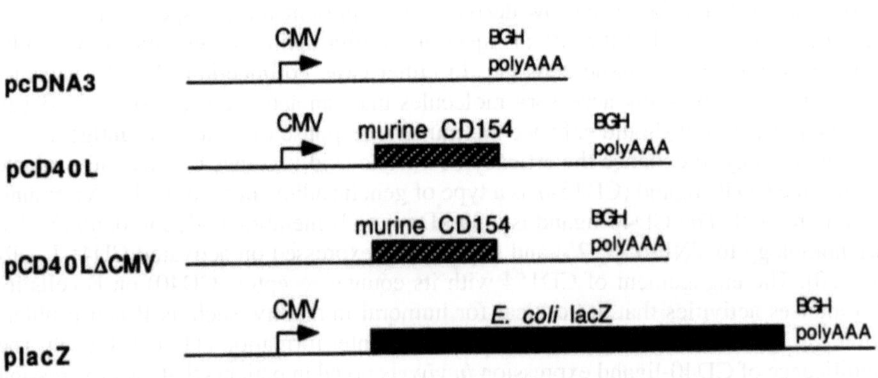

Fig. 2. Expression plasmids injected into mouse muscle and skin.

Immunization with pCD40L and the Induction of Immunity

pCD40L enhances the humoral immune response to β-galactosidase (β-gal)

The cDNA encoding the murine CD40-ligand (CD154) was isolated from activated BALB/c splenocytes and amplified via RT-PCR. This cDNA was inserted into pcDNA3 to generate pCD40L, a eukaryotic expression plasmid encoding CD154 under the control of the cytomegalovirus (CMV) promoter. Transfection of P3 cells with pCD40L resulted in stable, high level expression of CD154, as assessed by flow cytometry.

We evaluated the *in vivo* capacity of the CD40-ligand molecule to function as a genetic adjuvant thereby enhancing the immune response to β-gal, expressed from placZ – a pcDNA3-based vector encoding *E. coli* beta-galactosidase. BALB/c mice were administered four weekly injections of plasmids pcDNA3, pcDNA3 + placZ, pcDNA3 + pCD40L, or placZ + pCD40L (Fig. 2). Intramuscular injections into the right hindleg quadriceps consisted of a total of 100 (g plasmid DNA in 100 (l sterile saline. Serum samples were collected on alternate weeks (day 0, day 14, and day 28), via retro-orbital puncture, and assayed by ELISA for the presence of anti-β-gal immunoglobulin. Mice injected with either the unmodified pcDNA3 vector or pcDNA3 + pCD40L served as negative controls and did not induce antibodies to β-gal. However, the sera of animals co-injected with either placZ + pcDNA3 or placZ + pCD40L developed detectable anti-β-gal one week following the fourth and final injection, at day 28 (Fig. 3). In addition, mice injected with placZ + pCD40L had detectable serum anti-β-gal antibody one week following the second injection (day 14) (Fig. 3), and an eight-fold higher mean titer of anti-β-gal immunoglobulin at day 28 than mice given placZ + pcDNA3 [24]. The imtramuscular injection experiments outlined above were repeated using an intradermal route of immunization. The capacity of pCD40L to stimulate the immune response when injected into skin was similar to that achieved with the intramuscular injections. However, we were able to use half the amount of DNA (50 μg) when injecting into skin.

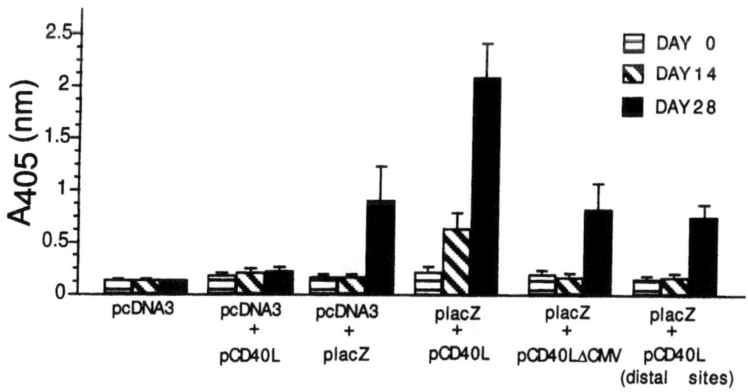

Fig. 3. DNA co-immunization with pCD40L enhances the immunoglobulin G response to β-gal in BALB/c mice. Groups of eight mice received intramuscular injections to the hind leg quadriceps of either 100 μg pcDNA3, 50 μg pcDNA3 + 50 μg pCD40L, 50 μg pcDNA3 + 50 μg placZ, 50 μg pCD40L + 50 μg placZ, 50 μg pCD40LΔCMV + 50 μg placZ, or 50 μg placZ (left hindleg) and 50 μg pCD40L (right hindleg). Mice were given a total of four weekly injections of plasmid DNA and bled on alternate weeks (d0, d14, and d28). The relative amounts of anti-β-gal present in the collected sera were determined via ELISA. The height of each bar depicts the mean OD of sera at a 1:40 dilution of each group ± SE.

The adjuvant effect of the pCD40L plasmid on the anti-β-gal antibody response was observed only when it was co-injected with placZ into the same quadriceps muscle (Fig. 3). Animals injected with placZ and pCd40L, into the left and right hind leg quadriceps, respectively, did not develop detectable anti-β-gal immunoglobulin until day 28. The levels of anti-(-gal in these mice at day 28 was similar to that of mice injected with placZ + pcDNA3.

The CD154 gene contains a six nucleotide sequence of AACGTT (nt 306-311). This sequence is similar to the PuPuCGPyPy motif that has been shown to exist in the ampR gene of bacterial expression vectors and reported to have immunostimulatory effects when co-injected with an antigen into mice [18, 31, 38]. To control for possible immunostimulatory effects due to the CpG motif in CD154, we manipulated pCD40L by deleting the CMV promoter to abolish expression of the CD40-ligand while retaining the AACGTT sequence. The plasmid pCD40LΔCMV was co-injected with placZ into BALB/c mice and did not enhance the production of anti-β-gal antibody to any greater extent than injections of pcDNA3 + placZ (Fig. 3).

Isotype analysis of the immune response

Despite enhancing the titer of the anti-β-gal antibody response, we found that the subclass of anti-(β-gal IgG induced by placZ was not altered by the co-injection of pCD40L. BALB/c mice injected with placZ developed primarily IgG_{2a} anti-β-gal antibody (Fig 4). Generally, Th1 immune responses in mice promote production of this

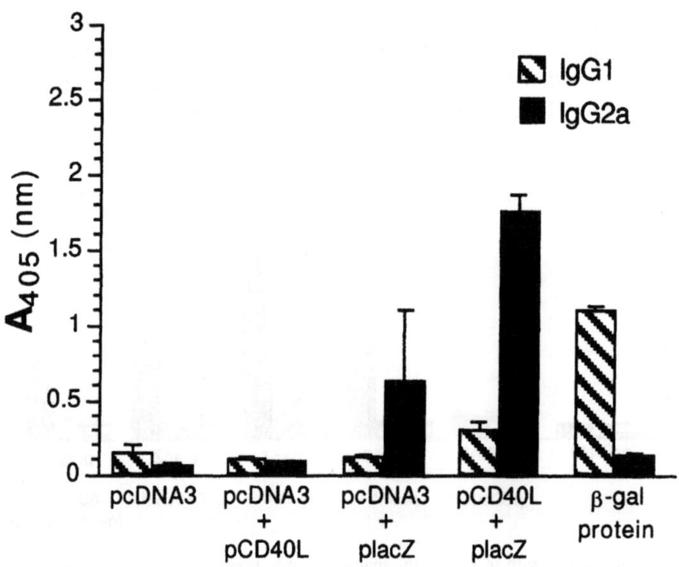

Fig. 4. Analysis of the IgG_1 and IgG_{2a} anti-β-gal antibody induced by the intramuscular plasmid DNA injections as indicated on the abscissa and in the legend to Fig. 3. The height of each bar depicts the mean O.D. measurements (± S.E.) of anti-β-gal IgG1 (striped bar) and anti-β-gal IgG_{2a} (solid bar) present in the post-immune sera (day 28). Also shown are the ELISA O.D. measurements of the day 28 sera of mice immunized with β-gal protein. The ELISA data depicted here are from serum samples diluted 1:40.

IgG subclass, whereas Th2 immune responses favor production of IgG_1 [9, 30]. Conceivably, the increased titers of anti-β-gal IgG of mice co-injected with placZ + pCD40L were due to production of IgG_{2a} and IgG_1 anti-β-gal antibody, reflecting recruitment of Th2-type helper activity. However, animals co-injected with placZ + pCD40L generated primarily IgG2a anti-β-gal Ab, with little or no detectable IgG_1 anti-β-gal Ab. In contrast, BALB/c mice injected with β-gal protein generated primarily IgG1 anti-β-gal antibody (Fig. 4), demonstrating that such mice are not obligate producers of IgG_2a anti-β-gal immunoglobulin. Collectively, these results suggest that pCD40L enhances, but does not alter, the Th1-type immune response induced by a co-administered DNA vaccine.

pCD40L enhances the generation of antigen-specific CTL

We examined whether injection of pCD40L could influence cellular immunity and enhance the generation of β-gal-specific cytolytic T lymphocytes (CTL). BALB/c mice were given four weekly intramuscular injections of pcDNA3, pcDNA3 + placZ, pcDNA3 + pCD40L, or pCD40L + placZ. Two weeks following the fourth injection, splenocytes were isolated from the immunized mice and co-cultured with IL-2 and irradiated P13.2 cells. P13.2 cells express the β-gal protein and are derived from the parent P815 mastocytoma cell line. The stimulated T lymphocytes were harvested and incubated in triplicate with either P13.2 or P815 cells at varying E:T ratios. Specific CTL activity was measured by quantifying the amount of lactate dehydrogenase released from the P13.2 target cells. At a 45:1 effector:target (E:T) ratio, the splenocyte effector cells from mice that received intramuscular injections of placZ + pcDNA3 achieved a 20% specific lysis of P13.2. In contrast, splenocytes from mice injected with placZ + pCD40L showed 75% specific lysis at a 45:1 E:T ratio and only required a 5:1 E:T ratio to achieve 20% lysis of the target cells. This result indicates that co-immunization with pCD40L is able to effect a 9-fold increase in cellular immunity. We repeated these studies by using an intradermal route of immunization and obtained similar results as obtained for the intramuscular injections (Table I). In both experiments, the splenocytes from mice co-injected with either pcDNA3 or pcDNA3 + pCD40L did not mediate specific lysis of P13.2 or P815.

Table I. Summary of the cellular and humoral immune responses induced by co-injection with placZ. Intramuscular injections consisted of 100 μg total DNA while the intradermal injections consisted of 50 μg total DNA. As a positive control for the IgG1 ELISA, a group of three mice each received one intramuscular injection of 10 μg β-gal protein in saline followed with an intraperitoneal injection two weeks later of 1 μg β-gal protein in Freund's Incomplete adjuvant.

	Intramuscular		Intradermal	
	Anti-β-gal	CTL	Anti-β-gal	CTL
pcDNA3	–	–	–	–
pcDNA3 + pCD40L	–	–	–	–
pcDNA3 + placZ	+	+	+	+
placZ + pCD40L	+++	+++	+++	+++
placZ + pCD40LΔCMV			+	
β-gal protein	++			

Discussion

Recent studies involving the development of nucleic acid vaccines have focused upon delineating the humoral and cellular immune responses of the vaccinated host – not only as a means to further understand the molecular mechanics of immunity, but also to progress toward the creation of therapeutic strategies that command manipulation of the immune response. Toward this end, we present evidence that the immune response against a target antigen (β-galactosidase) is enhanced by addition of the murine CD40 ligand expression vector to a genetic immunization protocol. Furthermore, utilization of the murine CD40L as a genetic adjuvant enhances both humoral and cellular immunity against the β-gal antigen.

That pCD40L can enhance the humoral and cellular response to placZ indicates that CD40-bearing cells are involved in the immune response to this DNA vaccine. Myocytes and T cells ordinarily do not express CD40 [34]. If myocytes presented antigen directly to T cells, then it would not be anticipated that local expression of CD154 would modify the immunogenicity of a transgene antigen. The effectiveness of pCD40L in augmenting the immune response to a transgene antigen argues in favor of the model proposing that the transgene antigen is presented by CD40-bearing APCs that are rendered more effective for cognate APC-T cell interactions through a CD40-dependent signal.

In addition to B cells, the CD40 receptor is also expressed on additional types of professional antigen presenting cells. CD40 is a 49 kDa glycoprotein that is a member of the TNF-receptor superfamily [22] and is expressed on dendritic cells [21], monocytes [1], endothelial cells [14, 39], and fibroblasts [13]. Cognate interactions between CD154 and CD40 involving these other cell types can induce antigen presenting cell functions that favor the development of a cellular, or Th1-mediated, immune response. The engagement of CD154 with CD40 can further induce the expression of immune accessory molecules such as CD80/CD86 (B7-1/B7-2) and IL-12 from B cells, macrophages and denedritic cells. In addition, cognate interactions between CD154:CD40 on T cells and endothelial cells can lead to the expression of the cell surface adhesion molecules ICAM-1 and VCAM-1 [28, 40].

Due to the large number of potential cell:cell interactions utilizing CD154:CD40 cross-linking, the many co-stimulatory molecules and cytokines that can be released from professional APCs is likely responsible for the 9-fold induction of humoral and cellular immunity in our experiments. Thus, a DNA immunization strategy utilizing CD154 as an adjuvant may be applicable for those antigens that are only weakly immunogenic. In addition, for those patients that lack expression of functional CD154 and develop hyper-IgM syndrome, it might be possible to provide CD154 in the form of a genetic vaccine to correct the disease condition.

Ordinarily, CD154 is transiently expressed by T cells upon lymphocyte activation and is rapidly down-modulated [4, 5, 20]. By placing CD154 under the control of the CMV promoter, expression of the gene is maintained at high levels by cells that take up the pCD40L plasmid, possibly accounting for the effectiveness of pCD40L as a genetic adjuvant. Conceivably, strategies that incorporate the gene transfer of CD154 under such strong promoters may enhance the response to other DNA or cellular vaccines, allowing for their more effective use in the prophylaxis of infections or the immune therapy of neoplastic disease.

Acknowledgments

This work was supported by the National Institutes of Health Grant CA66000. R. Mendoza is a recipient of the University of California President's Postdoctoral Fellowship.

References

1. Alderson MR, Armitage RJ, Tough TW, Strockbine L, Fanslow WC & Spriggs MK (1993). CD40 expression by human monocytes: regulation by cytokines and activation of monocytes by the ligand for CD40. J. Exp. Med. 178 : 669–674
2. Armitage RJ, Fanslow WC, Stockbrine L, Sato TA, Clifford KN, Macduff BM, Anderson DM, Gimpel SD, Davis-Smith T, Maliszewski CR, Clark EA, Smith CA, Grabstein KH, Cosman D & Spriggs MK (1992) Molecular and biologic characterization of a murine ligand for CD40. Nature 357 : 80–82
3. Banchereau J, Bazan F, Blanchard D, Briere F, Galizzi JP, van Kooten C, Liu YJ, Rousset F & Saeland S (1994) The CD40 antigen and its ligand. Annu. Rev. Immunol. 12 : 881–922
4. Cantwell MJ, T Hua, J Pappas and TJ Kipps. (1997) Acquired CD40-ligand deficiency in chronic lymphocytic leukemia. Nat. Med. 3 : 984
5. Castle BE, K Kishimoto, C Stearns, ML Brown and MR Kehry. (1993) Regulation of expression of the ligand for CD40 on T helper lymphocytes. J. Immunol. 151 : 1777
6. Clark EA & Ledbetter JA (1986) Activation of human B cells mediated through two distinct cell surface differentiation antigens, Bp35 and Bp50. Proc. Natl. Acad. Sci. USA 83 : 4494–4498
7. Corr M, Lee DJ, Carson DA & Tighe H (1996) Genetic vaccination with naked plasmid DNA: mechanism of CTL priming. J. Exp. Med. 184 : 1555–1560
8. Donnelly JJ, A Friedman, D Martinez, DL Montgomery, JW Shiver, SL Motzel, JB Ulmer and MA Liu (1995) Preclinical efficacy of a prototype DNA vaccine: enhanced protection against antigenic drift in influenza virus [see comments]. Nat. Med. 1 : 583
9. Finkelman FD, J Holmes, IM Katona, JF Urban, Jr., MP Beckmann, LS Park, KA Schooley, RL Coffman, TR Mosmann and WE Paul (1990) Lymphokine control of *in vivo* immunoglobulin isotype selection. Annu. Rev. Immunol. 8 : 803
10. Fooks AR, D Jeevarajah, A Warnes, GW Wilkinson and JC Clegg (1996) Immunization of mice with plasmid expressing the measles virus nucleoprotein gene. Viral Immunol. 9 : 65
11. Foy TM, Laman JD, Ledbetter JA, Aruffo A, Claassen E & Noelle RJ (1994) gp39-CD40 interactions are essential for germinal center formation and the development of B cell memory. J. Exp. Med. 180 : 157–163
12. Gonzalez Armas JC, CS Morello, LD Cramer and DH Spector (1996) DNA immunization confers protection against murine cytomegalovirus infection. J. Virol. 70 : 7921
13. Hess S, Rensing-Ehl A, Schwabe R, Bufler P & Engelmann H (1995) CD40 function in nonhematopoietic cells. Nuclear factor kappa B mobilization and induction of IL-6 production. J. Immunol. 155 : 4588–4595
14. Hollenbaugh D, Mischel-Petty N, Edwards CP, Simon JC, Denfeld RW, Kiener PA & Aruffo A (1995) Expression of functional CD40 by vascular endothelial cells. J. Exp. Med. 182 : 33–40
15. Iwasaki A, BJ Stiernholm, AK Chan, NL Berinstein and BH Barber (1997) Enhanced CTL responses mediated by plasmid DNA immunogens encoding costimulatory molecules and cytokines. J. Immunol. 158 : 4591
16. Kawabe T, Naka T, Yoshida K, Tanaka T, Fujiwara H, Suematsu S, Yoshida N, Kishimoto T & Kikutani H (1994) The immune responses in CD40-deficient mice: impaired immunoglobulin class switching and germinal center formation. Immunity 1 : 167–78
17. Kim JJ, V Ayyavoo, ML Bagarazzi, MA Chattergoon, K Dang, B Wang, JD Boyer and DB Weiner (1997) *In vivo* engineering of a cellular immune response by coadministration of IL-12 expression vector with DNA immunogen. J. Immunol. 158 : 816
18. Klinman DM, AK Yi, SL Beaucage, J Conover and AM Krieg (1996) CpG motifs present in bacterial DNA rapidly induce lymphocytes to secrete interleukin 6, interleukin 12, and interferon (. Proc. Natl. Acad. Sci. USA 93 : 2879
19. Lane P, Traunecker A, Hubele S, Inui S, Lanzavecchia A & Gray D (1992) Activated human T cells express a ligand for the human B cell-associated antigen CD40 which participates in T cell-dependent activation of lymphocytes. Eur. J. Immunol. 22 : 2573–2578

20. Lederman S, Yellin MJ, Inghirami G, Lee JJ, Knowles DM & Chess L (1992) Molecular interactions mediating T-B lymphocyte collaboration in human lymphoid follicles. Roles of T cell-B-cell activation molecule (5c8 antigen) and CD40 in contact-dependent help. J. Immunol. 149 : 3817–3826
21. Ludewig B, Graf D, Gelderblom HR, Becker Y, Kroczek RA & Pauli G (1995) Spontaneous apoptosis of dendritic cells is efficiently inhibited by TRAP (CD40-ligand) and TNF-alpha, but strongly enhanced by interleukin-10. Eur. J. Immunol. 25 : 1943–1950
22. Lynch F & Ceredig R 1989) Eur. J. Immunol 19 : 223–229
23. Martins LP, LL Lau, MS Asano and R Ahmed (1995) DNA vaccination against persistent viral infection. J. Virol. 69 : 2574
24. Mendoza R, MJ Cantwell and TJ Kipps (1997) Immunostimulatory effects of a plasmid expressing CD40 ligand (CD154) on gene immunization. J. Immunol. 159 : 5777–5781
25. Noelle RJ, Roy M, Shepherd DM, Stamenkovic I, Ledbetter JA, & Aruffo A (1992) A 39-kDa protein on activated helper T cells binds CD40 and transduces the signal for cognate activation of B cells. Proc. Natl. Acad. Sci. USA 89 : 6550–6554
26. Notarangelo LD, M Duse and AG Ugazio (1992) Immunodefic. Rev. 3 : 101–122
27. Pauli S, Ehlin-Henriksson B, Mellstedt H, Koho H, Ben-Aissa H & Perlmann P (1985) A p50 surface antigen restricted to human urinary bladder carcinomas and B lymphocytes. Cancer Immunol. Immunoth. 20 : 23–28
28. Ranheim EA & Kipps TJ (1993) Activated T cells induce expression of B7/BB1 on normal or leukemic B cells through a CD40-dependent signal. J. Exp. Med. 177 : 925–935
29. Raz E, A Watanabe, SM Baird, RA Eisenberg, TB Parr, M Lotz, TJ Kipps and DA Carson (1993) Systemic immunological effects of cytokine genes injected into skeletal muscle. Proc. Natl. Acad. Sci. USA 90 : 4523
30. Rizzo LV, RH DeKruyff, DT Umetsu and RR Caspi (1995) Regulation of the interaction between Th1 and Th2 T cell clones to provide help for antibody production *in vivo*. Eur. J. Immunol. 25 : 708
31. Sato Y, M Roman, H Tighe, D Lee, MP Corr, MD Nguyen, GJ Silverman, M Lotz, DA Carson and E Raz (1996) Immunostimulatory DNA sequences necessary for effective intradermal gene immunization. Science 273 : 352
32. Spriggs MK, Armitage RJ, Strockbine L, Clifford KN, Macduff BM, Sato TA, Maliszewski CR & Fanslow WC (1992) Recombinant human CD40 ligand stimulates B cell proliferation and immunoglobulin E secretion. J. Exp. Med. 176 : 1543–1550
33. Tsuji T, K Hamajima, N Ishii, I Aoki, J Fukushima, KQ Xin, S Kawamoto, S Sasaki, K Matsunaga, Y Ishigatsubo, K Tani, T Okubo and K Okuda (1997) Immunomodulatory effects of a plasmid expressing B7-2 on human immunodeficiency virus-1-specific cell-mediated immunity induced by a plasmid encoding the viral antigen. Eur. J. Immunol. 27 : 782
34. van Kooten C and J Banchereau (1996) CD40-CD40 ligand: a multifunctional receptor-ligand pair. Adv. Immunol. 61 : 1
35. Watanabe A, E Raz, H Kohsaka, H Tighe, SM Baird, TJ Kipps and DA Carson (1993) Induction of antibodies to kappa variable region by gene immunization. J. Immunol. 151 : 2871
36. Wolff JA, Malone RW, Williams P, Chang W, Acsadi G, Jani A & Felgner PL (1990) Science 247 : 1465
37. Xiang Z and HC Ertl (1995) Manipulation of the immune response to a plasmid-encoded viral antigen by coinoculation with plasmids expressing cytokines. Immunity 2 : 129
38. Yamamoto S, T Yamamoto, T Kataoka, E Kuramoto, O Yano and T Tokunaga (1992) Unique palindromic sequences in synthetic nucleotides are required to induce IFN and IFN-mediated natural killer activity. J. Immunol. 148 : 4072–4076
39. Yellin MJ, Brett J, Baum D, Matsushima A, Szabolcs M, Stern D & Chess L (1995) Functional interactions of T cells with endothelial cells: the role of CD40L-CD40-mediated signals. J. Exp. Med. 182 : 1857–1864
40. Yellin MJ, S Winikoff, SM Fortune, D Baum, MK Crow, S Lederman and L Chess (1995) Ligation of CD40 on fibroblasts induces CD54 (ICAM-1) and CD106 (VCAM-1) up-regulation and IL-6 production and proliferation. J. Leuk. Biol. 58 : 209–216

Gene immunization for the induction of antigen-specific, non MHC-restricted responses

Delphine J. Lee, Dennis A. Carson, Maripat Corr

Department of Medicine and The Sam and Rose Stein Institute for Research on Aging; University of California, San Diego; 9500 Gilman Drive; La Jolla, CA 92093-0663, USA.

Introduction

Injection of naked plasmid DNA encoding a specific antigen is capable of eliciting T cell responses which are restricted to Major Histocompatibility Complex (MHC) class I or MHC class II as well as antibody responses. Furthermore, the combination of plasmids expressing costimulator molecules along with antigen encoded plasmids can further augment certain responses. While immunization by standard protein injections allows the cells of the immune system to take up and present the foreign protein, gene immunization gives the added advantage of ectopically expressing membrane bound molecules such as potential antigen presenting molecules or costimulatory ligands which may alter the overall immune response. By injecting plasmids encoding murine CD1d1, B7.1, and ovalbumin, we can induce a CD1-restricted, ovalbumin-specific Cytotoxic T Lymphocyte (CTL) response.

The CD1 family

Classically, MHC class I or class II molecules are responsible for presenting peptide antigens to T cells. However, in both humans and mice, the non-MHC-encoded CD1 family of cell surface proteins have been implicated to also have antigen-presenting function [22, 42]. While MHC class I molecules mediate recognition of non-self or infected tissues by the immune system, the function of CD1 molecules is still unclear. Encoded outside of the MHC class I locus and unlike the MHC proteins, CD1 molecules are nonpolymorphic and have five isoforms in humans: CD1a, b, c, d, and e [36]. The isoforms are conserved in several mammalian species [19] and have been divided into two groups based on the sequences of their external domains [20]. CD1a, -b, -c and -e comprise group 1, while group 2 contains CD1d. Although all five isoforms are found in humans, only the group 2 isoforms are conserved from rodents to humans. Murine CD1 is comprised of two closely related genes, CD1D1 and CD1D2, and like the human CD1 family is also unlinked to the MHC locus.

CD1-antigen presentation

CD1 molecules share some characteristics with both MHC class I and MHC class II ligands. CD1 proteins bear some resemblance to the classical MHC class I proteins both in overall sequence homology, especially in the $\alpha 3$ domain, and by their usual association with β_2-microglobulin (β2m) [2, 20]. However, unlike MHC class I molecules, CD1 proteins have been reported to be expressed without β2m [3] and do not require the transporter proteins associated with antigen processing (TAP) for stable expression [17, 29, 50]. The mechanism of antigen processing for CD1 is more similar to that of MHC class II than class I [41, 43, 49]. Like MHC class II, human CD1b trafficks to endocytic compartments, including the specialized subset of endosomes where MHC class II proteins are believed to bind endocytosed antigens [38, 39, 45, 51].

Immunoelectron micrograph studies show human CD1b to colocalize with MHC II in dense multilamellar organelles, designated as MIIC. Furthermore, the intracytoplasmic tails of human CD1b and murine CD1 have a typical endosomal retrieval motif implying the potential recycling of the proteins from the cell surface to the endosome. The non-MHC encoded CD1 family of nonpolymorphic glycoproteins is therefore similar to, yet distinct from other antigen presenting molecules in its similarity to MHC class I by sequence, structural homology and association with β2m, as well as its similarity to MHC class II by its cellular localization and dependence on the endosomal compartment for presentation of exogenous antigens.

Unlike classical MHC, CD1 can present non-peptide ligands such as mycolic acid [5], lipoarabinomannan [47], mycobacterial lipid antigens [4] and glycosylceramide [30] to $\alpha\beta$ T cell receptor-bearing lymphocytes. The presentation of foreign non-peptide antigens by CD1 has been demonstrated for the human CD1b and CD1c as well as murine CD1d. However, by screening a synthetic phage display library, Castaño and colleagues have discovered that mCD1 can bind long peptides with hydrophobic and bulky amino acids [22]. Synthetic peptides of 15–20 amino acids bound CD1d1 with dissociation constants of 10^{-6} to 10^{-7} M. Furthermore, immunization of mice with CD1 transfected cells preincubated with peptide generated CD1-restricted, peptide-specific CTL. These data suggest that mCD1 may have antigen-presenting function by binding peptides with hydrophobic residues [22].

Development of a gene immunization strategy to induce a CD1-restricted response

To test the biological significance of mCD1 presentation of foreign protein antigens, we generated an antigen-specific, CD1-restricted response by plasmid DNA immunization [34]. Intradermal administration of plasmid DNA induces potent antigen-specific immune responses [44]. Chicken ovalbumin was selected as the test antigen as it contains a peptide with the reported mCD1 binding motif, F/W X X L/I/M X X W [22]. CD1 expression has been detected on hematopoietic cells, brain, thymus, liver, and spleen [2, 13, 16]. Reports of its expression on gastrointestinal epithelium are controversial [12, 16]. As murine CD1 is not prevalent in the dermis, a coinjection strategy was used to ectopically express the antigen presenting molecule (CD1d1) as well as the antigen, chicken ovalbumin. By using a combination of plasmids, DNA vaccination can therefore be used as a tool to prime a specific response not only to the antigen of interest, but also allows one to restrict the immune response to the desired antigen presenting molecule.

Additionally, plasmids encoding costimulatory molecules B7.1 or B7.2 were included to provide the responsive T cell with a nonspecific second signal in the same milieu as the cognate signal [15, 32, 46]. In other studies with two separate antigen systems (ovalbumin and β-galactosidase), gene immunization with combinations of plasmids expressing antigen and costimulators has proved to be effective in enhancing different arms of the immune system, with B7.1 useful for cytotoxic T cell priming and B7.2 to enhance antibody responses [24, 31]. The expression of the costimulator ligand appears to act locally as the enhancement of either CTL or antibody responses was dependent on the presence of the plasmid expressing the costimulator molecule at the same site as the antigen encoding plasmid.

Costimulation enhances priming a CD1-restricted, ovalbumin specific CTL response

Consequently, C57BL/6 mice were immunized two times, one week apart, with different combinations of plasmid DNA encoding mCD1D1 (pACB-CD1), chicken ovalbumin (nCMV-OVA), and costimulator molecules (nCMV-B7.1 or nCMV-B7.2). Mice were sacrificed at week 2, and after *in vitro* restimulation their splenocytes were assayed for their ability to lyse ovalbumin pulsed H-2^b CD1 transfected RMAS cells. In these experiments antigen loading of target cells was accomplished by incubating them with whole protein as recent reports suggest that CD1 antigen loading occurs through a TAP-independent endocytic mechanism [41, 43, 49]. The TAP independence of CD1 antigen processing made TAP deficient CD1 transfected RMAS cells preferred target cells [17, 50].

Mice immunized with a combination including B7.1-expressing plasmid repeatedly gave a higher specific lysis than mice immunized with a B7.2 encoding plasmid (Table 1). This gene immunization protocol using plasmids encoding CD1, B7.1, and the test antigen chicken ovalbumin raised a CD1-restricted ovalbumin-specific CTL response, demonstrating that protein antigen is recognized in the context of mCD1 and elicits a cellular immune response *in vivo*. Lysis by these cytotoxic lymphocytes are antigen and CD1 dependent, can be partially abrogated by anti-CD1 antibodies, and

Table 1. Recognition of ovalbumin by CD1d1-restricted CTL. Three mice per group were immunized with 50 μg of each plasmid at days 0 and 7. Two weeks after the first injection, mice were sacrificed and restimulated *in vitro* with CD1d1-transfected EL4 cells pulsed with ovalbumin protein for five days in the presence of 50 IU rIL-2. The specificity of the resulting pooled CTL was determined by measuring the lysis of CD1d1 transfected RMAS cells incubated with ovalbumin in triplicate. Mice were immunized with plasmids encoding the genes listed. The values plotted are average percent of maximum lysis of CD1-transfected RMAS cells pulsed with or without ovalbumin or RMAS cells pulsed with ovalbumin in triplicate. The values listed represent the lysis for the pooled splenocytes of three mice per group.

	Percent of Maximum Lysis		
Transgenes injected	RMA/s + OVA	RMA/s CD1D1 + OVA	RMA/s CD1D1
OVALBUMIN (OVA)	13.10	18.52	−1.23
CD1D1	−4.14	−0.38	−3.63
OVA + CD1D1	2.58	10.99	2.96
OVA + CD1D1 + B7.1	25.07	75.03	11.66
OVA + CD1D1 + B7.2	−5.25	12.31	−23.53

competitively inhibited by an established CD1-binding peptide. The *in vivo* requirement for adding a CD28 ligand is in contrast to *in vitro* studies with CD1b or CD1c-restricted human T cell hybridomas which utilize a pathway of costimulation outside of the interaction between CD28 and its counterreceptors [6].

Although the ovalbumin and CD1-restricted CTL response is greatly enhanced by the addition of the B7.1 costimulator in the priming immunization, it may not necessarily be required. Secondly, the role played by the expressed B7.1 protein in the induction of the CTL response is unclear (Fig. 1). B7.1 may actually be providing the second signal through CD28 on the CD1-restricted CTL precursor cell. Alternatively, since the ovalbumin encoded plasmid expresses the whole protein, MHC class I and class II epitopes are available for antigen processing, and it may be a MHC class I- or class II-restricted T cell that receives the costimulus. This activated ovalbumin-specific T lymphocyte may then in turn provide soluble factors in the vicinity of the CD1-restricted priming which could help stimulate the ovalbumin specfic, CD1-restricted lymphocytes.

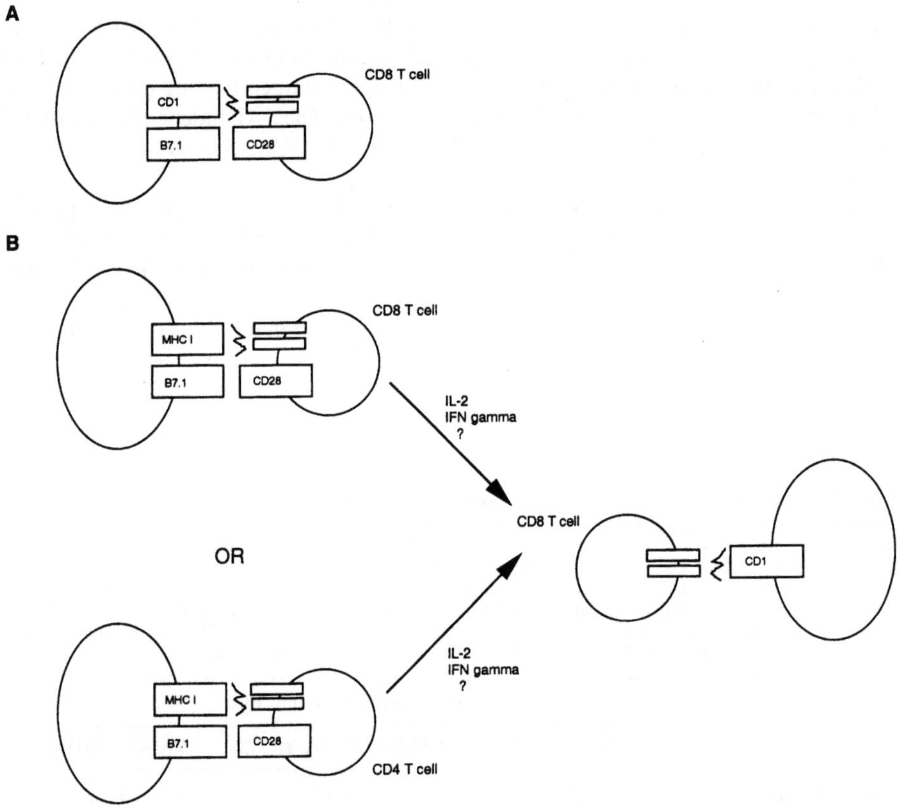

Fig. 1. Possible mechanisms of B7.1 enhancement of the CD1-restricted, ovalbumin specific CTL response. (A) B7.1 provides costimulation directly to the CD1-restricted T cell. (B) B7.1 costimulates either a MHC class I, ova-specific CD8+ T cell or a MHC class II, ova-specific CD4+ T cell which can then provide cytokines to enhance the priming of the CD1-restricted T cell.

Splenocytes from mice immunized with the combination of plasmids encoding ovalbumin, mCD1 and B7.1 were able to lyse MHC class I deficient, CD1$^+$ RMAS transfectants pulsed with ovalbumin more effectively than untransfected RMAS cells pulsed with ovalbumin. Although RMAS cells have very low levels of detectable CD1 expression on their surface by cytofluorometric analysis, augmenting the level of surface CD1 by transfection resulted in a three fold increase in cytotoxic lysis in the four hour period of the assays. The specificity of CD1 recognition was confirmed by antibody blocking studies. An antibody directed against MHC class I (H-2K^b/D^b) partially decreased lysis by 23%, while the anti-CD1 antibodies inhibited lysis by approximately 45% to 60%. None of the anti-CD1 antibodies were able to completely inhibit lysis at the concentrations used. In fact, the extent of inhibition varied between experiments, still, the 1H1 antibody was the most effective. This variation between the different anti-CD1 antibodies may reflect differences in their affinities for antigen or may represent different epitopes seen by mixed populations of T cells in each experiment.

To confirm that the CTL response was ovalbumin specific, we tested the CTL for lysis activity of CD1$^+$ RMAS cells pulsed with the p99 peptide previously described to bind murine CD1d1 [22]. The lysis of targets pulsed with p99 (16%) was not different from unpulsed targets (18%). Furthermore, p99 peptide competitively inhibited lysis of CD1$^+$ RMAS cells pulsed with ovalbumin protein, decreasing lysis from 82% to 37%. Hence DNA immunization elicited CTL which were both CD1 and antigen specific.

To further characterize the phenotype of the CD1-restricted CTL, blocking antibodies to CD4 and CD8 were used. Anti-CD8 repeatedly blocked lysis while anti-CD4 blocked lysis less consistently. The variation of inhibition between experiments by anti-CD4 implies a mixed effector population from the whole spleen preparations. Recently, Stenger and colleagues have identified two mechanisms of CD1-restricted cell-mediated cytotoxicity to contribute to the outcome of infection with intracellular pathogens [48]. CD1-restricted T cells which are CD4$^-$CD8$^-$ lysed targets through the Fas/Fas-ligand pathway while having no effect on intracellular bacterial survival, whereas CD8$^+$ effector cells used perforin and granzymes to kill the bacteria as well as their host cell. In our studies, antibodies against Fas-ligand had no effect on the lysis of CD1-transfected cells pulsed with ovalbumin.

CTL are not MHC dependent

Given that CD1 is nonpolymorphic, the same immunization protocol that was effective in generating CD1-restricted CTL in H-2^b mice should also generate CTL that recognize CD1 on cells of another MHC haplotype. Splenocytes from C57BL/6 (H-2^b) mice immunized with plasmids encoding mCD1D1 and B7.1 or mCD1D1, B7.1 and ovalbumin were tested for CTL activity to CD1D1-transfected P815 targets pulsed in the presence or absence of ovalbumin protein (Fig. 2). The high background lysis of CD1D1-transfected P815 in the absence of ovalbumin suggests a partial allogeneic response. However, H-2^b mice immunized with the three plasmids were able to mount a significant CTL response against both CD1D1-transfected, ovalbumin pulsed H-2^b RMAS cells and H-2^d P815 cells, when compared to the response of mice from the negative control group.

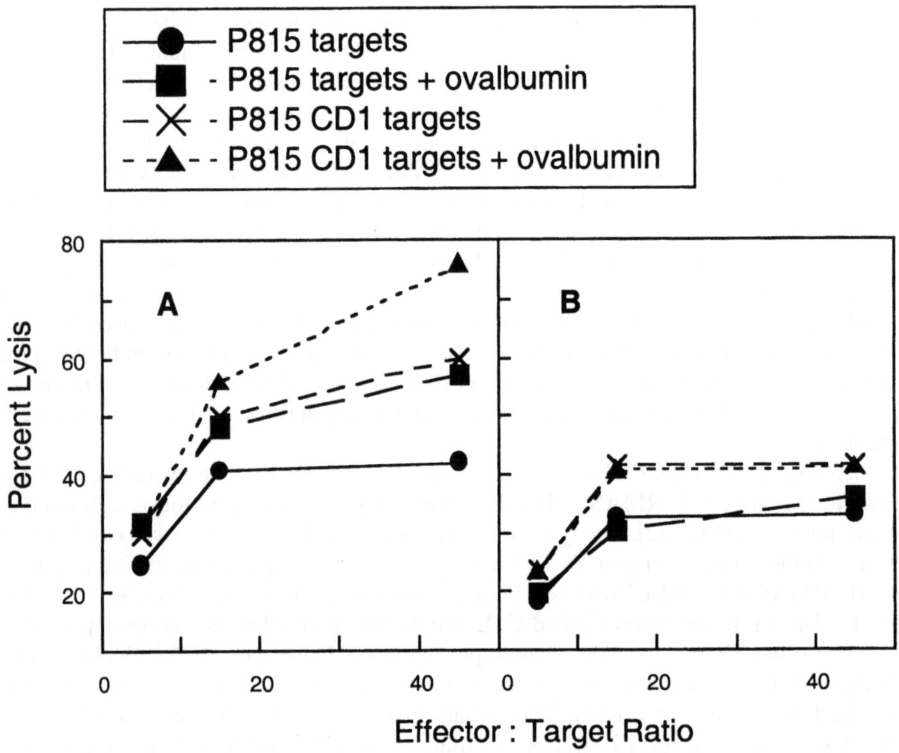

Fig. 2. Ovalbumin specific CD1-restricted CTL lysis of allogeneic targets. Ten C57BL/6 mice (H-2[b]) were immunized with plasmids encoding OVA, mCD1d1, and B7.1 (A) four mice with mCD1d1 and B7.1 (B) on days 0 and 10. Two weeks after the first injection, mice were sacrificed and restimulated *in vitro* with CD1d1-transfected RMAS cells pulsed with ovalbumin protein for five days in the presence of 50 IU/ml rIL-2. The specificity of the resulting CTL was determined by measuring the lysis of P815 cells (circles), P815 cells pulsed with ovalbumin (squares), CD1D1-transfected P815 cells (crosses), or CD1D1-transfected P815 cells pulsed with ovalbumin (triangles). The values plotted represent the average lysis.

In summary, T cells can be primed to recognize peptide antigens presented by murine non-MHC encoded CD1d (mCD1d) molecules by DNA immunization. Antigen specific, mCD1-restricted lymphocytes can be generated *in vivo* by immunizing normal mice with a combination of plasmids encoding chicken ovalbumin, murine CD1d, and costimulatory molecules. Expression of CD1 family members have been detected in a number of species including mice, rats, rabbits, sheep and humans [7, 19]. The highly conserved nature of CD1 proteins suggests that they may have evolved a specialized function to present non-peptidic ligands to T cells [42]. The crystal structure of CD1d1 reveals many differences from classical MHC molecules [54], including a deep and highly hydrophobic groove that would be structurally difficult to bind peptides in the manner of MHC molecules [14]. There remains, however, the possibility that CD1d may also present hydrophobic peptides which bind in a different configuration as suggested by the CD1d peptide binding motif and synthetic peptide binding studies [22]. Alternatively, CD1 may present lipoproteins by binding lipid portions of a molecule and presenting linked amino acid or carbohydrate residues to responsive lymphocytes. Moreover, lipids present in extracellular tissues may become oxidized over time [37] and covalently interact with exposed lysine residues. CD1 could presumably bind these lipids and present the haptenized peptides, using the lipid as a rudimentary nidus for binding antigenic fragments. The data presented here suggest that in addition to lipids and other non-peptidic molecules, endogenously generated polypeptides can be recognized as antigens in the context of CD1 *in vivo* to prime CTL that are antigen-specific.

CD1-responsive cells: possible immunoregulatory roles

Murine autoreactive CD1-restricted T cells have been identified in unimmunized mice [10, 21], however the physiological role of CD1 antigen presentation is unknown. One population in particular, the NK1$^+$ T cells [18, 28], have been shown to make IL-4 [10, 21] in response to CD1 or to anti-CD3 stimulation [35, 53]. These NK1$^+$ T cells have been reported to require CD1 for their development [8], mainly express a canonical T cell receptor and have either a CD4$^+$/CD8$^-$ or CD4$^-$/CD8$^-$ surface phenotype. The NK1$^+$ T cell receptor most often used is a single invariant TCR alpha, Vα14-Jα281, predominantly in association with Vβ8. Related cells exist which may not express the invariant alpha chain are still NK1$^+$ and CD1 specific [11].

In addition to *in vitro* observations of IL-4 production from NK1$^+$ T cells, a number of *in vivo* studies have suggested their unique regulatory functions. Transgenic mice overexpressing the canonical V alpha TCR produce increased levels of IL-4 when stimulated with mitogen *in vitro* and *vivo* [9]. Serum baseline levels of IgE and IgG1, Th2-regulated immunoglobulin isotypes, were also elevated. These studies suggest a potential regulatory role of the NK1$^+$ T cells in T helper cell differentiation, mainly in the induction of Th0 subset into a Th2 phenotype (Fig. 3). Unlike conventional CD4$^+$ T cells, the NK1$^+$ T cells do not require the presence of IL-4 at the time of stimulation to produce IL-4, as antibodies to IL-4 did not prevent their IL-4 generating capability

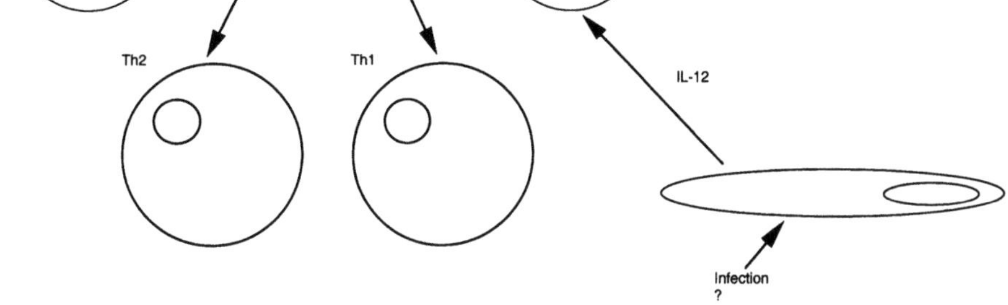

Fig. 3. Potential role of NK1$^+$ T cells. NK1$^+$ T cells may provide an early source of cytokines to affect the differentiation of T helper cells when stimulated through the TCR by CD1, MHC, or an unknown molecule.

[23]. However, NK1+ T cells can make a Th1 associated cytokine, interferon gamma upon NKR-P1 cross linking and murine CD4+NK1+ T cells purified from mouse splenocytes produce large amounts of both IL-4 and IFNγ upon activation with immobilized anti-CD3 monoclonal antibody [23]. Although IFNγ production was enhanced in the presence of IL-12, the NK1+ T cells made far less IFNγ in response to CD1-transfected L cells (L-CD1). On the other hand, IL-4 production in the presence of L-CD1 was comparable to the anti-CD3 treatment when NK1+ T cells had been restimulated with L-CD1. The differences in the timing and amounts of cytokine production from NK1+ T cells in comparison to conventional T cells suggest possible effects on the priming of CD4+ T helpers cells. However, the immunoregulatory roles may be more complex than simply as IL-4 providers in Th2 differentiation (Fig. 3).

The function of NK1+ T cells may be determined by the mode in which they are originally stimulated. For example, in mutant mice lacking MHC class II, NK1+ T cells make IL-2 in the setting of intracellular infection. While MHC class II^0 mice are relatively deficient in CD4+ cells, they have been described to contain greater numbers of CD4+ NK1+ T cells compared to wild-type mice [21]. As normal C57BL/6 mice, a fraction of autoreactive hybridomas generated from CD4+NK1+ T cells of MHC class II^0 mice were able to produce IL-4 or IFNγ in response to CD1 or other non-classical MHC molecules. However, upon infection of these mice *in vivo*, with the absence of MHC II-restricted CD4+ T cells, CD4+NK1++ cells appear to be important in providing help by serving as an early source of IL-2 in the priming of CD8+ CTL in the induction of resistance to infection by the intracellular parasite, *Toxoplama gondii* [26]. Moreover, RT-PCR analysis revealed sorted CD4+NK1+ T cells produce IL-4 mRNA when obtained from noninfected mice whereas they produced IL-2 mRNA from infected mice.

In addition to providing cytokines to influence T helper cell differentiation, NK1+ T cells have also been implicated to play a role in Th1 associated responses. A recent report by Cui and colleagues determined the importance of NK1+ T cells in mediating the antitumor effects of IL-12 [25]. Mice lacking the invariant Vα14-Jα281 T cell receptor were unable to suppress metastasis of two different tumor lines compared to wild-type control mice. Furthermore, IL-12 induced antitumor activity *in vitro* was impaired in splenocytes from the knock out mice.

The physiologic relevance of CD1 presentation of antigens remains unclear since T cells that recognize these molecules have been described as having similar effector functions as MHC class I and class II restricted T cells. The fact that a unique subset of CD1-responsive lymphocytes may play important roles by their cytokine secretion patterns, specific cytotoxic activities, or otherwise yet undetermined mechanisms suggest an immunological role for the CD1 gene family. It is important to note that studies in humans reveal a subset similar to the mouse NK1+ T cell population [33].

Human invariant Vα24+ T cells are analogous to the murine NK1+ T cells [27, 52]. Wilson and colleagues hypothesize that the loss of the ability to secrete IL-4 by Vα24+ T cells in type 1 diabetic patients may initiate Th1-cell mediated tissue damage. In this study, nine Vα24+ clones generated from an individual with type 1 diabetes specifically responded to CD1d. However, not all CD1-responsive cells found in humans are Vα24+ nor αβ TCR-bearing cells. CD4-/CD8- αβ+ T cell lines from the skin lesion of a leprosy patient and from the peripheral blood of a normal donor responded to sub-cellular fractions of mycobacteria in the presence of CD1-expressing antigen presenting cells [47]. In addition, γδ TCR-bearing and αβ TCR-bearing cytolytic T cell lines have been reported to recognize CD1c and CD1a, respectively [40].

Although the significance of CD1-restricted T cells has not yet been established, CD1-restricted T cells identified in human disease processes suggest a physiological role for CD1 antigen presentation.

Conclusions

DNA immunization gives rise to immune responses which can be skewed by the addition of plasmids encoding accessory molecules or alternative antigen presenting molecules. A combinination of plasmids encoding antigen, CD1 and B7.1 was an effective vaccine to elicit antigen-specific, CD1 restricted CTL. The CTL were predominantly $CD8^+$ and lysed targets in a Fas independent manner. Although several studies have demonstrated CD1-responsive cells in the mouse and human, the physiological role of CD1 antigen presentation is still unclear. Using DNA immunization techniques we may further investigate whether CD1-restricted T cells fulfill an ancillary, regulatory or completely independent role in the immune system.

Acknowledgment

The work was supported in part by grants A96192 from the American Federation for Research on Aging; AR07567, AR25443, and AR 41897 from the National Institutes of Health. We would like to thank N. Noon and J. Uhle for their assistance. D.J.L. is supported in part by grants from the Markey Charitable Trust and the National Institute of General Medical Sciences GM07198. M. Corr is an investigator of the Arthritis Foundation.

References

1. Arase H, N Arase, and T Saito (1996) Interferon gamma production by natural killer (NK) cells and $NK1.1^+$ T cells upon NKR-P1 cross-linking. J Exp Med 183 : 2391
2. Balk SP, PA Bleicher, and C Terhorst (1991) Isolation and expression of cDNA encoding the murine homologues of CD1. J Immunol 146 : 768–74
3. Balk SP, S Burke, JE Polischuk, ME Frantz, L Yang, S Porcelli, SP Colgan, and RS Blumberg (1994) Beta 2-microglobulin-independent MHC class Ib molecule expressed by human intestinal epithelium. Science 265 : 259–62
4. Beckman EM, A Melian, SM Behar, PA Sieling, D Chatterjee, ST Furlong, R Matsumoto, JP Rosat, RL Modlin, and SA Porcelli (1996) CDlc restricts responses of mycobacteria-specific T cells. Evidence for antigen presentation by a second member of the human CD1 family. J Immunol 157 : 2795-803
5. Beckman EM, SA Porcelli, CT Morita, SM Behar, ST Furlong, and MB Brenner (1994) Recognition of a lipid artigen by CD1-restricted alpha beta+ T cells [see comments]. Nature 372 : 691–4
6. Behar SM, SA Porcelli, EM Beckman, and MB Brenner (1995) A pathway of costimulation that prevents anergy in CD28-T cells: B7-independent costimulation of CD1-restricted T cells. J Exp Med 182: 2007–18
7. Bendelac A (1995) CD1: presenting unusual antigens to unusual T lymphocytes [comment]. Science 269 : 185–6
8. Bendelac A (1995) Positive selection of mouse $NK1^+$ T cells by CD1-expressing cortical thymocytes. J Exp Med 182 : 2091–6
9. Bendelac A, RD Hunziker, and O Lantz (1996) Increased interleukin 4 and immunoglobulin E production in transgenic mice overexpressing NK1 T cells. J Exp Med 184 : 1285–93
10. Bendelac A, O Lantz, ME Quimby, JW Yewdell, JR Bennink, and RR Brutkiewicz (1995) CD1 recognition by mouse $NK1^+$ T lymphocytes. Science 268 : 863–5

11. Bendelac A, MN Rivera, SH Park, and JH Roark (1997) Mouse CD1-specific NK1 T cells: development, specificity, and function. Annu Rev Immunol 15 : 535–62
12. Bleicher PA, SP Balk, SJ Hagen, RS Blumberg, TJ Flotte, and C Terhorst (1990) Expression of murine CD1 on gastrointestinal epithelium. Science 250 : 679–82
13. Bradbury A, KT Belt, TM Neri, C Milstein, and F Calabi (1988) Mouse CD1 is distinct from and co-exists with TL in the same thymus. Embo J 7 : 3081–6
14. Brenner M, and S Porcelli (1997) Antigen presentation: A balanced diet. Science 277 : 332
15. Bretscher P, and M Cohn (1970) A theory of self-nonself discrimination. Science 169 : 1042–9
16. Brossay L, D Jullien, S Cardell, BC Sydora, N Burdin, RL Modlin, and M Kronenberg (1997) Mouse CD1 is mainly expressed on hemopoietic-derived cells. J Immunol 159 : 1216–24
17. Brutkiewicz RR, JR Bennink, JW Yewdell, and A Bendelac (1995) TAP-independent, beta 2-microglobulin-dependent surface expression of functional mouse CD1.1. J Exp Med 182 : 1913–9
18. Budd RC, GC Miescher, RC Howe, RK Lees, C Bron, and HR MacDonald (1987) Developmentally regulated expression of T cell receptor beta chain variable domains in immature thymocytes. J Exp Med 166 : 577–82
19. Calabi F, KT Belt, CY Yu, A Bradbury, WJ Mandy, and C Milstein (1989) The rabbit CD1 and the evolutionary conservation of the CD1 gene family. Immunogenetics 30 : 370–7
20. Calabi F, JM Jarvis, L Martin, and C Milstein (1989) Two classes of CD1 genes. Eur J Immunol 19: 285–92
21. Cardell S, S Tangri, S Chan, M Kronenberg, C Benoist, and D Mathis (1995) CDl-restricted CD4+ T cells in major histocompatibility complex class II-deficient mice. J Exp Med 182 : 993–1004
22. Castano AR, S Tangri, JE Miller, HR Holcombe, MR Jackson, WD Huse, M Kronenberg, and PA Peterson (1995) Peptide binding and presentation by mouse CD1 [see comments]. Science 269 : 223–6
23. Chen H, and WE Paul (1997) Cultured NK1.1+ CD4+ T cells produce large amounts of IL-4 and IFN-gamma upon activation by anti-CD3 or CD1. J Immunol 159 : 2240–9
24. Corr M, H Tighe, D Lee, J Dudler, M Trieu, DC Brinson, and DA Carson (1997) Costimulation provided by DNA immunization enhances antitumor immunity. J Immunol 159 : 4999–5004
25. Cui J, T Shin, T Kawano, H Sato, E Kondo, I Toura, Y Kaneko, H Koseki, M Kanno, and M Taniguchi (1997) Requirement for Vα14 NKT cells in IL-12-mediated rejection of tumors. Science 278 : 1623–6
26. Denkers EY, T Scharton-Kersten, S Barbieri, P Caspar, and A Sher (1996) A role for CD4+ NKl.l+ T lymphocytes as major histocompatibility complex class II independent helper cells in the generation of CD8+ effector function against intracellular infection. J Exp Med 184 : 131–9
27. Exley M, J Garcia, SP Balk, and S Porcelli (1997) Requirements for CDld recognition by human invariant Vα24+ CD4-CD8- T cells. J Exp Med 186 : 109–20
28. Fowlkes BJ, AM Kruisbeek, H Ton-That, MA Weston, JE Coligan, RH Schwartz, and DM Pardoll (1987) A novel population of T-cell receptor alpha beta-bearing thymocytes which predominantly expresses a single V beta gene family. Nature 329 : 251–4
29. Hanau D, D Fricker, T Bieber, ME Esposito-Farese, H Bausinger, JP Cazenave, L Donato, MM Tongio, and H de la Salle (1994) CD1 expression is not affected by human peptide transporter deficiency. Hum Immunol 41 : 46–8
30. Kawano T, J Cui, Y Koezuka, I Toura, Y Kaneko, K Motoki, H Ueno, R Nakagawa, H Sato, E Kondo, H Koseki, and M Taniguchi (1997) CDld-restricted and TCR-mediated activation of Vα14 NKT cells by glycosylceramides. Science 278 : 1626–9
31. Kim JJ, ML Bagarazzi, N Trivedi, Y Hu, K Kazahaya, DM Wilson, R Ciccarelli, MA Chattergoon, K Dang, S Mahalingam, AA Chalian, MG Agadjanyan, JD Boyer, B Wang, and DB Weiner (1997) Engineering of in vivo immune responses to DNA immunization via codelivery of costimulatory molecule genes. Nat Biotechnol 15 : 641–6
32. Lafferty KJ, and AJ Cunningham (1975) A new analysis of allogeneic interactions. Aust J Exp Biol Med Sci 53 : 27–42
33. Lantz O, and A Bendelac (1994) An invariant T cell receptor alpha chain is used by a unique subset of major histocompatibility complex class I-specific CD4+ and CD4-8- T cells in mice and humane. J Exp Med 180 : 1097–106
34. Lee DJ, A Aberyratne, DA Carson, and M Corr (1998) Induction of an Antigen-specific, CD1-restricted Cytotoxic T Lymphocyte Response In Vivo. J Exp Med 187 : 433–438
35. Leite-de-Moraes MC, A Herbelin, F Machavoine, A Vicari, JM Gombert, M Papiernik, and M Dy (1995) MHC class I-selected CD4-8- TCR-alpha beta+ T cells are a potential source of IL-4 during primary immune response. J Immunol 155 : 4544–50

36. Martin LH, F Calabi, and C Milstein (1986) Isolation of CD1 genes: a family of major histocompatibility complex-related differentiation antigens. Proc Natl Acad Sci USA 83 : 9154–8
37. Palinski W, ME Rosenfeld, S Yla-Herttuala, GC Gurtner, SS Socher, SW Butler, S Parthasarathy, TE Carew, D Steinberg, and JL Witztum (1989) Low density lipoprotein undergoes oxidative modification in vivo. Proc Natl Acad Sci USA 86 : 1372–6
38. Peters PJ, JJ Neefjes, V Oorschot, HL Ploegh, and HJ Geuze (1991) Segregation of MHC class II molecules from MHC class I molecules in the Golgi complex for transport to lysosomal compartments [see comments]. Nature 349 : 669–76
39. Peters PJ, G Raposo, JJ Neefjes, V Oorschot, RL Leijendekker, HJ Geuze, and HL Ploegh (1995) Major histocompatibility complex class II compartments in human B lymphoblastoid cells are distinct from early endosomes. J Exp Med 182 : 325–34
40. Porcelli S, MB Brenner, JL Greenstein, SP Balk, C Terhorst, and PA Bleicher (1989) Recognition of cluster of differentiation 1 antigens by human CD4⁻CD8⁻ cytolytic T lymphocytes. Nature 341 : 447–50
41. Porcelli S, CT Morita, and MB Brenner (1992) CDlb restricts the response of human CD4⁻8⁻ T lymphocytes to a microbial artigen. Nature 360 : 593–7
42. Porcelli SA (1995) The CD1 family: a third lineage of antigen-presenting molecules. Adv Immunol 59: 1–98
43. Prigozy TI, PA Sieling, D Clemens, PL Stewart, SM Behar, SA Porcelli, MB Brenner, RL Modlin, and M Kronenberg (1997) The mannose receptor delivers lipoglycan antigens to endosomes for presentation to T cells by CDlb molecules. Immunity 6 : 187–97
44. Raz E, DA Carson, SE Parker, TB Parr, AM Abai, G Aichinger, SH Gromkowski, M Singh, D Lew, MA Yankauckas, and et al. (1994) Intradermal gene immunization: the possible role of DNA uptake in the induction of cellular immunity to viruses. Proc Natl Acad Sci USA 91 : 9519–23
45. Sanderson F, MJ Kleijmeer, A Kelly, D Verwoerd, A Tulp, JJ Neefjes, HJ Geuze, and J Trowsdale (1994) Accumulation of HLA-DM, a regulator of antigen presentation, in MHC class II compartments. Science 266 : 1566–9
46. Schwartz RH (1992) Costimulation of T lymphocytes: the role of CD28, CTLA-4, and B7/BB1 in interleukin-2 production and immunotherapy. Cell 71 : 1065–8
47. Sieling PA, D Chatterjee, SA Porcelli, TI Prigozy, RJ Mazzaccaro, T Soriano, BR Bloom, MB Brenner, M Kronenberg, PJ Brennan, and et al. (1995) CD1-restricted T cell recognition of microbial lipoglycan antigens [see comments]. Science 269 : 227–30
48. Stenger S, RJ Mazzaccaro, K Uyemura, S Cho, PF Barnes, JP Rosat, A Sette, MB Brenner, SA Porcelli, BR Bloom, and RL Modlin (1997) Differential effects of cytolytic T cell subsets on intracellular infection. Science 276 : 1684–7
49. Sugita M, RM Jackman, E van Donselaar, SM Behar, RA Rogers, PJ Peters, MB Brenner, and SA Porcelli (1996) Cytoplasmic tail-dependent localization of CDlb antigen-presenting molecules to MIICs. Science 273 : 349–52
50. Teitell M, HR Holcombe, L Brossay, A Hagenbaugh, MJ Jackson, L Pond, SP Balk, C Terhorst, PA Peterson, and M Kronenberg (1997) Nonclassical behavior of the mouse CD1 class I-like molecule. J Immunol 158 : 2143–9
51. Tulp A, D Verwoerd, B Dobberstein, HL Ploegh, and J Pieters (1994) Isolation and characterization of the intracellular MHC class II compartment [see comments]. Nature 369 : 120–6
52. Wilson SB, SC Kent, KT Patton, T Orban, RA Jackson, M Exley, S Porcelli, DA Schatz, MA Atkinson, SP Balk, JL Strominger, and DA Hafler (1998) Extreme Thl bias of invariant Vα24JαQ T cells in type 1 diabetes. Nature 391 : 177–81
53. Yoshimoto T, and WE Paul (1994) CD4pos, NKl.lpos T cells promptly produce interleukin 4 in response to in vivo challenge with anti-CD3. J Exp Med 179 : 1285–95
54. Zeng Z-H, AR Castano, BW Segelke, EA Stura, PA Peterson, and IA Wilson (1997) Crystal structure of mouse CD1: An MHC-like fold with a large hydrophobic binding groove. Science 277 : 339–345

DNA vaccines with rapid intracellular degradation are more effective for inducing CTL

Yunqi Wu, Thomas J. Kipps

UCSD Human Gene Therapy Program, Division of Hematology/Oncology, Department of Medicine, UCSD School of Medicine, La Jolla, CA 92093-0663, USA

Introduction

DNA vaccines have several advantages over conventional vaccines, such as ease of construction, low expense for mass production, high temperature stability, and ability to induce a full spectrum of exceptionally long-lasting immune responses, including cytolytic T lymphocytes (CTL) [6, 13]. Furthermore, because the transgene antigen is synthesized by cells of the host animal, it may be processed for immune recognition via a protein degradation pathway that is distinct from that of exogenous protein antigen.

Design of DNA vaccines that encode proteins that are not released from the cell or that do not induce antibodies against the transgene product may be advantageous. In some cases, release of the transgene antigen from the *in vivo* transfected cells may have deleterious consequences, such as allergic or inflammatory reactions. Moreover, released transgene product also may induce the antigen-specific antibodies that themselves could have undesirable side-effects, particularly if the antigen is a cell surface protein associated with a tumor or virus-infected cell. For example, such antibodies could effect the growth or survival of tumor cells if they are directed against a cell surface protein that functions as a growth-factor receptor. In addition, such antibodies may cause autoimmune pathology if they cross-react with other self proteins. For these reasons, consideration of the events within the cell leading to antigen presentation may lead to development of improved DNA vaccines.

Protein degradation pathways and antigen presentation

There are two major pathways of protein degradation in eukaryotic cells (Fig. 1). Endogenously synthesized protein antigens generally are cleaved by proteasomes into peptides that are translocated to the endoplasmic reticulum and ultimately bound by MHC class I molecules for presentation to CD8 T lymphocytes [9]. This pathway is mainly for the short-lived and mutated proteins. Exogenous proteins generally are

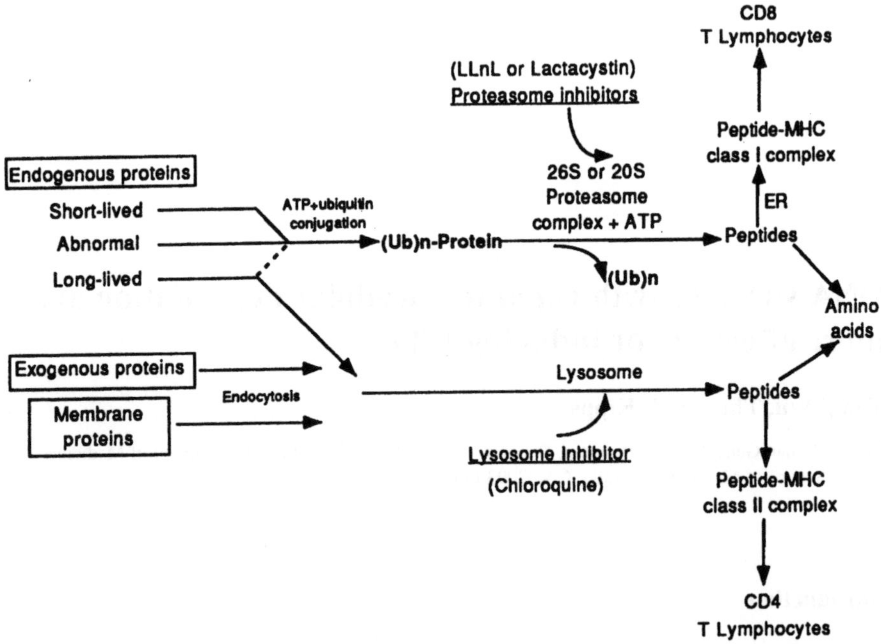

Fig. 1. Protein degradation pathways in eukaryotic cells. Endogenous proteins, mainly short-lived and abnormal proteins are conjugated with polyubiquitin molecules in the presence of ATP. The polyubiquitinated protein are targeted to the proteasome, leading to the generation of peptides and free polyubiquitin chains. These resultant peptides are transported into endoplasmic reticulum (ER) and bound to MHC class I molecules for presentation to CD8 T lymphocytes. Exogenous proteins enter the cells by endocytosis and degraded into peptides by lysosome. The peptides are presented on the cell surface in the context of MHC class II molecules.

taken up by endocytosis and then degraded in the lysosome by acid-optimal proteases (cathepsons) [1]. This pathway also involves in the degradation of membrane proteins and long-lived intracellular proteins. The processed peptides from such proteins generally bind to MHC class II molecules for presentation to CD4 T cells.

There are several inhibitors that can be used to determine which proteolysis pathway is involved for a given protein (Fig. 1). Peptide aldehyde N-acetyl-L-leucinyl-L-leucinal-L-norleucinal (LLnL) is a substrate-related inhibitor of the proteasome [19]. Lactacystin, *Streptomyces* metabolite that undergoes spontaneous conversion to *clasto*-lactacystin β-lactone [5, 7] is a more specific proteasome inhibitor. Chloroquine, a lysosomotropic agent inhibits lysosomal functions by elevating intralysosomal pH [20].

The pathways whereby polypeptides are processed into peptides that can be presented by MHC class I molecules involve intracellular proteolysis of the polypeptide into peptide fragments. A major candidate process for this pathway is that of polyubiquitination. Ubiquitination is an ATP-dependent process whereby the proteins lysine residues become coupled with ubiquitin, a 76-amino acid polypeptide [9, 19]. This directs the metabolism of the protein into peptides by the 20S proteasome, a large multi-catalytic protease core of the 26S proteasome.

Experiments in yeast and rabbit reticulocyte lysates have revealed that at least two factors determine the rate of polyubiquitination [2, 3, 10]. One factor is the identity of amino-terminal residue of the polypeptide, the so-called N-rule. Amino acids can be classified as being stabilizing or destabilizing residues, based upon their ability to influence the relative half-life of a polypeptide. The half-life of a given protein varies significantly (from 2 min to >20 h) depending on the identity of N-terminal amino acid [2, 10]. Another requirement is that the protein have accessible lysine residues for polyubiquitination [3].

DNA vaccines with enhanced intracellular degradation

Generation of vaccines that undergo proteasome-dependent degradation

Although it is clear that intracellular protein antigens generally must be processed into peptides for antigen presentation [8, 21, 22], it is not certain whether this process is mediated solely via the ubiquitin-proteasome pathway. Evidence that the ubiquitin-mediated proteolytic pathway provides all of the substrates for the proteasome has remained inconclusive from studies on temperature-sensitive UBE1 mutant cells [4, 15], or on proteins degraded through ubiquitin-independent pathways [12, 17]. Furthermore, studies using pairs of N-end rule substrates that varied in their intracellular stability provided evidence that the proteolytic turnover of endogenously synthesized proteins is not directly proportional to the generation of processed antigenic peptide/MHC class I complexes [11, 21]. Another study found that OVA with methylated lysine groups that were resistant to ubiquitination still could be presented by MHC class I molecules, albeit at a reduced amounts [16]. This indicates that there may be a ubiquitin-independent pathway(s) leading to the generation of peptides for MHC class I presentation.

We proposed that strategies that enhance the ubiquitin-proteasome degradation of a transgene product may result in improved DNA vaccines. We generated chimeric genes encoding ubiquitin (Ub), a fragment of lacI and beta-galactosidase (β-gal) with different intervening amino acids, allowing for production of processed protein products that have either stabilizing or destabilizing residues at their N-termini (Fig. 2). These vectors were termed pUb-X-lacZ, where X represents either methionine (Met), tyrosine (Tyr) or arginine (Arg). These amino acids represent either stabilizing (Met),

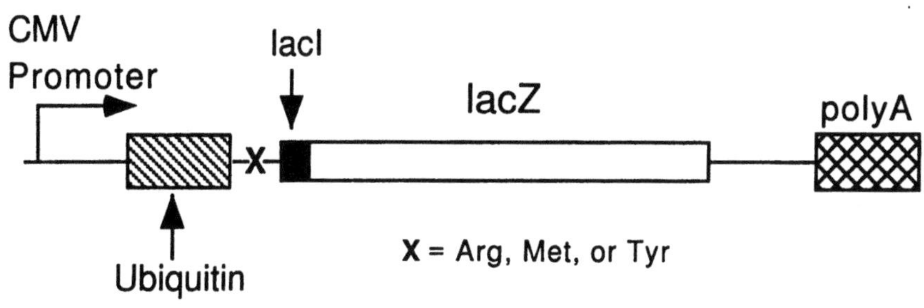

Fig. 2. Structure of pUb-X-lacI-lacZ. Chimeric genes Ub-X-lacI-lacZ were subcloned into pcDNA3 expression vectors that encode yeast ubiquitin (first repeat of UBI4), *E. coli* lacI segment (residues 1030-1149) and beta-galactosidase (β-gal) with different intervening amino acids (X). LacI has two lysine residues which serve as acceptors for ubiquitin. The 5 non-coding region of the ubiquitin cDNA was modified by inserting a Kozak sequence (GCCACC) to direct efficient translation of the chimeric gene transcripts in mammalian cells.

Table 1. Comparisons of β-Gal protein expression, activity and antigen presentation

Transfectants	β-Gal protein activity[a] control	LLnL	lactacystin	chloroquine	β-gal expression[b]	Antigen presentation[c]
pcDNA3	< 5	< 5	< 5	< 5	–	4 ± 1
pUB-Arg-lacZ	< 5	76	82	< 5	–	68 ± 4
pUB-Met-lacZ	85	87	92	66	+	59 ± 4
pUB-Tyr-lacZ	< 5	75	80	< 5	–	82 ± 3

[a] Four different P815 transfectants were treated with control, proteasome inhibitors LLnL or lactacystin, or lysosome inhibitor chloroquine at 100 μM each, for 2 h at 37°C. After incubation, the cells were loaded with the β-gal substrate, FDG, for 1 min at 37°C using hypotonic shock. β-gal activity were detected by flow cytometry. Data represent the proprotion of cells that have β-gal activity.

[b] β-gal protein expression from P815 transfectants were determined by immunoblot analysis with anti-β-gal antibody.

[c] P815 transfectants as target cells were incubated with 0805B, an H-2L^d-restricted β-gal-specific CTL clone. After 4 hours, specific lysis of the P815 transfectants was determined by measuring LDH release into the supernatant using the Cytotox-96 assay kit. These data are from a representative experiment of four experiments at a 2:1 effector:target ratio.

intermediate-destabilizing (Tyr), or destabilizing (Arg) residues, according to the N-end rule in yeast [2, 10]. These vectors were used to determine the effect of ubiquitin-proteasome pathway on protein degradation and antigen presentation *in vitro* and *in vivo*.

β-Gal protein expression in P815 transfectants

pUb-X-lacZ vectors were studied in vitro by transfecting into P815, a mouse mastocytoma cell line, by electroporation. After limited dilution, positive clones were examined for expression of β-gal by immunoblot analysis. The lysates of P815 cells transfected with pUb-Met-LacZ contained detectable amounts of the β-gal protein. Nevertheless, the lysates of P815 cells transfected with plasmids encoding β-gal with a destabilizing N-terminus, either pUb-Arg-lacZ or pUb-Tyr-LacZ did not have detectable expression of β-gal (Table 1).

Effect of ubiquitin-proteasome pathway on Ub-X-β-gal activity

β-Gal activity in each transfectant was also evaluated using flow cytometry. Consistent with the immunoblot analysis, pUb-Met-lacZ transfected cells had high levels of β-gal activity, whereas pUb-Arg-lacZ and pUb-Tyr-lacZ transfectants did not significantly have specific enzymatic activity greater than that of cells transfected with the negative control vector, pcDNA3 (Table 1).

However, over 76% or 75% of the cells transfected with pUb-Arg-lacZ or pUb-Tyr-lacZ, respectively, were found to express β-gal when treated with proteasome inhibitor LLnL. Similarly, after culturing the cells with lactacystin, we detected β-gal in 82% or 80% of the pUb-Arg-lacZ or pUb-Tyr-lacZ transfectants, respectively (Table 1). Moreover, such treatment increased the β-gal mean fluorescence intensity (MFI) of pUb-Tyr-lacZ- or pUb-Arg-lacZ- transfected cells by seven-fold or eight-fold, respectively [23]. In contrast, lysosomal inhibitor chloroquine or a specific calpain inhibitor E64d [14, 23], had no effect on the level of β-gal activity detected in any of the transfectants. On the other hand, none of the inhibitors caused much of a change in the already high percent numbers of pUb-Met-lacZ transfected cells (Table 1). These results indicate that the lack of detectable β-gal activity in the pUb-Arg-lacZ and pUb-Tyr-lacZ transfectants is due to the rapid intracellular degradation of this enzyme via the ubiquitin-proteasome pathway.

Effects of pUb-X-b-gal protein degradation on antigen presentation.

The ability of P815 transfectants to act as target cells was determined in a cytolytic T lymphocyte (CTL) assay with 0805B, an H-2L^d-restricted β-gal specific CTL clone [18]. Despite lacking detectable β-gal activity without proteasome inhibitors, the pUb-Arg-lacZ or pUb-Tyr-lacZ transfectants were as sensitive to cytolysis by 0805B as the pUb-Met-lacZ transfectant (Table 1) [23]. Moreover, these transfectants equally were able to inhibit the CTL activity of 0805B cell line against ^{51}Cr-labeled P13.2 cells when used as the cold targets in the CTL assay [23]. However, the transfectants treated with LLnL failed to inhibit the specific ^{51}Cr release of ^{51}Cr-labeled P13.2 in this same assay. These results suggest that the ubiquitin-proteasome pathway is involved processing of β-gal antigen and that the rapid processing of β-gal via the ubiquitin-proteasome pathway does not preclude these cells from generating sufficient numbers of peptides for recognition by class-I-restricted CTL.

Effect of increased pUb-X-lacZ degradation on immune responses in vivo

The effect of DNA vaccines with rapid intracellular processing on immune responses to β-gal were determined by muscular injection of pUb-X-lacZ (X = Arg or Met),

Table 2. Effect of increased pUb-X-lacZ degradation on immune response

	Anti-β-Gal antibody response[a]				
Vaccines	3 weeks	4 weeks	5 weeks	6 weeks	CTL activity[b]
pcDNA3	< 0.1	< 0.1	< 0.1	< 0.1	5 ± 1
placZ	0.4 ± 0.6	1.9 ± 1.5	2.6 ± 0.9*	2.1 ± 0.8*	17 ± 3*
pUB-Met-lacZ	< 0.1	< 0.1	< 0.1	0.1 ± 0.1	52 ± 4*
pUB-Arg-lacZ	< 0.1	< 0.1	0.3 ± 0.4	0.2 ± 0.2	87 ± 2*

Four BALB/s mice per group received i.m. injections of 100 μg of pcDNA3, placZ, pUb-Met-lacZ or pUb-Arg-lacZ each week for 4 consecutive wk. Immune responses were studied 3 weeks after the first DNA-injection.

[a] A 1:100 dilution of serum was assayed by ELISA for anti-β-gal antibodies. Data from 4 mice per group, represent the mean absorbance ±SD.

[b] Twelve weeks after the first injection, the splenocytes were stimulated *in vitro* for 7 days with P13.2, a lacZ transfectant of P815, and then assayed for cytolytic activity. Data from a representative experiment, represent the mean specific lysis ±SE of P13.2 cells minus lysis of negative controls, P815, at a 33:1 effector:target ratio.

* $P < 0.05$ between placZ or pUb-X-laxZ and control vector, Bonferroni's test.

placZ, or pcDNA3 into BALB/c mice (Table 2). In contrast to vectors encoding native β-gal plasmid vectors encoding β-gal with a destabilizing residue (Arg) did not significantly induce anti-β-gal antibodies over the course of study. This may reflect the rapid rate of intracellular protein turnover and/or poor release of native β-gal polypeptide from the *in vivo* transfected cells, precluding development of antibodies against the native protein. However, such vectors were significantly more effective than vectors encoding native β-gal or β-gal with a stabilizing residue, in stimulating CTL specific for P13.2, a lacZ transfectant of P815. As such, intramuscular injection of DNA vectors encoding β-gal with destabilizing amino termini may be better suited for inducing a cellular immune response to target antigens.

Conclusions

DNA vaccines encoding proteins with rapid rates of intracellular degradation via the ubiquitin-proteasome pathway are able to generate an enhanced cellular immune response. In addition, the response is limited to the cellular branch of the immune system and does not include the production of antibodies to the immunogen. Such vaccines and strategy may be especially useful in stimulating an immune response that can reject cancer cells or cells infected with virus. This may be particularly useful in the prevention or delay of the onset of de novo or recurrent cancer or in the treatment of viral infections.

The ability of such vectors to induce a cellular cytotoxic immune response against cells that express antigen without inducting antigen specific antibodies offers several advantages. In regard to antigens that are presented by tumor cells, the production of antibodies directed to these antigens have been hypothesized to inhibit cellular immune responses to such antigens. Also, such antibodies may effect the growth/survival of tumor cells expressing an antigen that is also a signal transducing receptor by acting as agonists of the receptor. Accordingly, incorporation of strategies that enhance proteasome-dependent protein degradation may generate DNA vaccines that prove more effective in inducing desired immune responses against tumors or cells infected with intracellular pathogens.

Acknowledgement.

This work was supported in part by the National Institutes of Health Grant CA66000 and the Susan Koman Breast Cancer Research Foundation. We wish to thank Dr. Jan Burger for technical assistance.

References

1. Allen PM, Babbitt BP, Unanue ER (1987) T-cell recognition of lysozyme: the biochemical basis of presentation. Immunol Rev 98 : 171
2. Bachmair A, Finley D, Varshavsky A (1986) In vivo half-life of a protein is a function of its amino-terminal residue. Science 234 : 179
3. Bachmair A, Varshavsky A (1989) The degradation signal in a short-lived protein. Cell 56:1019
4. Cox JH, Galardy P, Bennink JR, Yewdell JW (1995) Presentation of endogenous and exogenous antigens is not affected by inactivation of E1 ubiquitin-activating enzyme in temperature-sensitive cell lines. J Immunol 154 : 511
5. Dick LR, Cruikshank AA, Destree AT, Grenier L, McCormack TA, Melandri FD, Nunes SL, Palombella VJ, Parent LA, Plamondon L, Stein RL (1997) Mecanistic studies on the inactivation of the proteasome by lactacystin in cultured cells. J Biol Chem 272 : 182
6. Donnelly JJ, Ulmer JB, Liu MA (1997) DNA vaccines. Life Sci 60:163
7. Fenteany G, Standaert RF, Lane WS, Choi S, Corey EJ, Schreiber SL (1995) Inhibition of proteasome activities and subunit-specific amino-terminal threonine modification by lactacystin. Science 268 : 726
8. Germain RN (1994) MHC-dependent antigen processing and peptide presentation: providing ligands for T lymphocyte activation. Cell 76 : 287
9. Goldberg AL, Rock KL (1992) Proteolysis, proteasomes and antigen presentation. Nature 357 : 375
10. Gonda DK, Bachmair A, Wunning I, Tobias JW, Lane WS, Varshavsky A (1989) Universality and structure of the N-end rule. J Biol Chem 264 : 16700
11. Goth S, Nguyen V, Shastri N (1996) Generation of naturally processed peptide/MHC class I complexes is independent of the stability of endogenously synthesized precursors. J Immunol 157 : 1894
12. Jariel-Encontre I, Pariat M, Martin F, Carillo S, Salvat C, Piechaczyk M (1995) Ubiquitinylation is not an absolute requirement for degradation of c-Jun protein by the 26 S proteasome. J Biol Chem 270: 11623
13. McDonnell WM, Askari FK (1996) DNA vaccines. N Engl J Med 334 : 42
14. Mehdi S (1991) Cell-penetrating inhibitors of calpain. Trends Biochem Sci 16 : 150
15. Michalek MT, Grant EP, Gramm C, Goldberg AL, Rock KL (1993) A role for the ubiquitin-dependent proteolytic pathway in MHC class I-restricted antigen presentation. Nature 363 : 552
16. Michalek MT, Grant EP, Rock KL (1996) Chemical denaturation and modification of ovalbumin alters its dependence on ubiquitin conjugation for class I antigen presentation. J Immunol 157 : 617
17. Murakami Y, Matsufuji S, Kameji T, Hayashi S, Igarashi K, Tamura T, Tanaka K, Ichihara A (1992) Ornithine decarboxylase is degraded by the 26S proteasome without ubiquitination. Nature 360 : 597
18. Rammensee HG, Schild H, Theopold U (1989) Protein-specific cytotoxic T lymphocytes. Recognition of transfectants expressing intracellular, membrane-associated or secreted forms of beta-galactosidase. Immunogenetics 30 : 29
19. Rock KL, Gramm C, Rothstein L, Clark K, Stein R, Dick L, Hwang D, Goldberg AL (1994) Inhibitors of the proteasome block the degradation of most cell proteins and the generation of peptides presented on MHC class I molecules. Cell 78 : 761
20. Seglen PO (1983) Inhibitors of lysosomal function. Methods Enzymol 96 : 737
21. Townsend A, Bastin J, Gould K, Brownlee G, Andrew M, Coupar B, Boyle D, Chan S, Smith G (1988) Defective presentation to class I-restricted cytotoxic T lymphocytes in vaccinia-infected cells is overcome by enhanced degradation of antigen. J Exp Med 168 : 1211
22. Townsend AR, Gotch FM, Davey J (1985) Cytotoxic T cells recognize fragments of the influenza nucleoprotein. Cell 42 : 457
23. Wu Y, Kipps TJ (1997) Deoxyribonucleic Acid vaccines encoding antigens with rapid proteasome-dependent degradation are highly efficient inducers of cytolytic T lymphocytes. J Immunol 159 : 6037

Genetic vaccination against tuberculosis

Douglas B. Lowrie[1], Celio L. Silva[2], Ricardo E. Tascon[1]

[1] National Institute for Medical Research, The Ridgeway, Mill Hill, London NW7 1AA, UK
[2] University of Sao Paulo, Sao Paulo, Brazil

Abstract. New weapons are needed in the fight against tuberculosis. Recent research indicates that a vaccine better than BCG may be within reach. A diverse range of protein antigens can give encouragingly high levels of protective immunity in animal models when administered with adjuvants or as DNA vaccines. Accelerated arrest of bacterial multiplication followed by sustained decline in bacterial numbers are key parameters of protection and so the vaccine must target antigens produced by both actively multiplying and growth-inhibited bacteria. Consistent with this, the protective antigens have been found among secreted and stress proteins (e.g. Ag85, ESAT-6, hsp65, hsp70). Species-specific antigens are not needed, hence these remain available for diagnostic tests. Adoptive transfer of protection from vaccinated or infected mice into naive mice by transfer of purified T cells and clones shows that protection is expressed by antigen-specific cytotoxic T cells that produce interferon-γ and lyse infected macrophages. These cells are produced in response to endogenous antigen. DNA vaccination appears to be an excellent way of generating these cells and may be able to give long-lasting protection.

Introduction

Tuberculosis kills 3 million people every year [34]. The disease is due to respiratory infection with *Mycobacterium tuberculosis* and is curable. It is not getting cured because delivery of, and compliance with, the minimum of 6 months multidrug chemotherapy is difficult to achieve. The resultant incomplete drug treatment makes things worse because drug resistance emerges in the bacteria. Infections by drug-resistant bacteria are an increasing problem everywhere and patients with multidrug-resistant infection are essentially incurable. Furthermore, where HIV and tuberculosis coincide in a population, as is increasingly happening, the results are catastrophic. There is little sign of any radically new anti-tuberculosis drugs that might improve this situation, and even when these are devised, clinical implementation seems certain to be followed by re-emergence of drug resistance. Are the prospects for vaccination any better?

Correspondence to: D. B. Lowrie

Background

The bacille Calmette Guérin (BCG) vaccine is in widespread use but has doubtful impact on the global position. It is a live vaccine, derived from *Mycobacterium bovis*, a close relative of *M. tuberculosis*, by virulence attenuation during prolonged cultivation of the bacteria in the laboratory. It is used to vaccinate many millions of people every year. However, there are two main deficiencies: (1) it is known from numerous clinical studies to give very different levels of protection in different populations, from around 75% down to 0%; (2) an important diagnostic and epidemiological tool, skin test hypersensitivity, is difficult to use in subjects who have been vaccinated with BCG. Nevertheless, in contrast to the poor immediate prospects for major advances in chemotherapy, there are likely to be some substantially different vaccines competing for evaluation before long and these may overcome some of the limitations of BCG. Crucial to this development has been the application of recombinant DNA technology to the mycobacteria and this has surprisingly led to the prospect of DNA (genetic) vaccination against tuberculosis.

The subunit approach to making a better vaccine than BCG has a long and disappointing history. Dead BCG bacteria and purified antigenic fragments were found to evoke modest and transient protection in animal models and this could not be compensated by using larger doses [25]. It was reasoned that key protective antigens might be those that are secreted by the living vaccine bacteria and, therefore, are not present in adequate amounts in dead bacteria or extracts [1, 7, 75]. Although this concept has not been formally validated, in the sense that we still do not know by direct evidence what is secreted by the bacteria in the tissues, it is the case that many of the most immunogenic antigens are now known to be, or seem likely to be, secreted proteins [109]. Some of these antigens can generate encouragingly high levels of protective immunity when administered with adjuvants to guinea pigs [76] or when given as DNA vaccines to mice [51, 65]. The crucial question remains whether this protection can be long lasting. Before considering these findings further it is worth first of all briefly considering what we would like a new vaccine to achieve clinically and, therefore, in animal models.

The protective effects of vaccination are mediated by accelerated expression of acquired cell-mediated immunity, antibodies are not protective. Even in non-vaccinated individuals this response is usually able to control the infection at the primary focus in the lung, but not always before the infection has disseminated to other organs. It is this disseminated infection that subsequently causes disease in about 10% of the people initially infected [12]. The disease is usually extrapulmonary in children and predominantly confined initially to the upper lobes of the lung in adults. The accelerated cellular response in vaccinated individuals prevents disease by preventing this dissemination [12]; a replacement for BCG should have the same property. Aerosol infections of laboratory animals can be used to assess this directly. Any model which demonstrates earlier arrest of bacterial growth followed by decline in bacterial viability at initial sites of infection is likely to be a good guide. However, results with the same vaccine in different models can differ significantly, so a combination of test models is most appropriate [104].

Since disease is usually a consequence of regrowth of the bacteria at secondary sites of infection after dissemination, often after long periods of quiescence, a vaccine that minimizes persistence and reactivation of dormant bacteria is also desirable. Murine models in which this can be assessed have been developed [33, 61] and a monkey, *Macaca fascicularis*, which has a higher resistance to tuberculosis than the rhesus, may also be suitable [103]. Reactivation may require liquefaction of the caseous material that comprises an old lesion; rabbits may be the best model for this aspect [28, 30]. The kind of immune response needed to eliminate persistent bacteria and the kind needed to contain initial infection may be different. Furthermore, if the antigens produced by actively multiplying bacteria are different from those from dormant bacteria then the antigens required in the vaccine would also be different.

Clinical objectives

Obviously a new vaccine must be at least as good as BCG. For example, in the United Kingdom a single intradermal dose given to children of about 12–13 years of age protects against a subsequent airborne infection developing into the infectious cavitating pulmonary disease in young adults [43, 96]. Almost 80% of cases that would otherwise have occurred can be prevented by BCG vaccination, although protection probably only lasts for 15 years [43]. It is not known if there is a similar decline in protection in areas of the world where there is a much higher exposure to infections and environmental mycobacteria that might have a booster effect. Worldwide, a single BCG dose in newborn children significantly protects against the development of childhood forms of tuberculosis [83], although the impact on subsequent development of adult pulmonary disease is less clear [23]. A vaccine that works well in populations where BCG fails, such as those of South India [94], is obviously a major objective. Unfortunately the basis of BCG failure is not known with certainty so that any animal models and design strategies are necessarily speculative. The consensus view is that a major cause of BCG failure is pre-immunisation by exposure to environmental mycobacteria, although this is not proven and it is not clear how this interferes with vaccination [17, 27, 37, 97]. One possibility is that environmental mycobacteria and BCG can be equally good protective immunogens. Animal models suggest this to be the case [35, 54, 74, 77] and a comparison of human monocyte antimycobacterial activity before and 8 weeks after BCG vaccination, in London, UK and Chingleput, South India, was consistent with this interpretation [20]. If this is so, a better vaccine might result by engineering BCG, or some other non-pathogenic mycobacterium, to be more immunogenic by including antigens unique to *M. tuberculosis* such as crippled virulence determinants [52]. Alternatively, the environmental mycobacteria may subvert the immune response so that key elements of protective immunity are no longer evoked by BCG [97]. In this case a better vaccine would be one that can switch the protective responses back on, by changing the way the antigens are seen by the immune system rather than necessarily changing the antigens seen. For example, switching between predominantly cellular and predominantly antibody responses (the type 1 to type 2 cytokine profile switch) can be demonstrated to be reversible in mice [80]. It is noteworthy that a vaccine that is designed to do this might have a therapeutic role if, for example, a relative predominance of antibody over cellular responses in advanced tuberculosis has a causal relationship to disease progression. Such vaccines should, therefore, also be clinically evaluated as adjuncts to chemotherapy. Precedent for this approach exists in the killed *M. vaccae* vaccine that is currently being evaluated for therapeutic function [73, 84, 98].

A vaccine that does not interfere with diagnostic skin hypersensitivity testing is highly desirable. There is the same requirement in both man and domestic animals (principally cattle) to retain immunoreactivity as a diagnostic tool [21, 26] and for this a subunit approach is most appropriate. There is no evidence that specific antigens of *M. tuberculosis* are necessary for protection, so by using only some of the cross-reactive antigens in a vaccine the remainder, together with any specific ones, are available for skin testing. There was initially doubt that a subunit vaccine comprising only a handful of antigens could give a level of protection equal to that obtained with the whole live bacterium but these are being dispelled. Indeed it can be argued that the subunit approach has the potential to be superior to the live vaccine because of the removal of immunosuppressive effects of mycobacterial infection [60, 66, 81].

Vaccine candidate antigens

It is not difficult to obtain transient protective effects against tuberculosis by immunizing with antigenic components of mycobacteria. However, the effects do not last as long as those obtained by vaccinating with living BCG. The subunit approach, using purified proteins directly as a vaccine, has nevertheless resulted in identification of a number of antigens that are probably good candidates for inclusion in a new vaccine, provided that means can be found to create a long-lasting protective response. For example, culture filtrate that is collected during the early phase of mycobacterial growth and before bacterial lysis has occurred contains a large number of protein antigens [8, 36, 40, 76, 105]. Responses to culture filtrate antigens appear early during infection in mice [8] and humans [18], suggesting that some of these antigens at least are related to and probably identical to those released by live mycobacteria during the early stages of infection. It is possible that other antigens, released by bacteria growing in vivo but not in vitro, remain to be discovered since the environments are very different and radiolabelling studies indicate that the pattern of protein synthesis is also very different [62, 69]. Nevertheless, antigens in early culture filtrate have been found to elicit protective immunity when administered in suitable adjuvant to guinea pigs [76] and mice [5]. Protection was similar to the effect of BCG and lasted a few weeks. Protective antigens present in early culture filtrates have been identified as antigens 85A, 85B, superoxide dismutase, PhoS, MPT51 and MPT63 [7, 50] and ESAT-6 [6, 9, 18, 45, 95].

Diverse antigens that are not prominent in early culture filtrate but may be released later are also frequently recognised by T cells from tuberculosis patients [47]. These include a 19-kDa antigen [72] hsp10 [13, 68], PhoS, hsp65 and hsp70 [68]. The heat shock (or stress) proteins in particular have generated interest as potential protective antigens, largely on the basis of their prominence in the immune response in mice and humans at both antibody and T cell level [13, 55, 67, 110]. Furthermore, hsp65 appears to be produced in increased amounts by intracellular tubercle bacilli [62], presumably in response to the stress of intracellular existence, and a 17-kDa antigen that is a homologue of the α-crystallin stress protein becomes a dominant mycobacterial protein under such conditions [112]. It is intriguing that the α-crystallin homologue and hsp65 and hsp10 have been identified as prominent immunogens in a mycobacterial ribosomal preparation [99] that represents one of the more successful of the earlier subunit vaccines [108]. Thus, it seems likely that antigens such as stress proteins that are produced late in infection could also be good targets for a protective immune response, particularly if the development of bacterial persistence and dormancy are to be overcome, and even more so if there is to be a therapeutic vaccine.

Vaccination with naked DNA

Evidence that stress proteins are indeed among the important protective antigens has come from a series of studies in our laboratories. These studies established for the first time that a single mycobacterial antigen, hsp65, could generate protection similar to that obtained with live BCG [90] and then that this could be achieved by injecting bacterial plasmid DNA from which the antigen was subsequently expressed within the mouse tissues [100]. They have also led to important conclusions regarding the nature of the protective immune response [93]. We initially used tumour cells expressing *M. leprae* hsp65 because this was one of the first genes to become available; subsequent investigations with plasmid DNA expressing hsp65 or the 36-kDa proline-rich antigen showed that this approach has broad applicability. Other antigens have now been demonstrated to be protective when expressed from plasmid DNA [51, 100]. The implication of these and related findings is that a DNA vaccine against tuberculosis is now, unexpectedly, a realistic possibility and justifies a more detailed consideration.

Ex vivo transfected antigen-presenting cells

We first found that macrophage-like tumour cells expressing mycobacterial hsp65 from a retroviral vector were able to act as antigen-presenting cells (APC) to im-

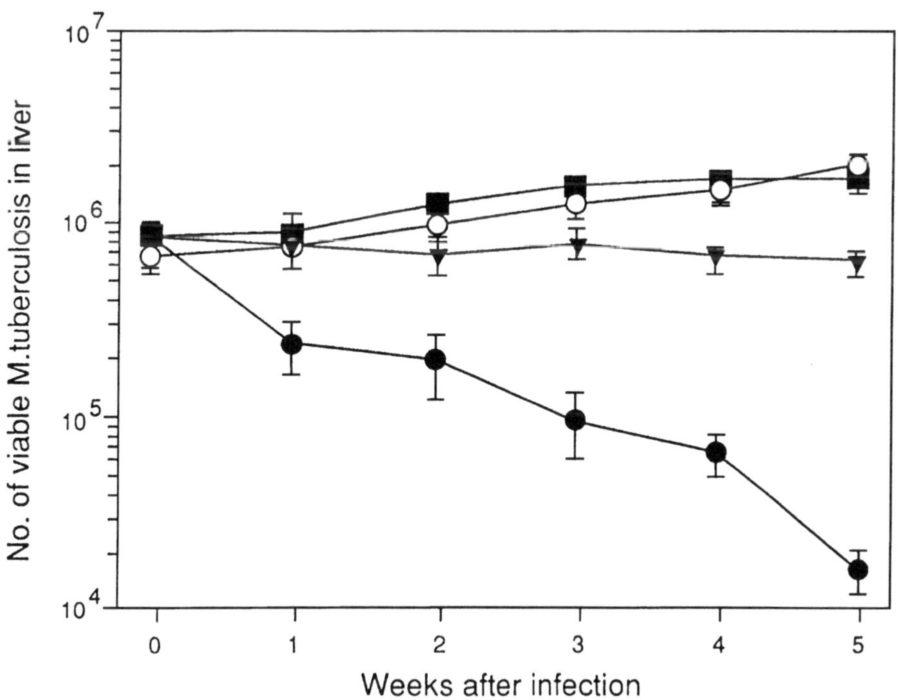

Fig. 1. Death of *Mycobacterium tuberculosis* in livers of J774-hsp65-vaccinated mice. Vaccination was either with J774-hsp65 tumour cells expressing the *M. Leprae* hsp65 gene (●), or with control tumour cells (○, ■), or with hsp65 protein in incomplete Freund's adjuvant (▲)

munise mice against challenge with large doses of virulent *M. tuberculosis*, whereas the protein and tumour cells separately were not (Fig. 1) [90]. This raised questions of specificity and mechanism. hsp65 is a highly conserved protein with immunological cross-reactivity with homologues not only in other microorganisms, including gut flora, but also in mammalian cells [110]. Background cross-reactivity to this protein may serve a normal function of alerting the immune system to stressed or damaged cells [32, 70, 71, 111]; it could also facilitate development of a protective response to this particular mycobacterial antigen. The specificity questions are largely resolved, since protection was found to be mediated by antigen-specific major histocompatibility complex (MHC)-restricted T cells [91, 93] and totally different antigens can be equally protective when delivered as DNA vaccines [51, 65]. Furthermore, the mechanisms involved in the generation and expression of protection with hsp65 have been clarified and seem likely to be applicable to other antigens.

Cytotoxicity

The key to the development of protection seems to be the presentation of the antigen to the immune system via the endogenous pathway and MHC class I for recognition by $CD8^+$ T cells. This can be achieved in various ways besides expressing the protein from a retroviral promoter in tumour cells. Protein expressed in transfected bone marrow cells was also effective [92], as was the use of positively charged liposomes to carry the antigen into cell cytosol (C.L. Silva, D.B. Lowrie, R.E. Tascon, V.M.F. Lima and V.L.D. Bonato; submitted for publication), or the injection of plasmid DNA (DNA vaccination) into muscle [100] or skin (R.E. Tascon and D.B. Lowrie, unpublished). These procedures all resembled BCG vaccination in that they gave protection against challenge with virulent *M. tuberculosis* and generated splenic T cell populations in which $CD8^+$ and $CD4^+$ cells were about equally increased, whereas protein in adjuvant or mixed with tumour cells did not protect and only increased $CD4^+$ cells selectively ([93] and C.L. Silva, D.B. Lowrie, R.E. Tascon, V.M.F. Lima and V.L.D. Bonato; submitted for publication). Analysis of the functions of purified T cell subpopulations or large numbers of T cell clones obtained from spleens after tumour-hsp65 or plasmid-hsp65 immunisation showed that $CD8^+$ cells had the greatest antimycobacterial activities in vitro and in vivo. Adoptive transfer of protective immunity to naive mice by transfer of T cell clones showed that the most protective T cells were those that produced interferon-γ and had the greatest cytolytic activity against infected macrophages. This was consistent with other evidence for both interferon-γ [39] and antigen-specific cytolysis [38, 41, 56, 101] playing important roles in protective immunity, although there is still much to be learned about how different T cell types function in protection, particularly in man [19].

Persistance

Protection by endogenous hsp65 was transient except after immunisation with plasmid DNA. After a series of intramuscular plasmid injections, protection equal to the effect of BCG persisted undiminished for at least 8 months (C.L. Silva, D.B. Lowrie, R.E. Tascon, V.M.F. Lima and V.L.D. Bonato; submitted for publication). Analysis of the splenic T cell populations indicated that this was associated with a progressive increase during the same period in numbers of cells with the hsp65-specific memory/activated phenotype ($CD44^{hi}/CD8^{+}$) that produced interferon-γ and antigen-specific cytotoxicity (unpublished); the other immunisation procedures did not achieve this. Plasmid DNA does not integrate into host cell DNA but persists episomally and can express encoded antigen for the lifetime of the injected mouse [106]. It may be relevant that the persistence of viable BCG has been argued to make a significant contribution to the persistence of protection after BCG vaccination [63]. Presumably the continued synthesis and presentation of endogenous hsp65 antigen may account for the persistent protection after DNA vaccination. This potentially important observation requires confirmation in other hands and with other antigens.

Type 1 cytokines

A striking difference between the immune response to DNA vaccination and the immune response to either BCG or *M. tuberculosis* infection is that DNA induces almost entirely a protective $CD44^{hi}$ type 1 cytokine response, whereas the mycobacterial infections have a major component of non-cytotoxic/$CD44^{lo}$ T cells that produce a type 2 cytokine response (V.L.D. Bonato, V.M.F. Lima, R.E. Tascon, D.B. Lowrie and C.L. Silva; submitted for publication). Clones of this phenotype obtained from *M. tuberculosis*-infected mice have virtually no protective capacity in adoptive transfer experiments and their role in the disease is unclear; do they primarily serve the purposes of the host or of the infectious agent? Since the type 1 and type 2 responses are mutually antagonistic, the type 2 is thought to be there to down-regulate the type 1 response to limit the tissue pathology on which the disease process depends [49, 87, 107]. However, on this basis it may also impede bacterial killing, since this also depends on the cytotoxicity (and interferon γ) of type 1 responding cells. Hence, the type 1 response that follows DNA vaccination may be preferable to the mixed response that follows BCG vaccination.

The hypothesis that inappropriate type 1/type 2 switching of the immune response might underly the failure of BCG in some human populations [85] has already been mentioned. Exposure to environmental mycobacteria might give a predominantly type 2 response to common mycobacterial antigens that stays that way despite subsequent BCG vaccination. While it is not clear what causes the mixed response seen in mycobacterial infection, the type 1 and type 2 responses are thought to tend to be self sustaining, through a combination of positive and negative feedback by cytokines in the local environment [29, 88]. It may be relevant, therefore, that DNA vaccination can reportedly switch an existing type 2 response into a type 1 response that is stable to subsequent boosting by exogenous antigen [80]. On that basis DNA might work where BCG fails, and could even have a therapeutic role. These possibilities are at present pure speculation but are amenable to experimentation in animal models.

Which antigens to include in a genetic vaccine

At this stage it is not possible to say which are the best antigens to encode in a practical vaccine except in general terms: they are those that are released in largest amount by the intracellular mycobacteria, that carry multiple or promiscuous epitopes and that are presented on MHC class I and MHC class II (for essential immunological help).

Those proven or reported to have at least some protective effect as DNA vaccines are hsp65, hsp70, 36-kDa PRA and ESAT-6 [65], MPT83 (R.E. Tascon, D.B. Lowrie, R.G. Hewinson and M.J. Colston; unpublished), PhoS [44, 113] and Ag85A [51]. The number of potential candidate antigens is large [3, 4, 109] and more are being described all the time. Some good candidates might be identified from current efforts to identify proteins produced in increased amounts by intracellular mycobacteria [62, 69, 86] or that carry secretory signals [64]. It is possible that others may be found by screening mycobacterial genome libraries as DNA vaccines in either a totally random fashion [14] or focused on putative genes identified through sequencing the whole genome [24].

It can be argued that microbial stress proteins do not make good candidates for inclusion in subunit vaccines because of the implication of the homologous mammalian proteins in autoimmune diseases [110]. However, there are possible alternatives to leaving these major antigens out of vaccines: the epitopes involved might be readily engineered out of the DNA (but such epitopes may be difficult to delimit) [10, 78, 102]; the formulation and delivery might be selected to direct the response away from a harmful and towards a beneficial type. Indeed, immunisation with mycobacterial heat shock proteins can either protect against or potentiate autoimmune disease, depending on how the antigens are encountered [2, 10, 15, 16, 22, 57]. We recently showed that DNA vaccination with mycobacterial hsp65 protected Lewis rats against induction of adjuvant arthritis [79]. This may be the best approach in the long run because, to the extent that an acquired immune response depends on recognition of 'altered self' rather than 'foreign', essentially all antigens may have the potential for autoimmune involvement.

Attractions of DNA as a vaccine

At the present state of the art, DNA vaccination is rather inefficient. Although nanogram amounts of plasmid coated on gold particles and fired by a compressed-gas gun into the skin can be enough to generate protection in some infection models [48, 53], by direct injection tens and even hundreds of micrograms of DNA are needed [11, 31]. Nevertheless, phase 1 clinical trials are underway in man against HIV and influenza and it has many attractions as a mode of vaccination [46, 59, 82, 89], not least of which are: an inherent adjuvanticity [42, 58], simplicity of production, stability of the product and extreme versatility. It is this versatility that is of most immediate interest in the context of tuberculosis, for using this technique we already know that about ten of the dozen or so tested mycobacterial protein antigens can be protective. DNA vaccination avoids the problems of purifying proteins without denaturing them and offers a way of rapidly testing different combinations and mixtures, selecting the best epitopes, omitting or modifying unwanted epitopes, targeting different antigen-presenting pathways, incorporating DNA encoding cytokines, etc. etc. All this can be done with almost no concern for vector constraints. The information obtained will be put to use, even if a different vector, such as a recombinant mycobacterium or virus, is ultimately preferred for clinical use. Although there are safety concerns with DNA vaccination that are as yet unresolved, these are not so great as to prevent phase 1 clinical trials that include healthy volunteers and so far there are no reports of adverse reactions [82]. Consequently, we would not discount the possibility of DNA vaccination against tuberculosis being clinically evaluated before long.

Acknowledgements. This work received financial support from the WHO Global Programme for Vaccines and Immunization (GPV), Fundação de Amparo à Pesquisa do Estado de São Paulo (FAPESP), Conselho Nacional de Desenvolvimento Científico e Tecnológico (CNPq) and Financiadora de Estudos e Projetos (FINEP).

References

1. Abou-Zeid C, Smith I, Grange JM, Ratliff TL, Steele J, Rook GAW (1988) The secreted antigens of *Mycobacterium tuberculosis* and their relationship to those recognized by the available antibodies. J Gen Microbiol 134 : 531
2. Adams E, Basten A, Rodda S, Britton WJ (1997) Human T-cell clones to the 70-kilodalton heat shock protein of *Mycobacterium leprae* define mycobacterium-specific epitopes rather than shared epitopes. Infect Immun 65 : 1061
3. Andersen AB (1994) *Mycobacterium tuberculosis* proteins – structure, function, and immunological relevance. Dan Med Bull 41 : 205
4. Andersen AB, Brennan P (1994) Proteins and antigens of *Mycobacterium tuberculosis*. In: Bloom BR (ed) Tuberculosis: pathogenesis, protection, and control. American Society for Microbiology, Washington, D.C., pp 307–332
5. Andersen P (1994) Effective vaccination of mice against *Mycobacterium tuberculosis* infection with a soluble mixture of secreted mycobacterial proteins. Infect Immun 62 : 2536
6. Andersen P (1994) The T cell response to secreted antigens of *Mycobacterium tuberculosis*. Immunobiology 191 : 537
7. Andersen P, Askgaard D, Ljungqvist L, Bennedsen J, Heron I (1991) Proteins released from *Mycobacterium tuberculosis* during growth. Infect Immun 59 : 1905
8. Andersen P, Askgaard D, Ljungqvist L, Bentzon MW, Heron I (1991) T-cell proliferative response to antigens secreted by *Mycobacterium tuberculosis*. Infect Immun 59 : 1558
9. Andersen P, Andersen AB, Sorensen AL, Nagai S (1995) Recall of long-lived immunity to *Mycobacterium tuberculosis* infection in mice. J Immunol 154 : 3359
10. Anderton SM, Zee R van der, Noordzij A, Eden W van (1994) Differential mycobacterial 65-kDa heat shock protein T cell epitope recognition after adjuvant arthritis-inducing or protective immunization protocols. J Immunol 152 : 3656
11. Babiuk LA, Lewis PJ, Cox G, Drunen Littel-van den Hurk S van, Baca-Estrada M, Tikoo SK (1995) DNA immunization with bovine herpes virus-1 genes. Ann NY Acad Sci 772 : 47
12. Balasubramanian V, Wiegeshaus EH, Smith DW (1994) Mycobacterial infection in guinea pigs. Immunobiology 191 : 395
13. Barnes PF, Mehra V, Rivoire B, Fong SJ, Brennan PJ, Voegtline MS, Minden P, Houghten RA, Bloom BR, Modlin RL (1992) Immunoreactivity of a 10-kDa-antigen of *Mycobacterium tuberculosis*. J Immunol 148 : 1835
14. Barry MA, Lai WC, Johnston SA (1995) Protection against mycoplasma infection using expression-library immunization. Nature 377 : 632
15. Billingham MEJ, Carney S, Butler R, Colston MJ (1990) A mycobacterial 65-Kd heat shock protein induces antigen-specific suppression of adjuvant arthritis, but is not itself arthritogenic. J Exp Med 171 : 339
16. Birk OS, Douek DC, Elias D, Takacs K, Dewchand H, Gur SL, Walker MD, Zee R van der, Cohen IR, Altmann DM (1996) A role of Hsp60 in autoimmune diabetes: analysis in a transgenic model. Proc Natl Acad Sci USA 93 : 1032
17. Bloom BR, Fine PEM (1994) The BCG experience: implications for future vaccines against tuberculosis. In: Bloom BR (ed) Tuberculosis: pathogenesis, protection, and control. American Society for Microbiology, Washington, D.C., pp 531–557
18. Boesen H, Jensen BN, Wilcke T, Andersen P (1995) Human T-cell responses to secreted antigen fractions of *Mycobacterium tuberculosis*. Infect Immun 63 : 1491
19. Boom WH (1996) The role of T-cell subsets in *Mycobacterium tuberculosis* infection. Infect Agents Dis 5 : 73
20. Cheng SH, Walker KB, Lowrie DB, Mitchison DA, Swamy R, Datta M, Prabhakar R (1993) Monocyte antimycobacterial activity before and after *Mycobacterium bovis* BCG vaccination in Chingleput, India, and London, United Kingdom. Infect Immun 61 : 4501

21. Cirillo JD, Stover CK, Bloom BR, Jacobs WR, Barletta RG (1995) Bacterial vaccine vectors and Bacillus Calmette-Guerin. Clin Infect Dis 20 : 1001
22. Cohen IR, Elias D (1996) Immunity to 60 kDa heat shock protein in autoimmune diabetes. Diabet Nutr Metab 9 : 229
23. Colditz GA, Berkey CS, Mosteller F, Brewer TF, Wilson ME, Burdick E, Fineberg HV (1995) The efficacy of bacillus Calmette-Guerin vaccination of newborns and infants in the prevention of tuberculosis: meta-analyses of the published literature. Pediatrics 96 : 29
24. Cole ST (1996) Why sequence the genome of *Mycobacterium tuberculosis*. Tuber Lung Dis 77 : 486
25. Collins FM (1991) Antituberculous immunity – new solutions to an old problem. Rev Infect Dis 13 : 940
26. Collins FM (1994) The immune response to mycobacterial infection: development of new vaccines. Vet Microbiol 40 : 95
27. Comstock GW (1994) Field trials of tuberculosis vaccines: How could we have done them better? Controlled Clin Trials 15 : 247
28. Converse PJ, Dannenberg AM, Estep JE, Sugisaki K, Abe Y, Schofield BH, Pitt MLM (1996) Cavitary tuberculosis produced in rabbits by aerosolized virulent tubercle bacilli. Infect Immun 64 : 4776
29. Croft M, Carter L, Swain SL, Dutton RW (1994) Generation of polarized antigen-specific CD8 effector populations: reciprocal action of interleukin (IL)-4 and IL-12 in promoting type 2 versus type 1 cytokine profiles. J Exp Med 180 : 1715
30. Dannenberg AM, Sugimoto M (1976) Liquefaction of caseous foci in tuberculosis. Am Rev Respir Dis 113 : 257
31. Davis HL, Michel ML, Mancini M, Schleef M, Whalen RG (1994) Direct gene transfer in skeletal muscle: plasmid DNA-based immunization against the hepatitis B virus surface antigen. Vaccine 12 : 1503
32. Denagel DC, Pierce SK (1993) Heat shock proteins in immune responses. Crit Rev Immunol 13 : 71
33. deWit D, Wootton M, Dhillon J, Mitchison DA (1995) The bacterial DNA content of mouse organs in the Cornell model of dormant tuberculosis. Tuber Lung Dis 76 : 555
34. Dolin PJ, Raviglione MC, Kochi A (1994) Global tuberculosis incidence and mortality during 1990–2000. Bull Who 72 : 213
35. Edwards KL, Goodrich JM, Muller D, Pollack A, Ziegler JE, Smith DW (1982) Infection with *Mycobacterium avium*-intracellulare and the protective effects of bacille Calmette-Guerin. J Infect Dis 145 : 733
36. Fifis T, Costopoulos C, Radford AJ, Bacic A, Wood PR (1991) Purification and characterization of major antigens from a *Mycobacterium bovis* culture filtrate. Infect Immun 59 : 800
37. Fine PEM (1995) Bacille Calmette-Guerin vaccines: a rough guide. Clin Infect Dis 20 : 11
38. Flynn JL, Goldstein MM, Triebold KJ, Koller B, Bloom BR (1992) Major histocompatibility complex class-I-restricted T-cells are required for resistance to *Mycobacterium tuberculosis* infection. Proc Natl Acad Sci USA 89 : 12 013
39. Flynn JL, Chan J, Triebold KJ, Dalton DK, Stewart TA, Bloom BR (1993) An essential role for interferon gamma in resistance to *Mycobacterium tuberculosis* infection. J Exp Med 178 : 2249
40. Gulle H, Fray LM, Gormley EP, Murray A, Moriarty KM (1995) Responses of bovine T cells to fractionated lysate and culture filtrate proteins of *Mycobacterium bovis* BCG. Vet Immunol Immunopathol 48 : 183
41. Gupta LK, Bhatnagar S, Ram GC, Bansal MP (1995) Role of cytotoxic lymphocytes in immunity against bovine tuberculosis. Med Sci Res 23 : 535
42. Halpern MD, Kurlander RJ, Pisetsky DS (1996) Bacterial DNA induces murine interferon-gamma production by stimulation of interleukin-12 and tumor necrosis factor-alpha. Cell Immunol 167 : 72
43. Hart PDA, Sutherland I (1977) BCG and vole bacillus vaccines in the prevention of tuberculosis in adolescence and early adult life: final report to the Medical Research Council. Br Med J 2 : 293
44. Haslov K, Andersen AB, Ljungqvist L, Bentzon MW (1990) Comparison of the immunological activity of 5 defined antigens from *Mycobacterium tuberculosis* in 7 inbred guinea pig strains. Scand J Immunol 31 : 503
45. Haslov K, Andersen A, Nagai S, Gottschau A, Sorensen T, Andersen P (1995) Guinea pig cellular immune responses to proteins secreted by *Mycobacterium tuberculosis*. Infect Immun 63 : 804
46. Hassett DE, Whitton JL (1996) DNA immunization. Trends Microbiol 4 : 307
47. Havlir DV, Wallis RS, Boom WH, Daniel TM, Chervenak K, Ellner JJ (1991) Human immune response to *Mycobacterium tuberculosis* antigens. Infect Immun 59 : 665
48. Haynes JR, Fuller DH, Eisenbraun MD, Ford MJ, Pertmer TM (1994) Accell(R) particle-mediated DNA immunization elicits humoral, cytotoxic, and protective immune responses. AIDS Res Hum Retroviruses 10 : S43

49. HernandezPando R, Orozcoe H, Sampieri A, Pavon L, Velasquillo C, Larriva Sahd J, Alcocer JM, Madrid MV (1996) Correlation between the kinetics of Th1/Th2 cells and pathology in a murine model of experimental pulmonary tuberculosis. Immunology 89 : 26
50. Horwitz MA, Lee BWE, Dillon BJ, Harth G (1995) Protective immunity against tuberculosis induced by vaccination with major extracellular proteins of *Mycobacterium tuberculosis*. Proc Natl Acad Sci USA 92 : 1530
51. Huygen K, Content J, Denis O, Montgomery DL, Yawman AM, Deck RR, DeWitt CM, Orme IM, Baldwin S, D'Souza C, Drowart A, Lozes E, Vandenbussche P, Van Vooren JP, Liu MA, Ulmer JB (1996) Immunogenicity and protective efficacy of a tuberculosis DNA vaccine. Nature Med 2 : 893
52. Jacobs WR, Tuckman M, Bloom BR (1987) Introduction of foreign DNA into mycobacteria using a shuttle phasmid. Nature 327 : 532
53. Johnston SA, Tang DC (1994) Gene gun transfection of animal cells and genetic immunization. Methods Cell Biol 43 : 353
54. Kamala T, Paramasivan CN, Herbert D, Venkatesan P, Prabhakar R (1996) Immune response and modulation of immune response induced in the guinea-pigs by *Mycobacterium avium* complex (MAC) and *M. fortuitum* complex isolates from different sources in the south Indian BCG trial area. Indian J Med Res 103 : 201
55. Kaufmann SHE (1990) Heat shock proteins and the immune response. Immunol Today 11 : 129
56. Kaufmann SHE (1993) Immunity to intracellular bacteria. Annu Rev Immunol 11 : 129
57. Kingston AE, Hicks CA, Colston MJ, Billingham MEJ (1996) A 71-kD heat shock protein (hsp) from *Mycobacterium tuberculosis* has modulatory effects on experimental rat arthritis. Clin Exp Immunol 103 : 77
58. Krieg AM (1996) An innate immune defense mechanism based on the recognition of CpG motifs in microbial DNA. J Lab Clin Med 128 : 128
59. Kumar V, Sercarz E (1996) Genetic vaccination: the advantages of going naked. Nature Med 2 : 857
60. Lagrange PH (1984) Cell-mediated immunity and delayed-type hypersensitivity. In: Kubica GP, Wayne LG (eds) The mycobacteria. A sourcebook. Dekker, New York, pp 681–720
61. Lecoeur H, Lagrange PH, Truffot C, Grosset J (1981) Microbial persistence and tuberculosis hypersensitivity after chemotherapy of the mouse experimental tuberculosis. Ann Immunol 132D : 237
62. Lee BY, Horwitz MA (1995) Identification of macrophage and stress-induced proteins of *Mycobacterium tuberculosis*. J Clin Invest 96 : 245
63. Lefford MJ, McGregor DD (1974) Immunological memory in tuberculosis. I. Influence of persisting viable organisms. Cell Immunol 14 : 417
64. Lim EM, Rauzier J, Timm J, Torrea G, Murray A, Gicquel B, Portnoi D (1995) Identification of *Mycobacterium tuberculosis* DNA sequences encoding exported proteins by using phoA gene fusions. J Bacteriol 177 : 59
65. Lowrie DB, Silva CL, Colston MJ, Ragno S, Tascon R (1997) Protection against tuberculosis by a plasmid DNA. Vaccine (in press)
66. Maes HH, Causse JE, Maes RF (1996) Mycobacterial infections: are the observed enigmas and paradoxes explained by immunosuppression and immunodeficiency? Med Hypotheses 46 : 163
67. Mehra V, Gong JH, Iyer D, Lin YG, Boylen CT, Bloom BR, Barnes PF (1996) Immune response to recombinant mycobacterial proteins in patients with tuberculosis infection and disease. J Infect Dis 174 : 431
68. Mendezsamperio P, Gonzalezgarcia L, Pinedafragoso PR, Ramossanchez E (1995) Specificity of T cells in human resistance to *Mycobacterium tuberculosis* infection. Cell Immunol 162 : 194
69. Monahan IM, Banerjee DK, Jacobs WR, Butcher PD (1996) Gene expression of *Mycobacterium bovis* BCG during interaction with macrophages. Abstracts of the 3rd International Conference on the Pathogenesis of Mycobacterial Diseases, 27–30 June, Stockholm. Swedish Institute for Infections Disease Control, Stockholm, abstr. no. 43
70. Murray PJ, Young RA (1992) Stress and immunological recognition in host-pathogen interactions. J Bacteriol 174 : 4193
71. Nomoto K, Yoshikai Y (1991) Heat-shock proteins and immunopathology – regulatory role of heat-shock protein-specific T-cells. Springer Semin Immunopathol 13 : 63
72. Oftung F, Mustafa AS, Husson R, Young RA, Godal T (1987) Human T cell clones recognise two abundant *Mycobacterium tuberculosis* protein antigens expressed in *Escherichia coli*. J Immunol 138 : 927

73. Onyebujoh PC, Abdulmumini T, Robinson S, Rook GAW, Stanford JL (1995) Immunotherapy with *Mycobacterium vaccae* as an addition to chemotherapy for the treatment of pulmonary tuberculosis under difficult conditions in Africa. Respir Med 89 : 199
74. Orme IM, Collins FM (1984) Efficacy of *Mycobacterium bovis* BCG vaccination in mice undergoing prior pulmonary infection with atypical mycobacteria. Infect Immun 44 : 28
75. Orme IM, Andersen P, Boom WH (1993) T-cell response to *Mycobacterium tuberculosis*. J Infect Dis 167 : 1481
76. Pal PG, Horwitz MA (1992) Immunization with extracellular proteins of *Mycobacterium tuberculosis* induces cell-mediated immune responses and substantial protective immunity in a guinea pig model of pulmonary tuberculosis. Infect Immun 60 : 4781
77. Palmer CE, Long MW (1966) Effects of infection with atypical mycobacteria on BCG vaccination and tuberculosis. Am Rev Respir Dis 94 : 553
78. Prakken ABJ, Eden W van, Rijkers GT, Kuis W, Toebes EA, DeGraeff Meeder ER, Zee R van der, Zegers BJM (1996) Autoreactivity to human heat-shock protein 60 predicts disease remission in oligo-articular juvenile rheumatoid arthritis. Arthritis Rheum 39 : 1826
79. Ragno S, Colston MJ, Lowrie DB, Winrow VR, Blake DR, Tascon R (1997) Immunization with naked DNA encoding mycobacterial hsp65 protects rats from adjuvant arthritis. Arthritis Rheum (in press)
80. Raz E, Tighe H, Sato Y, Corr M, Dudler JA, Roman M, Swain SL, Spiegelberg HL, Carson DA (1996) Preferential induction of a Th1 immune response and inhibition of specific IgE antibody formation by plasmid DNA immunization. Proc Natl Acad Sci USA 93 : 5141
81. Reiner NE (1994) Altered cell signaling and mononuclear phagocyte deactivation during intracellular infection. Immunol Today 15 : 374
82. Robertson JS (1996) The potential of DNA vaccines. J Biotech Healthcare 3 : 239
83. Rodrigues LC, Diwan VK, Wheeler JG (1993) Protective effect of BCG against tuberculosis meningitis and miliary tuberculosis: a meta-analysis. Int J Epidemiol 22 : 1154
84. Rook GAW, Hernandez Pando R (1994) T cell helper types and endocrines in the regulation of tissue-damaging mechanisms in tuberculosis. Immunobiology 191 : 478
85. Rook GAW, Onyebujoh P, Stanford JL (1993) TH1/TH2 switching and loss of $CD4^+$ T cells in chronic infections – an immunoendocrinological hypothesis not exclusive to HIV. Immunol Today 14 : 568
86. Russell WR, Pollock JM, Butcher PD, Hewinson RG (1996) The detection of *M. bovis* antigens expressed inside macrophages. Proceedings of the 2nd International Conference on *Mycobacterium bovis*: Tuberculosis in wildlife and domestic animals; 1996 Otago conference. University of Otago Press, Dunedin, pp 135–138
87. Sander B, Skansen Saphir U, Damm O, Hakansson L, Andersson J, Andersson U (1995) Sequential production of Th1 and Th2 cytokines in response to live bacillus Calmette-Guerin. Immunology 86 : 512
88. Seder RA, Paul WE (1994) Acquisition of lymphokine-producing phenotype by $CD4^+$ T cells. Annu Rev Immunol 12 : 635
89. Siegrist CA, Lambert PH (1996) DNA vaccines: what can we expect? Infect Agents Dis 5 : 55
90. Silva CL, Lowrie DB (1994) A single mycobacterial protein (hsp65) expressed by a transgenic antigen-presenting cell vaccinates mice against tuberculosis. Immunology 82 : 244
91. Silva CL, Silva MF, Pietro RCLR, Lowrie DB (1994) Protection against tuberculosis by passive transfer with T-cell clones recognizing mycobacterial heat-shock protein 65. Immunology 83 : 341
92. Silva CL, Pietro RLR, Januario A, Bonato VLD, Lima VMF, DaSilva MF, Lowrie DB (1995) Protection against tuberculosis by bone marrow cells expressing mycobacterial hsp65. Immunology 86 : 519
93. Silva CL, Silva MF, Pietro RCLR, Lowrie DB (1996) Characterization of T cells that confer a high degree of protective immunity against tuberculosis in mice after vaccination with tumor cells expressing mycobacterial hsp65. Infect Immun 64 : 2400
94. Smith PG (1994) BCG vaccination. In: Davies PDO (ed) Clinical tuberculosis. Chapman and Hall, London, pp 297–310
95. Sorensen AL, Nagai S, Houen G, Andersen P, Andersen AB (1995) Purification and characterization of a low-molecular-mass T-cell antigen secreted by *Mycobacterium tuberculosis*. Infect Immun 63 : 1710
96. Springett VH, Sutherland I (1990) BCG vaccination of school children in England and Wales. Thorax 45 : 83
97. Stanford JL, Rook GAW (1983) Environmental mycobacteria and immunization with BCG. In: Easmon CSF, Jeljaszewicz J (eds) Medical microbiology, vol 2; Immunization against bacterial disease. Academic Press, London, pp 43–69

98. Stanford JL, Stanford CA (1994) Immunotherapy of tuberculosis with *Mycobacterium vaccae* NCTC 11659. Immunobiology 191 : 555
99. Tantimavanich S, Nagai S, Nomaguchi H, Kinomoto M, Ohara N, Yamada T (1993) Immunological properties of ribosomal proteins from *Mycobacterium bovis* BCG. Infect Immun 61 : 4005
100. Tascon RE, Colston MJ, Ragno S, Stavropoulos E, Gregory D, Lowrie DB (1996) Vaccination against tuberculosis by DNA injection. Nature Med 2 : 888
101. Tsukaguchi K, Balaji KN, Boom WH (1995) CD4(+) α β T cell and γ δ T cell responses to *Mycobacterium tuberculosis* – Similarities and differences in Ag recognition, cytotoxic effector function, and cytokine production. J Immunol 154 : 1786
102. Van Eden W, Anderton SM, Zee R van der, Prakken ABJ, Rijkers GT (1995) Specific immunity as a critical factor in the control of autoimmune arthritis: the example of hsp60 as an ancillary and protective autoantigen. Scand J Rheumatol 101 : 141
103. Walsh GP, Tan EV, delaCruz EC, Abalos RM, Villahermosa LG, Young LJ, Cellona RV, Nazareno JB, Horwitz MA (1996) The Philippine cynomolgus monkey *(Macaca fascicularis)* provides a new nonhuman primate model of tuberculosis that resembles human disease. Nature Med 2 : 430
104. Wiegeshaus EH, Harding G, McMurray D, Grover AA, Smith DW (1971) A cooperative evaluation of test systems used to assay tuberculosis vaccines. Bull WHO 45 : 543
105. Wiker HG, Nagai S, Harboe M, Ljungqvist L (1992) A family of cross-reacting proteins secreted by *Mycobacterium tuberculosis*. Scand J Immunol 36 : 307
106. Wolffe JA, Ludtke JJ, Acsadi G, Williams P, Jani A (1992) Long-term persistence of plasmid DNA and foreign gene expression in mouse muscle. Hum Mol Genet 1 : 363
107. Yamamura M, Wang XH, Ohmen JD, Uyemura K, Rea TH, Bloom BR, Modlin RL (1992) Cytokine patterns of immunologically mediated tissue damage. J Immunol 149 : 1470
108. Youmans AS, Youmans GP (1965) Immunogenic activity of a ribosomal fraction obtained from *Mycobacterium tuberculosis*. J Bacteriol 89 : 1291
109. Young DB, Kaufmann SHE, Hermans PWM, Thole JER (1992) Mycobacterial protein antigens. – A compilation. Mol Microbiol 6 : 133
110. Young RA (1990) Stress proteins and immunology. Annu Rev Immunol 8 : 401
111. Young RA, Elliott TJ (1989) Stress proteins, infection, and immune surveillance. Cell 59 : 5
112. Yuan Y, Crane DD, Barry CE (1996) Stationary phase-associated protein expression in *Mycobacterium tuberculosis*: function of the mycobacterial α-crystallin homolog. J Bacteriol 178 : 4484
113. Zhu X, Venkataprasad N, Thangaraj H, Vordermeier HM (1996) Nucleic acid vaccination for protection against *M. tuberculosis*. Abstracts of the 3rd International Conference on the Pathogenesis of Mycobacterial Infections, 27–30 June, Stockholm. Swedish Institute for Infections Disease Control, Stockholm, abstr. no. 25

DNA gene vaccination for HIV

Jong J. Kim[1,2], David B. Weiner[2]

[1] Department of Chemical Engineering, University of Pennsylvania, 505 Stellar-Chance, 422 Curie Blvd., Philadelphia, PA 19104, USA
[2] Department of Pathology and Laboratory Medicine, University of Pennsylvania, 505 Stellar-Chance, 422 Curie Blvd., Philadelphia, PA 19104, USA

Introduction

The human immunodeficiency virus-1 (HIV-1) is a retrovirus which preferentially infects and kills $CD4^+$ T cells and macrophages, ultimately resulting in immune system failure and multi-pathogen infections. Recent breakthroughs in combination therapy using three different anti-retroviral agents have generated optimism regarding the ability to control viral replication in vivo [46]. However, this therapeutic regimen is costly, and it is too early to tell whether this approach can eradicate established infection [26, 46]. The costs and the stringent administration regimen requirements of these pharmaceutical agents make it clear that these drugs will only be effectively utilized in a limited part of the world population. Therefore, to address the worldwide problem of HIV-1 infection, there remains a need for a prophylactic vaccination strategy designed to control the epidemic through mass immunization campaigns [115].

Development of vaccines against HIV-1

The overall goal of any immunization strategy is to induce pathogen-specific immune responses which are both potent and durable, with the least number of immunizations over the lifetime of the immunized individual. More clinically efficacious vaccines should elicit pathogen-specific immune responses according to the correlates of protection known for the particular pathogen.

Obstacles opposing AIDS vaccine development

Major obstacles in the development of effective HIV-1 vaccines are the diversity of the virus and the uncertainty of protective correlates. HIV-1 is subject to a significant amount of sequence divergence over time because it is an RNA virus whose reverse

Correspondence to: D. B. Weiner

transcriptase lacks a proofing function, [108]. Divergence occurs not only within a subpopulation of infected individuals, but also along the geographic lines [39, 91].

Another significant obstacle in the development of a vaccine against HIV-1 is uncertainty regarding the exact immune correlates of protection [25]. Protective immune response could be provided by either the humoral or cellular arms of the immune system or both. Humoral immunity provides a significant contribution to protective responses in some successful viral vaccines. Antibodies are especially critical in preventing susceptible cells from becoming infected by blocking virus binding or entry to target cells. High-titer neutralizing antibodies have been correlated with efficacy in a number of viral diseases including hepatitis B and rabies. On the other hand, cellular immunity, especially in the form of $CD8^+$ cytotoxic T cells, has been shown to be protective against some viral infections. As a potent cellular immune response modulators, cytotoxic T lymphocytes (CTLs) target and destroy virus-infected cells by recognizing processed viral fragments presented on the infected cell surface associated with the host-specific class I major histocompatibility complex (MHC). CTLs can target not only the gene products present in the viral particle, but also all viral gene products expressed during viral replication. Targeting immune responses against viral proteins could aid in lowering viral load through the development of specific CTL responses which destroy viral factories.

In studies of long-term non-progressor groups of HIV-infected individuals, evidence supports the notion that correlates of protection against HIV-1 could be provided by humoral, cellular, or even both arms of immune response [19, 84]. High levels of neutralizing antibody have been observed in protected primates in some homologous challenge models [5, 6, 16, 17, 36]. The most important epitopes appear to be the hypervariable V3 loop and CD4 binding domain of gp120 as well as sites in gp41 [40, 92]. Although possibly important for protection, the presence of neutralizing antibody alone has not been clearly shown to protect primates from viral challenge [21, 53]. In addition, it is more difficult to neutralize clinical isolates of HIV-1 in comparison to long-term laboratory isolates [20]. Neutralizing antibodies are susceptible to antigenic diversity of HIV-1 envelope. Neutralizing antibodies developed against the V3 loop of a United States isolate, for example, were unable to neutralize African viral isolates, illustrating the type specificity of antibody-mediated protection [20].

Cytolysis induced by CTLs has also been shown to correlate with protection in some viral vaccine models including HIV-1. Because one of the hallmarks of HIV-1 disease progression is the loss of cellular immune function, the presence of strong cellular responses might be relevant for protection. Several reports point to HIV-specific-CTL responses as a potential mechanism of protection. In cases of acute HIV-1 infection studied by several investigators, viral clearance was associated with specific CTL activity in each case [10, 60]. In addition, a subset (7 of 20) of occupationally exposed health care workers who were not infected possessed transient HIV-1 specific CTL response [87]. HIV-1-specific CTLs were also found in a number of chronically exposed prostitutes in Gambia who continue to resist infection with HIV-1 [90]. Finally, HIV-specific CTL activity has been observed in an uninfected perinatally exposed child [89]. In spite of these studies supporting the role of neutralizing antibodies and CTLs in conferring immunity to infection, some vaccinated primates exhibiting both neutralizing antibody and CTL responses were not protected from subsequent viral challenge in the related simian immunodeficiency virus (SIV) model [51, 95]. Although an increasing number of reports address potential correlates, proving and understanding protective immunity against HIV-1 infection remains elusive.

Table 1. Potential advantages of DNA/genetic immunization

Efficacy	
	Induce both humoral and cellular immuno responses
Safety	
	Little risk for reversion to a disease-causing form
	No risk for secondary infection
Better design	
	DNA vaccines can be manipulated to present all or part of the genome
	Genes which lead to undesired immunological inhibition may be removed
Enhanced manufacturing and storage capability	
	Better stability and storage capability compared to traditional vaccine formulations
	Simpler and less expensive manufacturing process

DNA vaccines and unique characteristics

We originally and others recently have developed immunization strategies against HIV-1 using DNA/genetic inoculation for the production of in vivo immunity [14, 44, 58, 68, 82, 110]. This nucleic acid inoculation induces antigen-specific immune responses following injection of non-replicating plasmids directly into a host target tissue [13, 30, 35, 58, 101, 106, 110]. Once injected, these non-replicating transcription units drive the synthesis of specific foreign proteins within the inoculated host. These host-synthesized foreign proteins then become subject of immune surveillance, resulting in antigen-specific cellular and humoral immune responses without the associated risk of viral pathogenesis. This vaccination technique is being explored as an immunization strategy against a variety of pathogens, including HIV-1 [14, 44, 58, 68, 82, 110]. As summarized in Table 1, nucleic acid immunization may afford several potential advantages over traditional vaccination strategies such as whole killed or live attenuated virus and recombinant protein-based vaccines. Since DNA vaccines are non-replicating and the vaccine components are produced within the host cells, they can be constructed to function with the safety features as well as the specificity of a subunit vaccine. However, DNA vaccine cassettes produce immunological responses that are more similar to live vaccine preparations. By directly introducing DNA into the host cell, the host cell is essentially directed to produce the antigenic protein thus mimicking viral replication in host cells. This process has been demonstrated to generate both antibody and cell-mediated, particularly killer T cell-mediated immunity. Unlike alive attenuated vaccine, there is little risk from reversion to a disease-causing form with the injected DNA. Furthermore, there is no risk for secondary infection as the material injected is not live and not infectious. In addition, genes which lead to undesired immunological inhibition or cross-reactivity (autoimmunity) may be either altered or deleted altogether. Finally, DNA vaccines can be manipulated to present all or part of the genome of the organism of interest in non-replicating vectors. These unique features of nucleic acid immunization make it well suited as a vaccination strategy against HIV.

HIV genome and potential targets for DNA vaccination

Within the HIV genome, there are several potential immunological targets for DNA vaccination (Fig. 1). The HIV-1 genome is organized into three major structural and

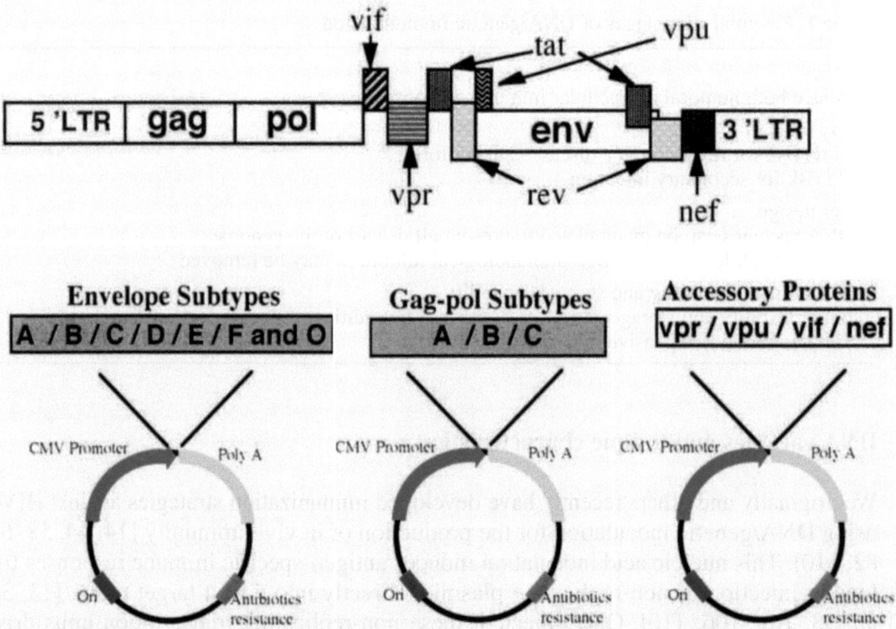

Fig. 1. Potential immunological targets for DNA vaccination against HIV-1. These targets include *env*, *gag*, and *pol* genes as well as the four accessory genes

enzymatic genes, two regulatory genes, and four accessory genes [29]. The first major gene target is *env* which codes for the outer viral envelope proteins. HIV enters the CD4+ cells via envelope-CD4 receptor and chemokine co-receptor complex (D'Souza MP, Harden VA (1996) Chemokines and HIV-1 second receptors. Confluence of two fields generates optimism in AIDS research. [Review]. Nature Med 2 : 1293). Following entry of HIV viral core, synthesis of a double-stranded DNA version of the HIV genome (called DNA provirus) begins by the viral DNA polymerase, reverse transcriptase (RT). The DNA provirus is then translocated to the nucleus as part of the protein-DNA pre-integration complex and is integrated into the host cell genome with the help of the viral integrase (Int) enzyme. The provirus then is carried along with the host DNA each time the cell divides. The gene *gag* codes for the core protein, and *pol* codes for the enzymatic proteins RT, Int, and Protease (Pro). In general, these enzymatic proteins remain somewhat conserved and preserve their catalytic functions. Accordingly, these proteins may be less divergent immune targets than envelope proteins for CTL-mediated responses [79].

The regulatory genes *tat* and *rev* affect HIV-1 gene expression. Viral transcription is increased several hundredfold by tat transactivation [29] making it an obvious target for therapeutic intervention. The rev protein increases the release of unspliced structural RNAs from the nucleus by displacing host splicing factors which otherwise prevent RNA transport from the nucleus to the cytoplasm [72]. In addition, rev is a critical component in the production of the structural proteins of HIV-1. Immune responses directed against rev could target this essential gene sequence and, thus, interfere with the viral life cycle.

In addition to the regulatory genes, HIV-1 carries an additional set of accessory genes, *vif* (virion infectivity factor), *vpr* (viral protein r), *vpu* (viral protein u), and *nef* (negative factor) which are potential targets for DNA immunization. These accessory genes can be deleted from the viral genome without eliminating replication in vitro, suggesting that these gene products play a secondary rather than primary role in viral infection. The vif protein is located in the plasma membrane and may be important for production of infectious virions [97]. In contrast to vif, vpu seems to facilitate the degradation of intracellular CD4 molecules [97]. The vpr protein is found in the viral particle in high amounts and appears to have several biological activities including the ability to increase viral transcription as well as to reactivate virus from cellular latency and arrest host cell division [63–65]. Nef has never been shown to be critical for viral infection of cell lines in vitro [59], although experiments performed with the related SIV found that rhesus macaques infected with virus having a deletion in *nef* had dramatically lower levels of viral replication [55]. Developing DNA vaccine constructs directed against these accessory genes could provide additional arsenal in our battle against HIV-1.

HIV subtypes represent a combination of the heterogeneity of the virus magnified by the geographic segregation of infected populations [1, 2]. A multiple subtype vaccine which includes both early macrophage tropic NSI isolates as well as later T cell tropic SI isolates may give broad protection. A DNA based approach is flexible enough to handle such complexity.

1. Cheng-Mayer C, Homsy J, Evans LA, Levy JA (1988) Identification of human immunodeficiency virus subtypes and distinct patterns of sensitivity to serum neutralization. Proc Natl Acad Sci – USA 85 : 2815
2. Saag M, Hahn BH, Gibbons JH, Li Y, Parks ES, Parks WP, Shaw GM (1988) Extensive variation of human immunodeficiency virus type-1 in vivo. Nature 334 : 440.

Progress of genetic immunization against HIV-1

Studies in small animals

A series of DNA envelope expression cassettes including pM160-HXB2, -MN and -Z6 envelopes were the first to be analyzed for immunogenicity [109, 110]. Studies demonstrated that the animals immunized with these envelope constructs produced antibodies specific to recombinant gp160, gp120, and gp41 proteins. These antisera also neutralized HIV-1 IIIB in vitro. Neutralization of homologous isolates has also been reported after immunization with constructs based on the HIV-1 NL4-3 isolate in the presence of relatively low anti-envelope IgG titers [68]. In addition, the pM160-MN construct not only demonstrated neutralization of homologous isolates but also showed lower, yet measurable neutralization of the heterologous HIV-1 Z6 isolate [112].

In addition to the humoral responses, cellular immune responses were observed from envelope inoculated mice. Induction of T helper cell proliferative response against recombinant gp120 protein was observed [110]. In addition, CTL responses have been observed against both targets infected with recombinant vaccinia expressing envelope protein and targets prepared with envelope peptides [44, 68, 109]. Cross-killing CTLs were also observed as MN envelope immunized animals were found to kill recombinant vaccinia-gp160HXB2 infected targets [49, 109].

In contrast to the sequence divergence observed in the envelope glycoproteins of HIV-1, the *gag* and *pol* gene sequences appear to be less variable immunological targets. Expression cassettes encoding for both gag and pol were constructed to immunize mice, and antigen-specific antibody responses were observed [58]. CTL response to specific CTL epitopes have been reported within both the gag and pol proteins, supporting the premise that cellular immunity may effectively target the virus through anti-gag-pol responses [22]. In addition to the DNA immunogen cassettes encoding envelope and gag/pol proteins, the DNA expression cassettes targeting nef and vif accessory proteins have been developed by our laboratory [3, 58].

Studies in primates

Primates represent the most relevant challenge system for HIV vaccine evaluation. However, primate models do have some limitations. Specifically, there are currently three different primate models for HIV vaccine studies. They are the SIV and chimeric (SIV)/HIV-1 (SHIV-1) challenge models in macaques and HIV challenge model in chimpanzees. The SIV model uses the related SIV which can replicate in vivo and cause disease in some macaques. This model does provide pathogenesis, however, it suffers from the fact that SIV and HIV are different viruses and that vaccines built for HIV-1 cannot be tested against SIV. The SHIV-1 also replicates in macaques. It differs from SIV in that the SIV envelope genes have been replaced by specific HIV-1 envelope genes. This represents an infectious challenge model for HIV-1 envelope based vaccines. However, the immunology and disease pathogenesis observed in the SIV or SHIV models dot not clearly mimic HIV-1 infection in humans. Furthermore, the SHIV model is limited to the testing of HIV-1 envelope genes. Similarly, the chimpanzee HIV-1 model has both positive and negative aspects. On the positive side, there are may similarities between the chimpanzee system and actual HIV infection in humans. Immunologically, humans and chimps are very similar. In fact, the vast majority of immunological reagents available for human studies are cross-reactive in the chimpanzee. In addition, HIV infection is similar; viral replication persists in both humans and chimps even in the face of neutralizing antibody responses and cellular immune responses. Recently, it has been reported that some chimpanzees can develop AIDS [80]. However, the frequency of this occurrence remains to be determined, and more work will be required to determine its relevance as a pathogenesis model. In addition, consideration should also be given to the limited numbers of these endangered animals which are available for study. Overall, however, the chimpanzee model allows for testing of vaccines against all of the open reading frames of the virus and is the most relevant HIV infection model.

Table 2 summarizes the success of various DNA immunization strategies in primates to date. DNA vaccines encoding both envelope (four different plasmids) and gag (one plasmid) genes of SIV were evaluated in macaques [69]. These monkeys were challenged

Table 2. Protection from viral challenge in primates

Primate type	DNA immunization	Immune reponses			Challenge virus	Challenge result
		AB	NAb	CTL		
Macaques	Four different envelope genes and gag/pol genes	+	+	+	SIV	No protection
Macaques	Envelope genes	+	+	+	SHIV-1	Partial protection
Chimpanzee	Envelope and gag/pol genes	+	+	+	HIV-1	Protection

Ab, antibodies; NAb, Neutralizing antibodies; CTL, cytotoxic T lymphocytes; SIV, simian immunodeficiency virus with SIVmac251 after their sixth immunization, but neither protection nor control of virus replication was observed in the vaccinated animals. In one primate study conducted by our group, four cynomolgus monkeys were immunized with two different HIV-1 envelope constructs (encoding subtypes B and D). Antigen-specific humoral responses comprising neutralizing antibodies and cellular responses including proliferative and cytotoxic responses were observed [27, 111]. One of four cynomolgus macaques vaccinated with envelope plasmid DNA was protected from intravenous challenge with 50 $TCID_{50}$ of a SHIV-1 HxB2 chimeric virus stock [12]. Viral replication appeared to be reduced in two of the other three vaccine recipients. This study demonstrated for the first time that DNA vaccination could lead to control of retroviral replication in vivo in primates.

Protective immunity in the chimpanzee model has also been observed. Three chimpanzees were also inoculated with an envelope construct and developed both specific cellular and humoral immune responses to envelope antigens [11]. These animals were later immunized with a gag/pol construct and one developed antibody responses to Pr55 core protein. Serum from all three immunized animals was able to neutralize HIV-1 MN in vitro, although with widely different titers. CTL activity was ultimately measured in two of the three immunized animals. One animal developed activity to both gag/pol and env targets, while the other showed CTL activity against gag/pol. These two chimpanzees and a non-vaccinated control chimpanzee were subsequently challenged intravenously with a high dose (250 chimpanzee ID_{50}) of a heterologous stock of HIV-1 SF2. While the control vector-immunized animal became infected by this viral challenge, the two immunized animals were protected. This result demonstrates that the use of multiple targets with both core and gp160 constructs was able to prevent the establishment of infection from a strain heterologous to the envelope construct. It is also interesting that of the two protected animals, one displayed substantial neutralization activity, while the other displayed superior CTL responses. This result is consistent with previous reports of protection in which the correlates of protection differed from animal to animal [37, 51, 53, 95].

Studies in humans

Several human studies are currently in progress. These include the first DNA vaccine studies to enter the clinic. Studies directed by R. R. MacGregor at the University of Pennsylvania tested the effects of the env/rev DNA vaccine in infected patients. Fifteen HIV-1-seropositive volunteers with more than 500 $CD4^+$ lymphocytes/ml were enrolled in this study. Patients in the trial receive three injections each separated by 10 weeks with escalating dosage (three dosage groups of five subjects) of envelope vaccine. Preliminary results reveal little clinical or laboratory adverse events measured in any of the three dosage groups (30, 100, 300 μg) [71]. The immunized individuals developed an increase in antibody responses to envelope proteins and peptides after receiving the 100 μg dose of pM160-MN [105]. Some increased cellular responses were also observed. These preliminary results demonstrate that the injection of even relatively low doses of a single immunogen DNA vaccine is capable of augmenting both existing humoral and cellular immune responses in humans. In addition to the initial human trials, a Phase I trial evaluating a gag/pol construct as a vaccine has been initiated through AVEG. Moreover, under the direction of J. Kovacs at the NIH a prophylactic DNA vaccine study for HIV enV has been initiated. This important study represents the first time that a gene therapy has been approved for testing in normal healthy individuals.

Taken together, these studies are dramatically expanding our knowledge of DNA vaccines for clinical use in humans.

New DNA immunization strategies: development of second generation DNA vaccines

The initial goal of the first generation DNA immunization was to demonstrate the ability of DNA vaccines to elicit humoral and cellular responses in vivo in a safe and well-

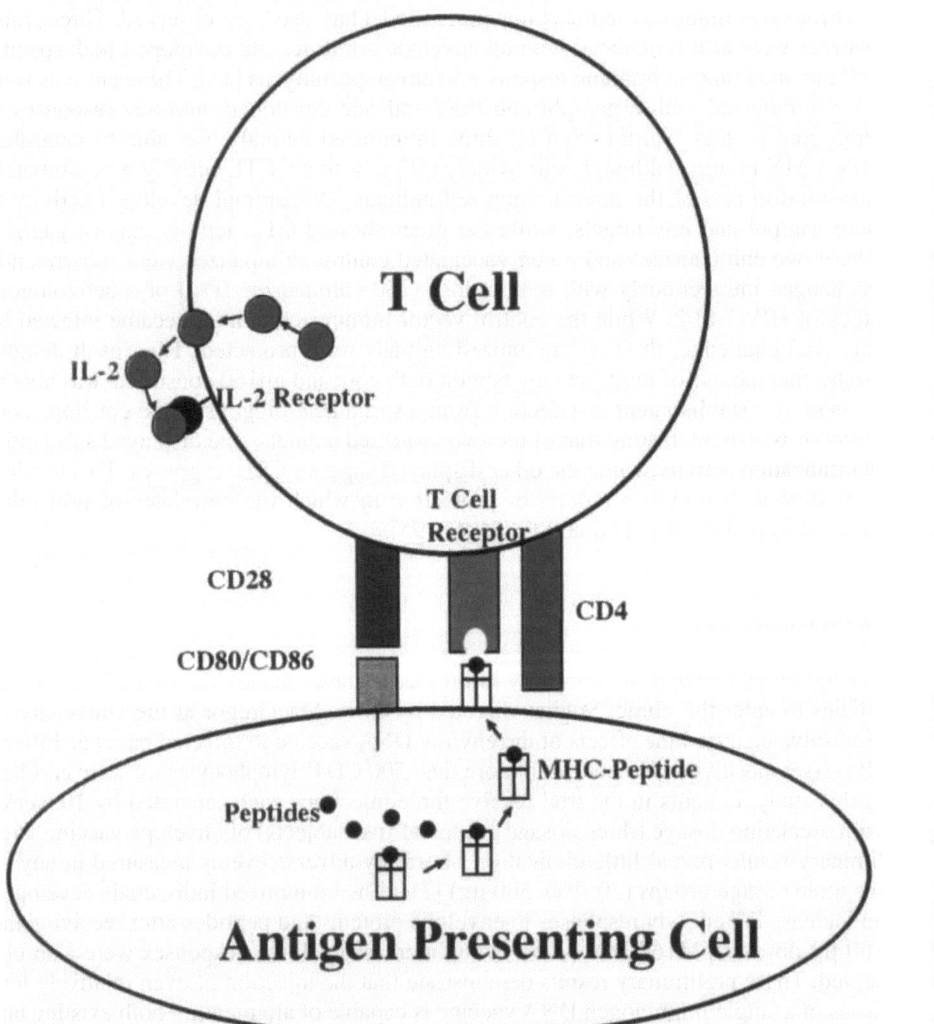

Fig. 2. Effective T cell activation by antigen-presenting cells (APCs). The interaction between antigen-major histocompatibility complex (*MHC*) and T cell receptor leads to the expression of interleuking-2 (*IL-2*) receptor. This T cell proliferates when the second signal is provided from APCs co-stimulatory proteins. CD28-CD80 ligation initiates the production of IL-2 production and leads to the proliferation of activated T cell

tolerated manner. As summarized above, these studies met and surpassed their original objectives. As we explore the next generation of DNA vaccines, our goal is to refine the current DNA vaccination strategy to elicit more clinically efficacious immune responses. The next generation vaccines may require control of the magnitude and direction (humoral or cellular) of the immune responses induced. Such refinement could be accomplished by co-delivering genes for immunologically important molecules, such as co-stimulatory molecules and cytokines. The strategies of co-administering co-stimulatory molecule and cytokine genes should be investigated because they play critical regulatory and signaling roles in immune expansion (Fig. 2). More specifically, they may be important in antigen presentation of the DNA vaccine.

The mechanism for antigen presentation following DNA immunization is currently being investigated [28, 32, 85], but is likely to be similar to traditional antigen presentation. In general, antigen must be processed and presented to T lymphocytes by professional antigen presenting cells (APCs) for efficient stimulation of an immune response. The ability of a professional APC to present antigen to T cells and provide efficient activation depends on several factors including interaction with matched MHC-antigen complexes and a reactive T cell receptor complex, surface-expressed co-stimulatory molecules, and the production of soluble cytokines [15]. Following intramuscular inoculation of plasmid DNA, a significant level of DNA is expressed in muscle [114], but muscle cells do not express requisite co-stimulatory molecules for immune expansion [47, 48]. Accordingly such muscle cells could provide expansion of an existing immune response, but should be poor initiators of an immune response. We postulate that the muscle cells could be engineered to serve as potent APCs through the co-administration of co-stimulatory molecule and cytokine genes along with DNA immunogen cassettes.

Importance of co-stimulatory molecules

Effective T cell activation by APCs requires two stimuli (Fig. 2): the first signal originates from the binding of antigen-MHC and T cell receptor molecules which confers specificity; the second signal is from co-stimulatory proteins on APCs [52]. The co-stimulatory signal seems to be required for the clonal expansion and differentiation of T cells, and blocking this co-stimulatory signal leads to T cell anergy (Fig. 3) [93]. The most potent co-stimulatory proteins are CD80 and CD86 which belong to the B7 co-stimulatory molecule family [62, 66]. CD80 is a surface glycoprotein expressed by dendritic cells, activated B cells, monocytes, macrophages, T lymphocytes and natural killer (NK) cells [34]. CD86 is expressed by the same cell types as CD80, but it is also constitutively expressed by resting human monocytes [4].

Recent studies indicate that CD80 and CD86 may play different roles in directing CD4 T cells into divergent immunological pathways. Kuchroo et al. [61] showed that interleukin (IL)-4 production of murine T lymphocytes increases when anti-CD80 is added, thus increasing the production of Th2 cells, while the addition of anti-CD86 led to greater interferon (IFN)-γ production and, thus, increased production of Th1 cells [61]. They also found that daily injections with CD80 antibodies ameliorated experimental allergic encephalomyelitis (an autoimmune disease of mice induced by Th1 cells) and increased the number of Th2 cells, while anti-CD86 antibodies exacerbated the disease. Simultaneous injection of antibodies to IL-4 and CD80 abolished the beneficial effect of CD80. This suggests that the relative amounts of CD80 and CD86

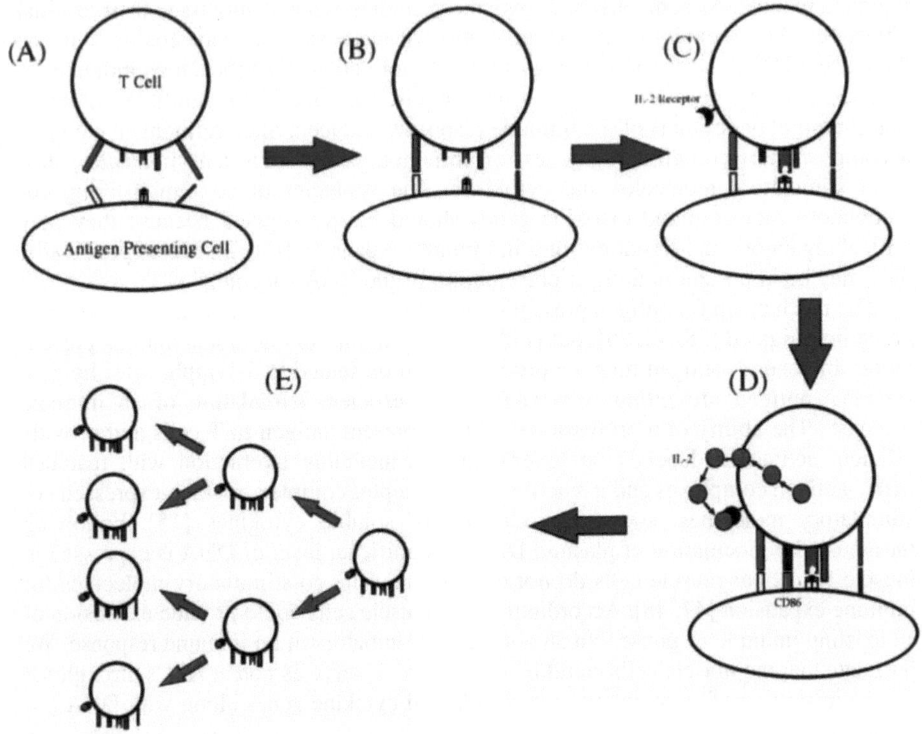

Fig. 3A–E. Proliferation of activated T cells. The co-stimulatory signal is required for the clonal expansion and differentiation of T cells (**D** and **E**)

determine whether the newly activated Th0 cells will differentiate to Th1 or Th2 cells, and this is partially mediated by IL-4. Since CD80 does not induce IL-4 production, it leaves the stimulated cells open to other influences, such as IL-12 produced by macrophages. Thus, CD80 and CD86 play important roles in initiating Th1/Th2 determination, but their actions seem to be more permissive than directive. It is not known how CD80 and CD86 generate different signals in directing CD4+ T cells to Th1 or Th2 pathways because each is currently thought to be recognized by the same receptors. Whatever the mechanism, the recognition of a role in differentiation for the co-stimulatory proteins has considerable experimental value and may lead to new strategies for therapeutic intervention. However, the mechanism(s) responsible these interventions remains to be elucidated.

Studies have also shown that B7 co-stimulation may be critical for the initiation of a cytotoxic CD8+ T cell response in vivo and in vitro [45, 94]. In addition, it has been observed that the expression of CD80 on tumor cells led to the activation of cytotoxic CD8+ T cells [45, 102]. Tan et al. [100] have shown that blocking the B7-CD28 interaction by anti-CD28 antibodies inhibited the in vitro activation of alloreactive and antigen-specific CTLs [100]. CD8+ T cells can also be directed to proliferate and exhibit cytotoxic activity when provided with co-stimulation by CD80 [100]. Guerder et al. [42] found that the CD80/CD86 co-stimulation leads to the accumulation of granzymes required for cytotoxic functions in addition to the production of IL-2 by CD8+ T cells.

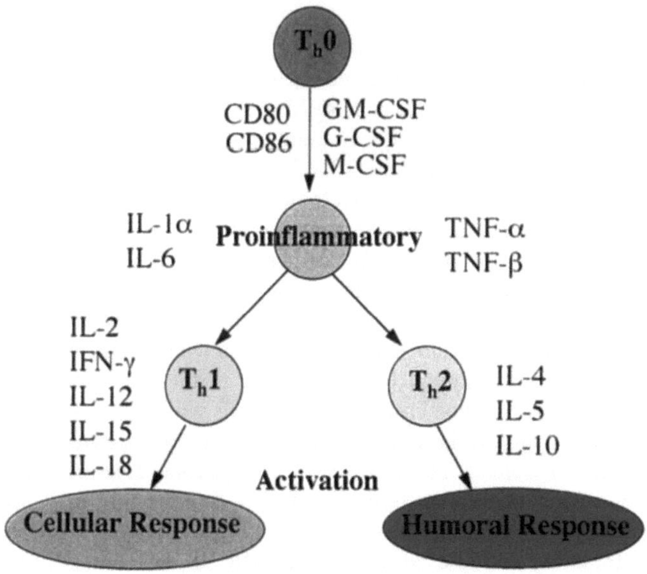

Fig. 4. Cytokines as immune response regulators. Cytokines play critical roles in the immune and inflammatory responses. Based upon their specific function in the immune system these cytokines could be further grouped as proinflammatory, Th1, and Th2 cytokines. Along with co-stimulatory molecules, these cytokines also play important roles in the activation and proliferation of T and B cells (*G*, granulocyte; *M*, macrophage; *CSF*, colony-stimulating factor; *TNF*, tumor necrosis factor; *IFN*, interferon

Importance of cytokines

Another group of valuable immune modulators is represented by cytokines. Cytokines play important roles in the immune and inflammatory responses as the initiators and regulators of the immune network (Fig. 4). Based upon their specific function in the immune system these cytokines could be further grouped as proinflammatory, Th1, Th2, and hematopoietic cytokines.

Proinflammatory cytokines

Proinflammatory cytokines IL-1, tumor necrosis factor (TNF)-α and TNF-β play important role as the initiator of the host responses to injury and infection [78]. IL-1 indirectly activates T cells by inducing the production of IL-2 and up-regulating the IL-2 receptor (IL-2R) on these cells [54]. IL-1 also influences B cells by inducing their differentiation, growth, and synthesis of IgGs [67]. TNF-α and TNF-β are closely related proteins (about 30% amino acid residue homology) which bind to the same cell surface receptors [8, 113]. TNF-α is produced by activated macrophages and monocytes neutrophils, activated lymphocytes, and NK cells, while TNF-β is produced by lymphocytes [107]. TNF-α and TNF-β are also implicated in septic shock following infection by Gram-negative bacteria [103] and in rheumatoid arthritis [117]. Furthermore, TNF-α has been suggested to play a pivotal role in regulating the synthesis of other proinflammatory cytokines [2].

Thl cytokines

Thl cytokines regulate the cellular or T cell-mediated arm of the immune response. IFN-γ, a prototypical Th1-type cytokine, is produced by Th1, CD8+, and NK cells, and has been shown to have antiviral effects as well as immunomodulatory effects such as the up-regulation of MHC class I and II antigens [75, 83]. IL-12 is also an important inducer and enhancer of Th1-type response and cytotoxic activities. IL-12 is heterodimeric cytokine (p35 and p40 chains) produced by macrophages and B cells; it induces IFN-γ production and plays a role in the enhancement of both NK and CD8+ T lymphocyte cytotoxic activities [104]. A new cytokine, IFN-γ-inducing factor or IL-18, has been found to enhance the production of IFN-γ, while inhibiting the production of IL-10 in stimulated peripheral blood mononuclear cells (PBMC) [81]. IL-18 also augments NK cell activity in cultures of human PBMC, similar to the structurally unrelated cytokine IL-12 [81]. IL-2 is produced primarily by T cells which have been activated by external stimulation and it is critical for the proliferation and clonal expansion of antigen-specific T cells [77]. IL-2 serves this pivotal role in T cell activation by its interaction with a receptor system consisting of three chains, α, β, and γc chains [43]. IL-15, a newly identified homologue of IL-2, is a pleiotropic cytokine which possesses T cell stimulatory activities similar to IL-2 [18, 38, 99].

Th2 cytokines

Th2 cytokines regulate the humoral or antibody-mediated arm of the immune response. Touted as a prototypical Th2-type cytokine, IL-4 synergizes with IL-2 to stimulate B cell growth [94]. It is a major regulator of immunoglobulin isotype expression. IL-4 induces IgE and IgG1 production and decreases IgG2b and IgG3 production by lipopolysaccharide (LPS)-stimulated B cells [86]. IL-4 also suppresses cytokine production by Th1 cells, resulting in the suppression of cellular immune responses [86]. IL-5 is a dimeric cytokine that controls the differentiation of B cells into antibody-producing plasma cells [98]. It has been shown to induce antigen-specific IgA production by murine and human B cell [7, 74]. IL-5 also promotes the growth and proliferation of eosinophils [9]. IL-10 was shown initially to be produced by Th2 T cell clones, but is also produced by B cells and monocytes [31, 33]. IL-10 has been shown to inhibit the production of such cytokines as IL-1α, IL-6, IL-8, and TNF-α by mitogen-activated monocytes [33] as well as to inhibit the macrophage-activating effects of IFN-γ [50]. IL-10 also has been reported to play a role in HIV-1 infection; IL-10 mRNA was up-regulated and increased levels of IL-10 were observed from PBMC from asymptomatic HIV-positive individuals compared with PBMC from uninfected individuals [24]. Furthermore, IL-10 has been shown to decrease viral replication in human macrophages in vitro [1].

Hematopoietic cytokines

In addition to these cytokines, granulocyte(G)-macrophage(M) colony-stimulating factor (CSF), G-CSF, and M-CSF are important growth factors for hematopoietic cells. GM-CSF is a which stimulates neutrophil, monocyte/macrophage, and eosinophil colony formation [76]. G-CSF plays an important role in the activation and differentiation of hematopoietic cells of neutrophilic granulocyte lineage [76]. Similarly, the primary function of M-CSF has been shown to be the regulation of the growth and differentiation of mononuclear phagocytes [96].

Co-administration of genetic adjuvant cassettes can modulate immune responses

We have co-immunized these immunologically important genes along with DNA immunogens for HIV-1 and observed that the immune responses could be modulated [56–58].

Co-immunization with co-stimulatory molecule gene expression cassettes

We developed expression cassettes for CD80 and CD86 genes and co-immunized them along with DNA immunogen cassettes expressing HIV-1 envelope and gag/pol into the BALB/c mice [57]. A negligible effect on the level of antigen-specific humoral response was observed. On the other hand, we observed that co-injection with CD86, not CD80 resulted in a dramatic increase in antigen-specific T helper cell proliferative responses. Furthermore, while the co-immunization with CD80 seemed to have minimal effect on the level of CTLs, the co-immunization with CD86 resulted in a significant augmentation of the CTL response which were restricted by MHC class I and $CD8^+$ T cells. These experiments demonstrate that the muscle cells can be engineered to function as APCs by enabling the expression of CD86, a key component for antigen presentation. By expressing co-stimulatory molecules through co-administration, one interpretation of these studies is that muscle cells can be engineered to serve as potent APCs through the MHC class I pathway available in these cells.

Co-immunization with cytokine gene expression cassettes

We co-injected genes for IL-12 and GM-CSF along with DNA vaccine cassettes for HIV-1 into mice [58]. We analyzed the immunological effects of the co-immunization with these cytokine expression cassettes on the magnitude and direction of antigen-specific immune responses. A moderate level of reduction in humoral response was seen with IL-12 co-delivery, while an enhancement of humoral response was observed with GM-CSF co-immunization. An increase in antigen-specific T helper cell proliferation was seen with either IL-12 or GM-CSF co-immunization. Importantly, we observed a significant enhancement of CTL response in vivo with the co-administration of murine IL-12 genes with four different HIV-1 DNA immunogens (*gag/pol, envelope, vif,* and *nef*), which were $CD8^+$ T cell and MHC class I restricted. In contrast, almost no effect on CTL induction was observed with the genes for GM-CSF in these studies.

In addition to our report on immune modulation following co-immunizations with DNA vaccines and IL-12 and GM-CSF genes, others have reported on the effects of delivering cytokine genes to elicit immune responses in vivo or in vitro. Raz et al. [88] reported that intramuscular injections of plasmids encoding IL-2, IL-4, or transforming growth factor (TGF)-β1 modulated immune responses to transferrin delivered at a separate site. IL-2 immunization resulted in an enhancement of antibody and T helper proliferative responses, while TGF-β1 immunization reduced anti-transferrin responses. Xiang and Ertl [116] reported that intramuscular co-inoculation of plasmid expressing the glycoprotein of rabies virus and plasmid encoding mouse GM-CSF enhanced the B and T helper cell activity to rabies virus, while co-inoculation with plasmid expressing IFN-γ resulted in a decrease of these responses. Chow et al. [23] reported that either injection of plasmid co-expressing hepatitis B surface antigen (HBsAg) and IL-2 or co-injection of IL-2 genes with plasmid expressing HBsAg resulted in the enhancement of both antibody and T helper cell responses [23].

Potential clinical applications of co-immunization strategy

Taken together, these results demonstrate that the direction and magnitude of immune responses induced by DNA vaccines could be modulated by the co-administration of cytokine genes. We postulate that a further control of immune responses could be conducted by co-immunizing with the co-stimulatory and cytokine genes discussed above. In Table 3, we summarize the potential modulation of immune responses by this genetic adjuvant strategy. For instance, a co-delivery of Th1 cytokines could lead to an enhancement of T cell-mediated immunity, while a co-delivery of Th2 cytokines could lead to an enhancement of antibody-mediated immunity. In addition, the co-administration of proinflammatory cytokine or co-stimulatory molecule genes could result in the enhancement of both the cellular and humoral arms of the immune system.

This co-administration strategy could lead to the development of a new generation of vaccines which are more clinically efficacious. For instance, in the case of infection by respiratory syncytial virus, T cell-mediated immune response is paramount, but the humoral response may not be needed or even be harmful [41]. In such cases, IL-12 or CD86 genes could be chosen as the immune modulator to be co-immunized with a specific DNA immunogen. On the other hand, for building vaccines to target extracellular bacteria, for example, Th2 cytokine genes could be co-immunized. Furthermore, in cases such as herpes where both $CD4^+$ T helper cells and antibodies play more important roles in protection, GM-CSF could be co-immunized [73]. Lastly, in cases where all three arms of immune responses are critical proinflammatory cytokines may be co-administered to give a combined enhancement of antibody, T helper cell, and CTL responses.

Table 3. Potential effects of genetic adjuvant strategy

Genetic adjuvant groups	Effect on immune response		
	Ab	Th	CTL
Co-stimulatory molecules	$\leftrightarrow$	$\Big\uparrow$	$\Big\uparrow$
Proinflammatory cytokines	$\uparrow$	$\uparrow$	$\uparrow$
Hematopoietic cytokines	$\uparrow$	$\Big\uparrow$	$\leftrightarrow$
Th1 cytokines	$\downarrow$	$\Big\uparrow$	$\Big\uparrow$
Th2 cytokines	$\Big\uparrow$	$\uparrow$	$\downarrow$

Ab, antibodies; *Th,* T helper cells; *CTL,* cytotoxic T lymphocytes

The development of this genetic adjuvant network underscores a new level of control in the induction of specific immune responses to tailor the vaccination programs more closely to the correlates of protection which vary from disease to disease. Controlling the magnitude and direction of the immune response should be advantageous in a wide variety of vaccine strategies. In infectious targets such as HIV-1, where the correlates of protection are uncertain, a vaccination strategy could be utilized to identify them. For example, humoral or cellular immune responses could be specifically increased by co-administering cytokine genes. The correlate of protection could then be analyzed by pathogen challenge. This finer control of vaccine and immune therapies was previously unattainable. These findings demonstrate the establishment of this strategy as the basis of optimizing current DNA immunization programs and a new generation of rationally designed vaccines and immunotherapies.

Conclusions

Developing successful vaccines for HIV-1 will likely involve targeting multiple antigenic components of the virus to direct and empower the immune system to protect the host from viral infection. DNA immunization holds great promise for providing safe and inexpensive vaccines for many infectious pathogens, including HIV-1. The direct injection of foreign genes by genetic immunization has resulted in specific immune responses that exhibit characteristics of protective immunity against a number of infectious agents in small animal models as well as in primate studies. Genetic vaccination cassettes targeting each of HIV-1's three major genes, two regulatory genes, or four accessory genes have been developed and studied in small animals, primates, and humans. Such a collection of immunization cassettes should be capable of stimulating broad immunity against both humoral and cellular epitopes, thus giving a vaccine the maximum ability to deal with viral immune escape. Furthermore, the power of the genetic adjuvant co-administration (consisting of co-stimulatory molecule or cytokine genes) to dramatically direct and enhance the antigen-specific humoral and cellular immune responses induced by DNA immunogens is analogous to the potential demonstrated by the combination therapy consisting of three different anti-retroviral agents for the control of HIV pathogenesis. We theorize that a successful immunization strategy against HIV infection could also involve a combination of such DNA vaccine cassettes. Specifically, a "right" combination of DNA expression cassettes coding for env, gag/pol, accessory proteins, co-stimulatory molecules, or cytokines may provide effective protection against one of the most feared viruses in the history of mankind.

References

1. Akridge RE, Oyafuso LK, Reed SG (1994) IL-10 is induced during HIV-1 infection and is capable of decreasing viral replication in human macrophages. J Immunol 153:5782
2. Arend WP, Dayer JM (1995) Inhibition of the production and effects of interleukin-1 and tumor necrosis factor a in rheumatoid arthritis. Arthritis Rheum 38:151
3. Ayyavoo V, Nagashunmugam T, Boyer JD, Sundarasamy M, Fernandes LS, Lee P, Lin J, Nguyen C, Chattergoon MA, Goedert JJ, Friedman H, Weiner DB (1997) Development of genetic vaccines for pathogenic genes: construction of attenuated Vif DNA immunization cassettes (in press)
4. Azuma M, Ito D, Yagita H, Okumura K, Phillips JH, Lanier LL, Somoza C (1993) B70 antigen is a second ligand for CTLA-4 and CD28. Nature 366:76

5. Barrett N, Eder G, Dorner F (1991) Characterization of a vaccinia-derived recombinant HIV-1 gp160 candidate vaccine and its immunogenicity in chimpanzees. Biotech Therapeut 2:91
6. Berman P, Gregory TJ, Riddle L, Nakamura GR, Champe MA, Porter JP, Wurm FM, Hershberg RD, Cobb EK, Eichberg JW (1990) Protection of chimpanzees from infection by HIV-1 after vaccination with recombinant glycoprotein gp120 but not gp160. Nature 345:622
7. Bertolini JN, Bertolini J, Thean E, Benson EM (1992) Human low molecular weight B cell growth factor induces surface IgM+/A- B cells to express and secrete IgA. J Immunol 149:1771
8. Beutler B, Greenwald D, Hulmes JD, Chang M, Pan YC, Mathison J, Ulevitch R, Cerami A (1985) Identity of tumour necrosis factor and the macrophage-secreted factor cachectin. Nature 316:552
9. Blom M, Tool AT, Kok PT, Koenderman L, Roos D, Verhoeven AJ (1994) Granulocyte-macrophage colony-stimulating factor, interleukin-3 (IL-3), and IL-5 greatly enhance the interaction of human eosinophils with opsonized particles by changing the affinity of complement receptor type 3. Blood 83:2978
10. Borrow P, Lewicki H, Hahn BH, Shaw GM, Oldstone MB (1994) Virus-specific $CD8^+$ cytotoxic T-lymphocyte activity associated with control of viremia in primary human immunodeficiency virus type-1 infection. J Virol 68:6103
11. Boyer J, Wang B, Ugen KE, Srikantan V, Gilbert L, Kudchokar S, Javadian MA, Dang K, Merva M, Newman M, Carrano R, Coney L, Weiner DB (1995) Induction of humoral and cellular immune responses to HIV-1 in cynomologus Macaques and chimpanzees by in vivo DNA inoculation. In: Brown F, Chanock RM, Ginsberg HS, Norrby E (eds) Vaccines 95: Molecular approaches to the control of infectious diseases. Cold Spring Harbor Laboratory Press, Cold Spring Harbor
12. Boyer J, Wang B, Ugen K, Agadjanyan MG, Javadian MA, Frost P, Dang K, Carrano R, Ciccarelli R, Coney L, Williams WV, Weiner DB (1996) In vivo protective anti-HIV immune responses in non-human primates through DNA immunization. J Med Primatol 25:242
13. Boyer JD, Wang B, Ugen K, Agadjanyan MG, Javadian MA, Frost P, Dang K, Carrano R, Ciccarelli R, Coney L, Williams WV, Weiner DB (1996) Protective anti-HIV immune responses in non-human primates through DNA immunization. J Med Primatol 25:242
14. Boyer JD, Ugen KE, Wang B, Agadjanyan MG, Gilbert L, Bagarazzi M, Chattergoon M, Frost P, Javadian A, Williams WV, Refaeli Y, Ciccarelli RB, McCallus D, Coney L, Weiner DB (1997) Protection of chimpanzees from high-dose heterologous HIV-1 challenge by DNA vaccination. Nature Med (in press)
15. Brodsky FM, Guagliardi LE (1991) The cell biology of antigen processing and presentation. Annu Rev Immunol 9:707
16. Bruck C, Thiriart C, Delers A, et al (1993) Comparison of vaccine protection in chimpanzees immunized with two different forms of recombinant HIV-1 envelope glycoprotein. AIDS Res Hum Retroviruses 9:S110
17. Bruck C, Thiriart C, Fabry L, et al (1993) HIV-1 envelope elicited neutralizing antibody titres correlate with protection and virus load in chimpanzees. J Cell Biochem 17:88
18. Burton JD, Bramford RN, Peters C, Grant AJ, Kurys G, Goldman CK, Brennan J, Roessler E, Waldmann TA (1994) A lymphokine, provisionally designated interleukin T and produced by a human adult T-cell leukemia line, stimulates T-cell proliferation and the induction of lymphokine-activated killer cells. Proc Natl Acad Sci USA 91:4935
19. Cao Y, Qin L, Zhang L, Safrit J, Ho DD (1995) Virologic and immunologic characterization of long-term survivors of human immunodeficiency virus type-1 infection. N Engl J Med 332:201
20. Cheingsong-Papov R, Callow D, Beddows S, et al (1992) Geographic diversity of human immunodeficiency virus type 1: serologic reactivity *env* epitopes and relationship to neutralization. J Infect Dis 165:256
21. Cheng-Mayer C, Homsy J, Evans LA, Levy JA (1988) Identification of human immunodeficiency virus subtypes and distinct patterns of sensitivity to serum neutralization. Proc Natl Acad Sci USA 85:2815
22. Choppin J, Guillet JG, Levy J-P (1992) HLA class I binding regions of HIV-1 proteins. Criti Rev Immunol 12:1
23. Chow Y-H, Huang W-L, Chi W-K, Chu Y-D, Tao MH (1997) Improvement of hepatitis B virus DNA vaccines by plasmids coexpressing hepatitis B surface antigen and interleukin-2. J Virol 71:169
24. Clerici M, Wynn TA, Berzofsky JA, Blatt SP, Hendrix CW, Sher A, Coffman RL, Shearer GM (1994) Role of interleukin-10 in T helper cell dysfunction in asymptotic individuals infected with the human immunodeficiency virus. J Clin Invest 93:768
25. Cohen J (1993) AIDS Research: the mood is uncertain. Science 260:1254

26. Condra JH, Holder DJ, Schleif WA, et al (1996) Genetic correlates of in vivo viral resistance to indinavir, a human immunodeficiency virus type 1 protease inhibitor. J Virolo 70:8270
27. Coney L, Wang B, Ugen KE, Boyer JD, McCallus D, Srikantan V, Agadjanyan MG, Pachuk CJ, Herold K, Merva M, Gilbert L, Dang K, Moelling K, Newman M, Williams WV, Weiner DB (1994) Facilitated DNA inoculation induces anti-HIV-1 immunity in vivo. Vaccine 12:1545
28. Corr M, Lee DJ, Carson DA, Tighe H (1996) Gene vaccination with naked plasmid DNA: mechanism of CTL priming. J Exp Med 184:1555
29. Cullen B, Greene WC (1990) Functions of the auxiliary gene products of the human immunodeficiency virus type 1. Virology 178:1
30. Davis H, Michel ML, Whalen RG (1993) DNA-based immunization induces continuous secretion of hepatitis B surface antigen and high levels of circulating antibody. Hum Mol Genet 2:1847
31. De Waal-Malefyt R, Abrams J, Bennett B, Figdor CG, de Vries J (1991) Interleukin 10 (IL-10) inhibits cytokine synthesis by human monocytes: an autoregulatory role of IL-10 produced by monocytes
32. Doe B, Selby M, Barnett S, Baenzinger J, Walker CM (1996) Induction of cytotoxic T lymphocytes by intramuscular immunization with plasmid DNA is facilitated by bone marrow-derived cells. Proc Natl Acad Sci USA 93:8578
33. Fiorentino DF, Bond MW, Mosmann TR (1989) Two types of mouse T helper cell. IV. Th2 clones secrete a factor that inhibits cytokine production by Th1 clones. J Exp Med 170:2081
34. Freeman GJ, Freedman AS, Segil JM, Lee G, Whitman JF, Nadler LM (1989) B7 a new member of the Ig superfamily with unique expression on activated and neoplastic B cells. J Immunol 143:2714
35. Fynan E, Webster R, Fuller D, Haynes J, Santoro J, Robinson H (1993) DNA vaccines: protective immunizations by parenteral, mucosal, and gene-gun inoculations. Proc Natl Acad Sci USA 90:11478
36. Girard M, Kieny MP, Pinter A, et al (1991) Immunization of chimpanzees confers protection against challenge with human immunodeficiency virus. Proc Natl Acad Sci USA 88:542
37. Girard M, Meignier B, Barre-Sinoussi F, Kieny M-P, Matthews T, Muchmore E, Nara PL, Wei Q, Rimsky L, Weinhold K, Fultz PN (1995) Vaccine-induced protection of chimpanzees against infection by a heterologous human immunodeficiency virus type-1. J Virol 69:6239
38. Grabstein KH, Eisenman J, Shanebeck K, Rauch C, Srinivasan S, Fung V, Beers C, Richardson J, Schoenborn MA, Ahdieh M, Johnson L, Alderson MR, Watson JD, Anderson DM, Giri JG (1994) Cloning of a T cell growth factor that interacts with the β chain of the interleukin-2 receptor. Science 264:965
39. Graham B, Wright PF (1995) Candidate AIDS Vaccines. N Engl JMed 333:1331
40. Graham B, Keefer MC, McElrath MJ, Gorse GJ, Schwartz DH, Weinhold K, Matthews TJ, Esterlitz JR, Sinangil F, Fast PE, NIAID AVEG (1996) Safety and immunogenicity of a candidate HIV-1 Vaccine in healthy adults: recombinant (RGP) 120. A randomized, double-blind trial. Ann Intern Med 125:270
41. Groothuis JR (1994) Rolc of antibody and use of respiratory syncytial virus (RSV) immune globulin to prevent severe RSV disease in high-risk children. J Pediatr 124:S28
42. Guerder S, Carding SR, Flavell RA (1995) B7 co-stimulation is necessary for the activation of the lytic function in cytotoxic T lymphocyte precursors. J Immunol 155:5167
43. Hatakeyama M, Tsudo M, Minamoto S, Kono T, Doi T, Miyata T, Miyasaka M, Taniguchi T (1989) Interleukin-2 receptor beta chain gene: generation of three receptor forms by cloned human alpha and beta chain cDNA's. Science 244:551
44. Haynes J, Fuller DH, Eisenbraun MD, Ford MJ, Pertmer TM (1994) AccellÆ particle-mediated DNA immunization elicits humoral, cytotoxic and protective responses. AIDS Res Hum Retroviruses 10:S43
45. He XS, Chen HS, Chu K, Rivkina M, Robinson WS (1996) Costimulatory protein B7-1 enhances the cytotoxic T cell response and antibody response to hepatitis B surface antigen. Proc Natl Acad Sci USA 93:7274
46. Ho DD (1996) Therapy of HIV infections: problems and prospects. Bull N Y Acad Med 73:37
47. Hohlfeld R, Engel AG (1990) Induction of HLA-DR expression on human myoblasts with interferon-gamma. Am J Pathol 136:503
48. Hohlfeld R, Engel AG (1994) The immunobiology of muscle. Immunol Today 15:269
49. Hom RC, Finberg RW, Mullaney S, Ruprecht RM (1991) Protective cellular retroviral immunity requires both $CD4^+$ and $CD8^+$ immune T cells. J Virol 65:220
50. Hsu DH, Moore KW, Spits H (1992) Differential effects of interleukin-4 and -10 on interleukin-2 induced interferon-γ synthesis and lymphokine-activated killer activity. Int Immunol 4:563

51. Hulskotte EG, Geretti A-M, Siebelink KH, Amerongen G van, Cranage MP, Rud EW, Norley SG, Vries P de, Osterhaus AD (1995) Vaccine-induced virus neutralizing antibodies and cytotoxic T cells do not protect macaques from experimental infection with Simian immunodeficiency virus $SIV_{mac32H(J5)}$. J Virol 69:6289
52. June C, Bluestone JA, Nadler LM, Thompson CB (1994) The B7 and CD28 receptor families. Immunol Today 15:321
53. Katzenstein D, Vujcic LK, Latif A, et al (1990) Human immunodeficiency neutralizing antibodies in sera from North Americans and Africans emergence of neutralization. J Acquir Immune Defic Syndr 3:810
54. Kaye J, Gillis S, Mizel B, Shevach EM, Malek TR, Dinarello CA, Lachman LB, Janeway CA (1984) Growth of a cloned helper T-cell line induced by a monoclonal antibody specific for the antigen receptor: interleukin-1 is required for the expression of receptors for interleukin-2. J Immunol 133:1339
55. Kestler H, Ringler DJ, Mori K, Panicalli DL, Sehgai PK, Daniel MD, Desrosiers RC (1991) Importance of the *nef* gene for maintenance of high virus loads and for the development of AIDS. Cell 65:651
56. Kim J, Ayyavoo V, Bagarazzi ML, Chattergoon M, Boyer JD, Wang B, Weiner DB (1997) Development of a multi-component candidate vaccine for HIV-1. Vaccine 15 : 879–883
57. Kim J, Bagarazzi ML, Hu Y, Trivedi N, Chattergoon MA, Dang K, Agadjanyan MG, Mahalingam S, Boyer JD, Wang B, Weiner DB (1997) Engineering of in vivo immune responses to DNA immunization via co-delivery of costimulatory molecule genes. Nat Biotechn 15 : 641–645
58. Kim JJ, Ayyvoo V, Bagarazzi ML, Chattergoon MA, Dang K, Wang B, Boyer JD, Weiner DB (1997) In vivo engineering of a cellular immune response by co-administration of IL-12 expression vector with a DNA immunogen. J Immunol 158:816
59. Kim S, Ikeuchi K, Byrn R, Groopman J, Baltimore D (1989) Lack of a negative influence on viral growth by the *nef* gene of human immunodeficiency virus type 1. Proc Natl Acad Sci USA 86:9544
60. Koup R, Safrit JT, Cao Y, et al (1994) Temporal association of cellular immune responses with the initial control of viremia in primary human immunodeficiency virus type-1 syndrome. J Virol 68:4650
61. Kuchroo VK, Das MP, Brown JA, Ranger AM, Zamvil SS, Sobel RA, Weiner HL, Nabavi N, Glimcher LH (1995) B7-1 and B7-2 co-stimulatory molecules activate differentially the Th1/Th2 developmental pathways: application to autoimmune disease therapy. Cell 80:707
62. Lanier LL, O'Fallon S, Somoza C, Phillips JH, Linsley PS, Okumura K, Ito D, Azuma M (1995) CD80 (B7) and CD86 (B70) provide similar co-stimulatory signals for T cell proliferation, cytokine production, and generation of CTL. J Immunol 154:97
63. Levy DN, Fernandes LS, Williams WV, Weiner DB (1993) Induction of cell differentiation by human immunodeficiency virus 1 vpr. Cell 72:541
64. Levy DN, Refaeli Y, MacGregor RR, Weiner DB (1994) Serum vpr regulates productive infection and latency of human immunodeficiency virus type 1. Proc Natl Acad Sci USA 91:10873
65. Levy DN, Refaeli Y, Weiner DB (1994) Extracellular vpr protein increases cellular permissiveness to HIV replication and reactivates virus from latency. J Virol 69:1243
66. Linsley PS, Clark EA, Ledbetter JA (1990) The T cell antigen, CD28, mediates adhesion with B cells by interacting with activation antigen, B7/BB-1. Proc Natl Acad Sci USA 87:5031
67. Lipsky PE, Thompson PA, Rosenwasser LJ, Dinarello CA (1983) The role of interleukin-1 in human B-cell activation: inhibition of B-cell proliferation and the generation of immunoglobulin secreting cells by antibody against human leukocytic pyrogen. J Immunol 130:2709
68. Lu S, Santoro JC, Fuller DH, Haynes JR, Robinson HL (1995) Use of DNAs expressing HIV-1 *env* and non-infectious HIV-1 particles to raise antibody responses in mice. Virology 209:147
69. Lu S, Arthos J, Montefiori DC, Yasutomi Y, Manson K, Mustafa F, Johnson E, Santoro JC, Wissink J, Mullins JI, Haynes JR, Letvin NL,Wyand M, Robinson HL (1996) Simian immunodeficiency virus DNA vaccine trial in Macaques. J Virol 70:3978
70. Reference deleted
71. MacGregor R, Gluckman S, Lacy K, Kaniefski B, Boyer JD, Wang B, Bagarazzi ML, Williams WV, Francher D, Ginsberg R, Higgins T, Weiner DB (1997) First human trial of a facilitated DNA plasmid vaccine for HIV-1: safety and host response. XI International Conference on AIDS, Vancouver 1 : 23
72. Malim M, Hauber J, Le SY, Maizel JV, Cullen BR (1989) The HIV-1 *rev trans*-activator acts through a structured target sequence to activate a nuclear export of unspliced viral mRNA. Nature 338:254
73. Manickan E, Rouse RJ, Yu Z, Wire WS, Rouse BT (1995) Genetic immunization against herpes simplex virus. Protection is mediated by $CD4^+$ T lymphocytes. J Immunol 155:259

74. Matsumoto S, Matsumoto M, Mita S, Hitoshi Y, Ando M, Araki S, Tominaga A, Takatsu K (1989) IL-5 induces maturation but not class switching of surface IgA-positive B cells into IgA-secreting cells. Immunology 66:32
75. Mogensen SC, Virelizier JL (1987) The interferon-macrophage alliance [Review]. Interferon 8:55
76. Moore MAS (1991) The clinical use of colony stimulating factors. Annu Rev Immunol 9:159
77. Morgan DA, Ruscetti FW, Gallo R (1976) Selective in vitro growth of T lymphocytes from normal human bone marrows. Science 193:1007
78. Nakane A, Minagawa T, Kato K (1988) Endogenous tumor necrosis factor (cachetin) is essential to host resistance against Listeria monocytigenes infection. Infect Immun 56:2563
79. Nixon D, Townsend AR, Elvin JG, Rizza CR, Gallwey J, McMichael AJ (1988) HIV-1 gag-specific cytotoxic T lymphocytes defined with recombinant vaccinia virus and synthetic peptides. Nature 336:484
80. Novembre FJ, Saucier M, Anderson DC, Klumpp SA, O'Neil SP, Brown CR II, Hart CE, Guenthner PC, Swenson RB, McClure HM (1997) Development of AIDS in a chimpanzee infected with human immunodeficiency virus type 1. J Virol 71:4086
81. Okamura HHT, Komatsu T, Yutsudo M, Hakura A, Tanimoto T, Torigoe K, Okura T, Nukada Y, Hattori K, Akita K, Namba M, Tanabe F, Konishi K, Fukuda S, Kurimoto M (1995) Cloning of a new cytokine that induces IFN-gamma production by T cells. Nature 378:88
82. Okuda K, Bukawa H, Hamajima K, Kawamoto S, Sekigawa K-I, Yamada Y, Tanaka S-I, Ishii N, Aoki I, Nakamura M, Yamamoto H, Cullen BR, Fukushima J (1995) Induction of potent humoral and cell-mediated immune responses following direct injection of DNA encoding the HIV type 1 *env* and *rev* gene products. AIDS Res Hum Retroviruses 11:933
83. Paliard X, De Waal-Malefyt R, Yssel H, Blanchard D, Chretien I, Abrams J, Vries J de, Spits H (1988) Simultaneous production of IL-2, IL-4, and IFN-gamma by activated human CD4+ and CD8+ T cell clones. J Immunol 141:849
84. Pantaleo G, Menzo S, Vaccarezza M, et al (1995) Studies in subjects with long-term nonprogressive human immunodeficiency virus infection. N Engl J Med 332:209
85. Pardoll DM, Beckerleg AM (1995) Exposing the immunology of naked DNA vaccines. Immunity 3:165
86. Paul W (1991) Interleukin-4: a prototypic immunoregulatory lymphokine. Blood 77:1859
87. Pinto L, Sullivan J, Berzofsky JA, Clerici M, Kessler HA, Landay AL, Shearer GM (1995) Env-specific cytotoxic T lymphocyte responses in HIV seronegative health care workers occupationally exposed to HIV-contaminated body fluids. J Clin Invest 96:867
88. Raz E, Watanabe A, Baird SM, Eisenberg RA, Parr TB, Lotz M, Kipps TJ, Carson DA (1993) Systemic immunological effects of cytokine genes injected into skeletal muscle. Proc Natl Acad Sci USA 90:4523
89. Rowland-Jones S, Nixon DF, Aldhous MC (1993) HIV-specific cytotoxic T-cell activity in an HIV-exposed but uninfected infant. Lancet 341:860
90. Rowland-Jones S, Sutton J, Ariyoshi K, Dong T, Gotch F, McAdam S, Whitby D, Sabally S, Allimore A, Corrah T, Takiguchi M, McMichael A, Whittle H (1995) HIV-specific T-cells in HIV-exposed but uninfected Gambian women. Nature Med 1:59
91. Saag M, Hahn BH, Gibbons JH, Li Y, Parks ES, Parks WP, Shaw GM (1988) Extensive variation of human immunodeficiency virus type-1 in vivo. Nature 334:440
92. Schwartz D, Gorse G, Clements ML, Belshe R, Izu A, Duliege A-M, Berman P, Twaddell T, Stablein D, Sposto R, Siliciano R, Matthews T (1993) Induction of HIV-1 neutralising and syncytium-inhibiting antibodies in uninfected recipients of HIV-1(IIIB) rpg120 subunit vaccine. Lancet 342:69
93. Schwartz RH (1992) Costimulation of T lymphocytes: the role of CD29, CTLA-4, and B7/BB1 in interleukin-2 production and immunotherapy. Cell 71:1065
94. Seder RA, Paul WE (1994) Acquisition of lymphokine-producing phenotype by CD4+ T cells. Annu Rev Immunol 12:635
95. Sheppard H, Bridges SH, Mathieson BJ, Walker MC, Weinhold K (1994) Conference on Advances in AIDS Vaccine Development-1993 Summary:cCorrelates of HIV immunity working group. AIDS Res Hum Retroviruses 10:S171
96. Sherr C (1990) Colony-stimulating factor-1 receptor. Blood 75:1
97. Strebel K, Dauherty D, Clouse K, Cohen D, Folks T, Martin MA (1987) The HIV "A" (sor) gene product is essential for virus infectivity. Nature 328:728
98. Swain SL, Dutton RW (1982) Production of a B cell growth-promoting activity, (DL)BCGF, from a cloned T cell line and its assay on the BCL1 B cell tumor. J Exp Med 156:1821

99. Tagaya Y, Bamford RN, DeFillipis AP, Waldman TA (1996) A pleiotropic cytokine with diverse receptor signalling pathways whose expression is controlled at multiple levels. Immunity 4:329
100. Tan R, Teh SJ, Ledbetter JA, Linsley PS, Teh HS (1992) B7 costimulates proliferation of CD4-CD8+ T lymphocytes but is not required for the deletion of immature CD4+CD8+ thymocytes. J Immunol 149:3217
101. Tang D, DeVit M, Johnston S (1992) Genetic immunization is a simple method for elicting an immune response. Nature 356: 152
102. Townsend SE, Allison JP (1993) Tumor rejection after direct co-stimulation of CD8+ T cells by B7-transfected melanoma cells. Science 259:368
103. Tracey K, Fong Y, Hesse DG, Manogue KR, Lee AT, Kuo GC, Lowry SF, Cerami A (1987) Anti-cachectin/TNF monoclonal antibodies prevent septic shock during lethal bacteraemia. Nature 330:662
104. Trinchieri G (1995) Interleukin-12: a proinflammatory cytokine with immunoregulatory functions that bridge innate persistance and antigen-specific adaptive immunity. Annu Rev Immunol 13:251
105. Ugen K, Boyer JD, Wang B, Gluckman S, Williams WV, Nyland S, Carmack B, Agadjanyan MG, Bagarazzi ML, Higgins T, Coney L, Ciccarelli R, Ginsberg R, MacGregor RR, Weiner DB (1997) Facilitated nucleic acid vaccination of humans with an HIV-1 expressing DNA boosts immune responses against the envelope glycoprotein. In: Brown F, Chanock RM, Ginsberg HS, Norrby E (eds) Vaccines 97: molecular approaches to the control of infectious diseases. Cold Spring Harbor Laboratory Press, Cold Spring Harbor (in press)
106. Ulmer J, Donnelly J, Parker SE, et al (1993) Heterologous protection against influenza by injection of DNA encoding a viral protein. Science 259:1745
107. Vilcek J, Lee TH (1991) Tumor necrosis factor. New insights into the molecular mechanisms of its multiple actions [Review]. J Biol Chem 266:7313
108. Walker BD (1994) The rationale for immunotherapy in HIV-1 infection. J Acquir Immune Defic Syndr 7:S6
109. Wang B, Boyer JD, Srikantan V, Coney L, Carrano R, Phan C, Merva M, Dang K, Agadjanyan MG, Ugen KE, Williams WV, Weiner DB (1993) DNA inoculation induces neutralizing immune responses against human immunodeficiency virus type 1 in mice and non-human primates. DNA Cell Biol 12:799
110. Wang B, Ugen KE, Srikantan V, Agadjanyan MG, Dang K, Refaeli Y, Sato A, Boyer J, Williams WV, Weiner DB (1993) Gene inoculation generates immune responses against human immunodeficiency virus type 1. Proc Natl Acad Sci USA 90:4156
111. Wang B, Boyer JD, Srikantan V, Ugen KE, Gilbert L, Phan C, Dang K, Merva M, Agadjanyan MG, Newman M, Carrano R, McCallus D, Coney L, Williams WV, Weiner DB (1995) Induction of humoral and cellular immune responses to the human immunodeficiency type-1 virus in non-human primates by in vivo DNA inoculation. Virology 211:102
112. Wang B, Boyer JD, Ugen KE, Srikantan V, Ayyavoo V, Agadjanyan MG, Williams WV, Newman M, Coney L, Carrano R, Weiner DB (1995) Nucleic acid-based immunization against HIV-1: induction of protective in vivo immune responses. AIDS 9:S159
113. Williams TW, Granger GA (1968) Lymphocyte in vitro cytotoxicity: lymphotoxins of several mammalian species. Nature 219:1076
114. Wolff JA, Malone RW, Williams P, Chong W, Acsadi G, Jani A, Felgner PL (1990) Direct gene transfer into mouse muscle in vivo. Science. 247:1465
115. WorldBank (1993). Investing in Health. World Development Report 1993. Oxford University Press, Oxford, p 62
116. Xiang Z, Ertl HC (1995) Manipulation of the immune response to a plasmid-encoded viral antigen by coinoculation with plasmids expressing cytokines. Immunity 2:129
117. Yocum D, Esparza L, Dubry S, Benjamin J, Volz R, Scuderi P (1989) Characteristics of tumor necrosis factor production in rheumatoid arthritis. Cell Immunol 122:131

DNA-based immunization against hepatitis B virus

Heather L. Davis[1,2], Cynthia L. Brazolot Millan[1]

[1] Loeb Research Institute, Ottawa Civic Hospital, 1053 Carling Avenue, Ottawa, Canada K1Y 4E9
[2] Faculties of Health Sciences & Medicine, University of Ottawa, Ottawa, Canada

Introduction

Hepatitis B infection

Hepatitis B virus (HBV) poses a widespread and serious international health problem that is not completely managed by the current vaccines due to issues of availability, affordability and their effectiveness in inducing the appropriate immune responses. This is especially true with respect to chronic carriers of HBV for whom a cellular immune response, not achieved with the current vaccines, is required.

There are approximately 250 million chronic HBV carriers worldwide. These make up less than 0.5% of the population in Europe and North America, but the prevalence rate is 10–20% in areas where HBV is endemic (i.e., China, Southeast Asia and sub-Saharan Africa). Although some of these individuals are healthy carriers without liver pathology, approximately 70% remain in a state of chronic hepatitis and are particularly susceptible to developing cirrhosis and hepatocellular carcinoma later in life [18, 49]. It is estimated that one million deaths per year can be attributed to complications arising as a result of chronic HBV infection.

With acute HBV infection approximately 80% of individuals exhibit subclinical, often undetected infection from which they recover fully. Medical management may be required for the 20% of individuals who develop acute hepatitis. A very low proportion (< 1%) of infected individuals present with fulminant hepatitis which can be fatal in the absence of liver transplant. Regardless of the clinical course, some proportion of infected individuals will fail to launch the appropriate immune responses to clear infection and will become chronic HBV carriers.

In HBV endemic regions, viral transmission is frequently horizontal among young children (Africa) or vertical from a chronically infected mother to her newborn (Asia). Up to 95% of neonatal infections will progress to a chronic carrier state. By comparison, where HBV is not endemic, transmission is usually horizontal between adults, by transfer of blood products (e.g., needle-stick injuries) or other body fluids (e.g., sexual contact). Most individuals infected as adults recover completely; however, 5–10% become chronic carriers.

Correspondence to: H. L. Davis

HBV thus represents a serious problem. The World Health Organization (WHO) Expanded Programme on Immunization recommended, and the World Health Assembly endorsed, universal prophylactic immunization by 1995 in areas where HBV is endemic, and in all countries by 1997 [23]. Largely due to the expense of available vaccines, these goals have not been met.

The hepatitis B virus

HBV consists of a lipoprotein envelope enclosing a core protein (capsid) and the viral genome, which contains only four genes: S, C, P and X; surface (HBs), core (HBc), pol and X proteins, respectively. The surface and core proteins are structural, whereas pol functions in transcription. The function of the X protein is unclear but it may have transcription-activating properties and as such increase viral viability in the host [13, 16].

The HBV envelope protein gene is a single large open reading frame terminating in a solitary stop codon, but which contains three in-frame ATG start codons. These divide the gene into three domains; pre-S1, pre-S2 and S, from 5' to 3'. Transcription initiates from any of these start sites, resulting in three polypeptides; small or major (S),

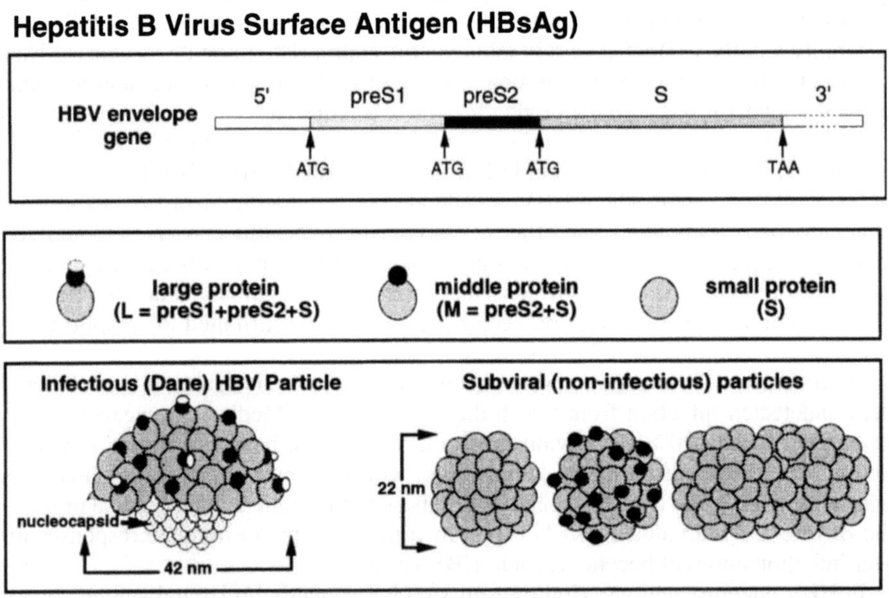

Fig. 1. HBsAg is encoded by a single gene which is divided into S, pre-S2 and pre-S1 regions by three ATG start codons. Three polypeptides are thus encoded by this gene: the small or major (*S*), middle (*M = pre-S2 + S*) and large (*L = pre-S1 + pre-S2 + S*) surface proteins. A messenger RNA transcript containing all three ATG codons has the ability to produce all three forms of the protein since internal initiation can take place. The envelope of infectious viral particles (Dane particles) contains all three forms of HBsAg, but with a predominance of the small (S) protein. Also found in the serum of acutely or chronically infected individuals are empty viral envelope particles containing only the small (S) protein or particles containing S protein or mixtures of the S + M envelope proteins. Similar particles are produced in yeast [51] or mammalian cells [33] for use as a recombinant protein hepatitis B virus (HBV) vaccine

middle (M; pre-S2 + S) and large (L; pre-S1 + pre-S2 + S) (see [49]). The envelope of the infectious 42-nm HBV particle (Dane particle) contains all forms, with a predominance of S and variable amounts of M and L proteins (Fig. 1). Serum of infected individuals also contains large numbers of smaller (22-nm) empty subviral particles composed solely or predominantly of S and sometimes small amounts of M protein [49].

Several B and T cell epitopes have been identified on both the S and pre-S domains, and are known collectively as HBV surface antigen (HBsAg). The S domain encodes the major protective B cell epitope, the HBV group-specific determinant "*a*". Also associated with S are two other determinants, one of which has either "*d*" or "*y*" specificity, and the other which has either "*w*" or "*r*" specificity. Combination of determinants thus results in four subtypes: *adw*, *adr*, *ayw* and *ayr* [16].

Immunogenicity of HBV

Both humoral and cell-mediated immunity (CMI) may result from natural HBV infection. However, the exact role of cytotoxic T lymphocytes (CTL) and CMI in protecting against HBV is unknown. After natural infection, antibodies are detected against HBsAg (anti-HBs) and viral core antigen (HBcAg; anti-HBc). Protein-based HBV vaccines, which contain alum as an adjuvant, induce only antibodies. Nevertheless, in the case of HBV, antibodies alone are clearly sufficient to confer protective immunity and all HBV vaccines have been designed to elicit this. The common clinical standard for anti-HBs antibody levels is milli-International Units/ml (mIU/ml) and in humans a level of 10 mIU/ml is considered sufficient to confer protection [5].

The role for anti-HBc in conferring protection is less clear. HBcAg is highly immunogenic and immunization to HBcAg alone has been shown to protect chimpanzees against challenge with live HBV [22, 35]. However, high titers of maternal anti-HBc fail to protect infants of chronically infected mothers from infection [22]. It is possible that CMI is responsible for protection in the HBcAg-immunized chimpanzees.

HBV vaccines: why we need another vaccine

HBV vaccines used to date in humans have been subunit vaccines consisting of 22-nm empty subviral particles composed solely of HBV envelope protein. Initially these were purified from the plasma of chronic carriers [3, 30, 40, 42], but their use was restricted by a limited supply of chronically infected human plasma and persistent but unfounded concerns about their safety [20, 29, 41, 46]. Today, most HBV vaccines contain recombinant HBsAg protein [14] produced in stably transfected yeast [50] or Chinese hamster ovary cells [31]. The recombinant protein vaccines are very effective but expensive to produce, and this factor alone precludes widespread use in many of those areas of the world where HBV vaccines are most needed. Subunit vaccines also have the disadvantages that two to three doses are required and they require a "cold-chain", increasing their cost in areas of the world where refrigeration is not commonplace. Cost of delivery is further increased in endemic areas where transmission is vertical since vaccination must be initiated within the first few weeks of life, making the immunization schedule asynchronous with that for other vaccines recommended by the WHO [23].

Shortcomings of the subunit vaccines, in addition to cost, include the problem of non-response (no detectable level of anti-HBs) or hypo-response (< 10 mIU/ml anti-HBs) despite a series of three to four injections and increased vaccine dose [19]. This is particularly worrisome for individuals at risk of HBV exposure (e.g., health care workers, blood product recipients or partners of chronic HBV carriers). In immunocompetent individuals, incidence of non- or hypo-response is less than 5% for young adults, but increases to 30–50% with advancing age. The problem of non-response is, at least in some cases, HLA-linked and several non-responsive haplotypes have been identified [25]. Other factors (e.g., HIV infection, kidney dialysis and immunosuppression) can increase the incidence of non-response to as high as 80%.

Finally, there is an urgent need for a therapeutic vaccine which could be used to treat HBV chronicity. Presently, chronic carriers may be treated with interferon-α (IFN-α); however, this helps only a proportion of those treated and even then it does not necessarily constitute a cure.

Attempts to develop effective yet less expensive vaccines have met with limited success. It is not possible to produce whole killed or live attentuated vaccines owing to the difficulty of growing HBV in culture. HBsAg-expressing vaccinia and adenoviral vectors could protect chimpanzees against viral challenge, but were not good candidates for mass vaccination since antibody titers induced were significantly lower than those induced with the recombinant vaccines [26, 34]. Furthermore, live viral vectors are undesirable owing to the potential for untoward reactions, especially in immunocompromised individuals. Synthetic peptide vaccines, while safe, were also found to be poorly immunogenic in chimpanzees [15, 48], probably owing to loss of the major B cell epitopes which are conformational.

Thus, there is still a need to develop an inexpensive HBV vaccine which is as safe and efficacious as the plasma-derived and recombinant subunit vaccines. In addition, even where cost is not prohibitive, there is a need for novel vaccination strategies which could circumvent non- or hypo-responsiveness to HBsAg and can be used to treat the chronic carrier state. Based on results obtained to date in animal models, a DNA vaccine against HBV has the potential to meet these challenges.

DNA-based immunization against HBsAg in mice

Potential of DNA vaccines for HBV

Many of the generic benefits of DNA vaccines could prove beneficial for application to HBV. The efficient induction of strong immune responses owing to in vivo synthesis of antigen and the potent self-adjuvanting nature of the DNA (owing to unmethylated CpG motifs) [24, 44], could overcome the problem of hypo- or non-response and reduce the number of required doses, which in turn would reduce the cost. In addition, the strong cell-mediated immunity and Th1-type responses induced by DNA vaccines might allow immunotherapeutic application to chronic carriers of HBV. Furthermore, the ease and low cost of production, ease of quality control, and the ability to transport and store at ambient temperature, are all important advantages for developing areas of the world, where the need for HBV vaccines is also the greatest.

HBV DNA vaccine model

Skeletal muscle has been found to have relatively high efficiency of uptake and expression of plasmid DNA [51] and intramuscular injection of HBsAg-expressing plasmid DNA is a highly effective method for inducing HBV-specific immune responses in mice and other animals [7]. In experiments described below, four vectors expressing one or more of the HBV envelope proteins are used. Three of the vectors utilize the immediate early promoter of cytomegalovirus (CMV) to drive expression of the S (pCMV-S), pre-S2 + S (pCMV-S2.S) or pre-S1 + pre-S2 + S (pCMV-S1.S2.S) envelope gene. A fourth vector uses the endogenous HBV promoter within the pre-S1 domain to drive expression (pHBV-S2.S) [7, 32] (Fig. 2).

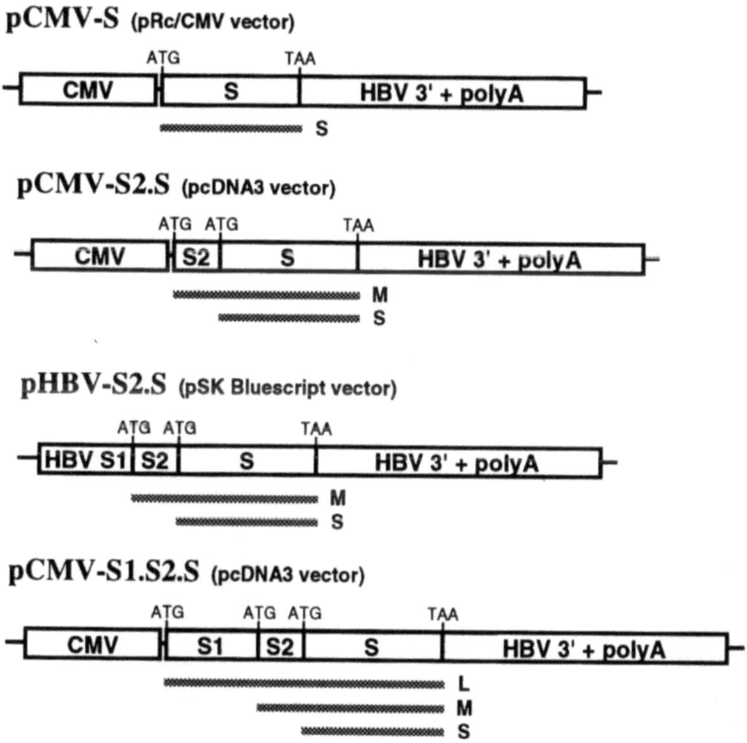

Fig. 2. Schematic diagram of the four HBV envelope expression vectors used. The plasmid backbone used for each construct is given in *parentheses* after the vector designation. The sequences encoding the pre-S1, pre-S2 and S sequences are indicated, along with the three in-frame ATG initiator codons and the TAA stop codon. The remainder of the viral sequences located 3' to the envelope-coding sequences contain the viral transcription termination and poly-adenylation signals. Three vectors use the human cytomegalovirus (CMV) promoter coming from the pRc/CMV or pcDNA3 plasmids, and the fourth uses the endogenous HBV promoter embedded in the pre-S1 coding sequences. The expected protein products are indicated as *thick gray lines* below the respective coding sequences and represent the major surface protein (S) as well as the middle (M) and large (L) envelope proteins [32] [reprinted with permission: Proc Natl Acad Sci USA (1995) 92: 5308]

In vivo synthesis of HBsAg

Intramuscular injection of 50 μg of HBsAg-expressing DNA into the tibialis anterior muscle (TA) of the mouse results in transfection of approximately 1–2% of muscle fibers (i.e., 30–60 fibers), which can be detected by immunofluorescent label [12]. Detection antibodies recognize conformational epitopes, indicating that the expressed HBsAg adopts a conformation similar to that of proteins resulting from natural infection or recombinant proteins as used in the subunit vaccines.

Transfected fibers retain a normal histological appearance 5 days after DNA injection, but are seen to fragment at about 10 days and disappear completely by 30 days. Disappearance of HBsAg-expressing muscle fibers is likely due to attack by HBsAg-specific CTL (see below) since similarly transfected fibers are spared in mice with severe combined immunodeficiency [12].

Low levels of circulating antigen (≤ 1 ng/ml) are detected only at early time points (2–4 weeks after DNA injection) (Fig. 3) and a lack of detectable HBsAg in the serum at later times probably reflects neutralization of antigen by antibodies (Fig. 3; see below) as well as reduced synthesis with the destruction of expressing fibers.

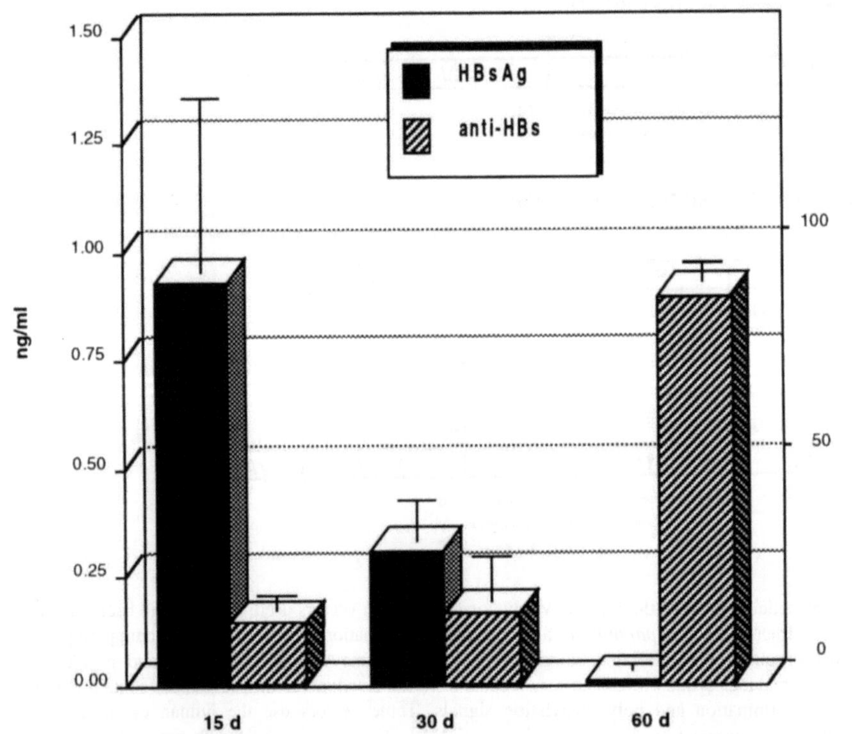

Fig. 3. Amounts of HBsAg and anti-HBs in plasma of mice following direct intramuscular injection of 100 μg [unilateral tibialis anterior muscle (TA)] of pure plasmid DNA encoding HBsAg (pCMV-S) into regenerating (5 days after cardiotoxin-induced degeneration) TA muscles. Significant amounts of both HBsAg and anti-HBsAg were detected at 15 days (n = 6). With longer periods (30 and 60 days, n = 4) levels of HBsAg decreased, while those for anti-HBs increased

Humoral response

Kinetics and specificity of anti-HBs. Anti-HBs antibodies may be detected as early as 1 week after injection of HBsAg-expressing DNA. The kinetics, antibody isotype and fine specificity of the subsequent humoral response are comparable to those seen following natural infection. For example, the earliest detectable antibodies are principally of the IgM isotype but soon undergo a class shift to the IgG isotype. Isotype switching of autoreactive B cells strongly suggests that DNA-based immunization triggers $CD4^+$ T helper cells.

Antibodies specific to both group (*a*) and subtype (*y*) determinants of HBsAg may be detected, as well as anti-pre-S2 antibodies for those vectors expressing pre-S2 (i.e., pCMV-S2.S, pCMV-S1.S2.S, pHBV-S2.S). With S-encoding DNA, there is a predominance of group-specific (*a*) antibodies, which, in humans, could provide cross-protection against heterologous strains of HBV. When present, antibodies to the pre-S2 domain predominate, especially in the early period as is seen following natural HBV infection [36]. Pre-S2 specific antibodies may be beneficial for prophylactic vaccination as alone they can confer protective immunity in chimpanzees [21, 37]. In addition, anti-pre-S2 antibodies are a marker of virus clearance from the liver under infection conditions and are absent in individuals who progress to a chronic carrier state [1].

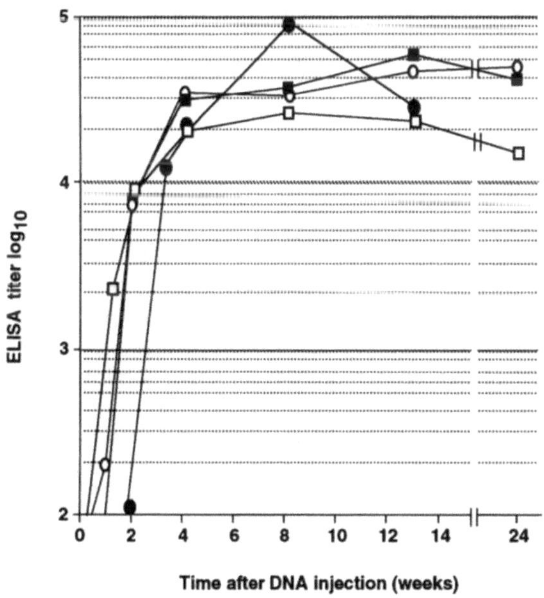

Fig. 4. Kinetics of total IgG anti-HBs response in mice immunized with different HBV envelope-expressing plasmids. The vectors used were pCMV-S (○), pCMV-S2.S (□), pCMV-S1.S2.S (■) and pHBV-S2.S (●). Sera were taken at different times after a single DNA injection and pools were made from all sera taken at a single time point. Antibodies were detected by ELISA using a solid phase made up of S-containing HBsAg of a homologous (*ay*) or heterologous subtype (*ad*), as well as HBsAg containing approximately 30% of the middle (pre-S2+S) protein of the *ay* subtype. Bound antibodies were detected in the second step by addition of peroxidase-labeled goat anti-mouse IgG. End-point titers were defined as the highest serum dilution that resulted in an absorbance value two times greater than that of sera from non-immunized or control immunized (irrelevant DNA) mice, with a cut-off value of 0.05

The humoral response is similar for all vectors used, with minor differences in kinetics being observed (Fig. 4). The more precocious response observed for vectors which include the pre-S2 sequences corresponds well with the kinetics of the response observed following natural infection. This is most likely due to the presence of B and T helper cell epitopes, which have been identified on the pre-S2 polypeptide. On the other hand, a delay in the appearance of antibodies following the use of vectors which include the pre-S1 sequence may be due to the known poor secretion of the L protein [32]. Thus, vector design may play an important role for a DNA vaccine against HBV for humans. An early and strong immune response such as that elicited by pCMV-S2.S may be critical for vaccination of infants born to chronically infected mothers. In other cases, the vector which ultimately induces the highest antibody titers may be more desirable.

Dose response. The precocity and strength of the humoral response following DNA-based immunization is dose dependent. With a single injection of 1 μg DNA into normal muscle, seroconversion (defined arbitrarily as > 1 mIU/ml) of all mice is not evident until 8 weeks post-immunization, whereas 100% seroconversion is observed by 4 and 2 weeks following injection of 10 or 100 μg HBsAg-expressing DNA, respectively. Antibody titers are higher with greater amounts of DNA but not in a directly proportional manner. Those induced with 100 μg DNA are only about 2.5-fold higher than those with 10 μg DNA [8]. This may reflect saturation of DNA at the injection site since some increase in antibody titer can be attained if the equivalent dose of DNA is delivered to several sites (Brazolot Millan and Davis, unpublished results).

Transfection efficiency, and in turn the immune response, for a given amount of DNA can be increased up to 10-fold by injecting the DNA into regenerating muscle (obtained by first inducing degeneration with a necrotizing agent such as snake-venom-derived cardiotoxin [6]) or somewhat less by injecting the DNA with a local anesthetic such as bupivacaine (Brazolot Millan and Davis, unpublished results).

Longevity of response. In mice immunized with HBsAg-expressing DNA, peak antibody titers are reached by 4–8 weeks after injection of DNA and persist at near maximal levels for up to 17 months without boost. This is remarkable since there is no synthesis of new antigen after about 2 weeks, when transfected muscle fibers are destroyed, presumably by CTL. Sustained high antibody titers suggest that antigen is still presented to the immune system, perhaps by association with follicular dendritic cells in regional lymph nodes.

Despite the high sustained response, antibody levels may be further increased approximately 10-fold with a second DNA injection, or about half as much by injection of recombinant HBsAg protein, even when the amount of antigen injected is approximately 1000 times more than would be synthesized in situ in the DNA-boosted animals [10].

Cell-mediated responses

DNA-based immunization using HBsAg-expressing plasmid DNA results in very strong CTL. Mice immunized with vectors expressing any of the three forms of the HBsAg protein (pCMV-S, pCMV-S2.S, pCMV-S1.S2.S) gave rise to high levels of both CTL and their precursors [9]. After specific restimulation in vitro for 5 days with HBsAg-expressing cells, spleen cells from DNA-immunized mice were capable of specific lysis of 80–90% at effector:target ratios as low as 2.5:1, indicating high levels of CTL precursors. Pre-existing mature CTL can be detected after nonspecific stimulation *in vitro*. Spleen cells incubated overnight with interleukin-2 (IL-2) exhibited 40% specific lysis at effector:target ratios of 200:1. CTL activity developed between 3 and 6 days after DNA injection, reached maximal levels by 12 days and peak activity was maintained for at least several months [9].

In contrast to most other proteins, HBsAg supplied in an exogenous form can induce CTL, provided it is injected in the absence of adjuvant [45]. However, in comparison to HBsAg synthesized *in situ* from plasmid DNA, injection of a much larger amount of recombinant HBsAg induces only low levels of precursors and no detectable mature CTL [9].

DNA overcomes haplotype restricted non-response to HBsAg

Certain strains of mice are known poor responders to the B cell epitopes of the S protein unless the pre-S2 and/or pre-S1 domains of the envelope gene are also present [33]. This hypo-responsiveness is genetically linked to the H-2 haplotype. Comparison of the humoral response in congenic strains of mice of different H-2 haplotypes immunized with either S-expressing DNA or recombinant S protein with adjuvant showed that a single injection of DNA is superior to a single injection of protein (Brazolot Millan, Michel, Mancini, Whalen and Davis, unpublished results). Indeed, in some poorly responding strains of mice, seroconversion was induced by a single administration of DNA but the protein antigen failed to induce anti-HBs without boost. This is particularly impressive considering that the amount of HBsAg synthesized in vivo in the DNA-immunized mice would be approximately one thousand times less than that injected as recombinant protein. The superiority of the DNA approach in these animals may by due to the sustained synthesis of antigen, which might facilitate the stimulation of low-affinity epitopes, and the direct effects of CpG immunostimulatory motifs in the DNA on B cells.

The finding that DNA based immunization can overcome haplotype-restricted non-responsiveness to HBsAg has clinical significance for non- or hypo-responsiveness to HBsAg in humans. Approximately 10% of adults immunized against HBV with the current protein-based HBV vaccines fail to respond and in at least one-quarter of these cases this is HLA linked [25].

DNA breaks tolerance to HBsAg in transgenic mice

Transgenic (Tg) mice constitutively expressing HBsAg in the liver can be used as a model for the chronic HBV carrier. One such Tg mouse line carries a copy of the HBV genome with the core gene deleted [2]. In these mice, HBV envelope proteins are expressed from before birth, principally in the liver, under the control of an endogenous HBV promoter. There is no HBsAg accumulation within hepatocytes, nor liver pathology. However, HBsAg is secreted into the serum, which contains up to 9,000 ng/ml in the form of subviral particles. These mice are tolerant to high levels of circulating antigen and do not produce anti-HBs.

Intramuscular injection of pCMV-S2.S into these Tg mice results in rapid appearance of anti-HBs antibodies. By 2 weeks after DNA injection significant titers are detected and by 8–12 weeks antibody levels are as high as those induced in normal mice after DNA-based immunization. Antibody isotypes induced are the same as seen in normal mice; early IgM, then IgG; predominantly IgG2 as well as IgG1 with some IgG3. The antibody isotypes, along with the profile of cytokines secreted by spleen-derived cells (see below) indicates that primarily a Th1 response was induced, although the presence of IgG1 indicates that at least a weak Th2 response was also induced [28].

A loss of circulating antigen accompanies the appearance of anti-HBs. In most animals circulating HBsAg is undetectable by 8 weeks after DNA injection. This loss persists for at least 20 weeks and is due in part to neutralization by antibodies, but is also due to a complete disappearance of HBV mRNA in the liver. Following DNA immunization of Tg mice with initially the highest levels of circulating HBsAg, levels of circulating HBsAg and liver HBV mRNA are seen to reduce greatly.

Down-regulation of transgene expression is likely mediated by HBsAg-specific T cells since it can be induced in naive Tg mice by passive transfer of T but not B cells from normal HBsAg-DNA-immunized mice. There is no elevation of liver enzymes in the blood nor histological evidence of liver necrosis at the time that circulating HBsAg is rapidly decreasing. The T cell effect thus appears to be mediated through a non-cytolytic, probably cytokine-mediated mechanism. Specifically, stimulated cultured spleen cells from DNA-immunized Tg mice produce predominantly IFN-γ and low levels of IL-2 and tumor necrosis factor-α (TNF-α). In a similar Tg model it has been shown that passive transfer of HBsAg-specific $CD8^+$ CTL into non-immunized Tg mice caused a transient down-regulation of the HBV transgene expression which was also mediated in a predominantly non-cytolytic fashion by IFN-γ and TNF-α [17].

Since the immunizing DNA encodes an identical gene product as the transgene in these Tg mice it is difficult to explain how DNA-based immunization breaks tolerance or anergy to HBsAg. Injection of pure recombinant HBsAg protein has no effect on these mice unless it contains a heterologous epitope (e.g., HIV V3 loop) as a fusion protein, or is from a heterologous strain [27], indicating that epitopes must appear different or be associated with unrelated helper epitopes to induce immune responses. HBsAg expressed from muscle is possibly somewhat different than that expressed in the liver or may result in a different mode of presentation of the envelope protein antigens if different antigen-presenting cells (APC) are involved. Another possibility is that the danger signal provided by CpG motifs in the DNA results in presentation of antigen in association with co-stimulatory molecules and this would in turn break tolerance previously induced by HBsAg expressed in the liver in the absence of co-stimulatory molecules [43]. Support for this possibility is provided by the finding that recombinant HBsAg given in Freund's complete adjuvant is capable of breaking tolerance in these Tg mice [28].

Regardless of the mechanism, these results with DNA-based immunization of Tg mice may have important clinical significance for immunotherapeutic treatment of HBV chronic carriers.

Neonatal immunization

Immunization of newborn mice (aged 1 or 7 days) from HBsAg-naive mothers is successful with HBsAg-expressing DNA but not recombinant HBsAg protein. DNA-immunized mice attained anti-HBs titers of $> 10^3$ which were maintained for at least 25 weeks (Brazolot Millan, Davis, unpublished results). Protein-immunized animals elicited no detectable humoral response, nor were they tolerized, as a second administration of protein given once they were adult did elicit a typical primary humoral response.

Neonates born to previously immunized, anti-HBs-positive mothers have significant levels of serum anti-HBs until 10–12 weeks of age. Neither DNA nor protein immunization of these mice (at 1 or 7 days of age) results in persistence of anti-HBs beyond this period of maternally derived anti-HBs. Detectable humoral responses can be induced by a second injection of DNA or protein, but only those previously receiving DNA exhibit an anamnestic response to HBsAg, indicating that immune priming can occur with the DNA vaccine despite the presence of high levels of circulating maternally derived anti-HBs (Brazolot Millan, Davis, unpublished results).

These findings suggest that DNA may be superior to protein for immunization of newborn humans and that DNA but not protein vaccines may be effective even in the presence of maternal antibodies. This will prove to be particularly critical in regions where HBV is endemic.

DNA-based vaccination of chimpanzees against HBV

The chimpanzee is the best animal model to evaluate DNA vaccines for their potential use in humans. It is similar to man with respect to susceptibility to HBV infection and antibody titer required for protection. Furthermore, it is the only animal which can be challenged with human HBV [38].

Humoral response

Intramuscular immunization of chimpanzees using pCMV-S2.S DNA resulted in an HBsAg-specific humoral response. High anti-HBs levels (> 100 mIU/ml) were induced in a female chimpanzee immunized with 2 mg DNA, however at least two boost injections of DNA were required to prevent antibody levels from diminishing over time. Nevertheless, extremely high titers were ultimately attained (> 14,000 mIU/ml), with high levels being sustained for at least 1 year. In a second chimpanzee (male) injected with a lower dose of DNA (400 μg), no anti-HBs was detected until after the second injection of DNA. Although antibody titers of 60 mIU/ml were eventually attained these were transient even after three DNA boosts. Despite loss of detectable anti-HBs, this chimpanzee showed a strong anamnestic response to injection of recombinant HBsAg given 1 year after the initial DNA injection [11]. The weaker response in the second animal may be due to the lower dose and possibly also the fact that immune responses to HBsAg are often weaker in male than female chimpanzees and humans [4, 52].

As observed in mice, DNA-based vaccination of chimpanzees induces HBsAg-specific antibodies. Initially of IgM isotype, these subsequently shift to IgG antibodies, which are predominantly IgG1. This is consistent with a Th1 and/or Th2 response. The antibodies induced are predominantly against the pre-S2 domain but are also specific to the group and subtype determinants of the S protein.

Comparison of DNA to other HBV vaccines

A comparison of the DNA vaccine with commercial or experimental HBV vaccines used in chimpanzees favorably highlights DNA-based immunization. Mean titers of anti-HBs attained following vaccination with live recombinant viral vector (vaccinia or adenovirus) or peptide (S or pre-S2) plus adjuvant vaccines are ≤ 10 mIU/ml, but are about 6,000 mIU/ml with recombinant HBsAg plus adjuvant. The antibody titers induced by the DNA vaccine in the better responding chimpanzee were as high as the best response induced by the commercial recombinant subunit vaccine, and those in the poorer responding chimpanzee are at least as good as the other experimental vaccines.

Levels of anti-HBs and amount of protection afforded correlate well for both humans and chimpanzees. Titers greater than 10 mIU/ml almost always protect against both infection and hepatitis, whereas titers of 1–10 mIU/ml rarely protect against infection but protect against hepatitis in about half the cases. Based on this, the female chimpanzee receiving the higher DNA dose would have been protected against HBV infection by only a single DNA injection. The male receiving the lower dose was probably not protected against infection; however the rapid and strong anamnestic response to the recombinant vaccine indicates hepatitis would not have developed in the event of infection [11].

Neonatal immunization

Two chimpanzees born to HBsAg-naive mothers were immunized on the day of birth and at 6 and 24 weeks with 500 μg pCMV-S [39]. Although only transient and low levels of anti-HBs were detected (26 and 41 mIU/ml), both animals were protected from subsequent live viral challenge. Neither HBsAg nor anti-HBc, indicative of HBV infection, were detected.

Conclusions: potential for HBV DNA vaccine for humans

Results following intramuscular injection of HBsAg-encoding plasmid DNA in animal models indicate that DNA vaccines should be feasible for vaccination of humans against HBV. A DNA vaccine may be superior to recombinant HBsAg for prophylactic vaccination, especially in cases of non- or hypo-responsiveness, or for the induction of a very rapid humoral response in infants born to chronic carrier mothers. In addition, a DNA vaccine may be effective therapeutically for HBV chronic carriers, possibly because of the induction of strong CTL.

Despite encouraging results obtained in animal models, it would be preferable for economic and safety reasons that the approach be optimized such that lower doses of DNA than were used in the chimpanzees could be used in humans. Such optimization could involve increasing (i) the efficiency of gene transfer, by for example other routes of administration or targeted delivery, (ii) improving the level of gene expression such as through vector design, and/or (iii) increasing the immune response to the expressed antigen by appropriate use of CpG immunostimulatory motifs or other adjuvants or co-expressing the antigen with costimulatory molecules or cytokines.

Acknowledgements. We are grateful to all of our colleagues who have graciously collaborated with us on the studies reported here: M.-L. Michel and M. Mancini (INSERM U163, Pasteur Institute, Paris, France), R.H. Purcell (NIAID, NIH, Bethesda, MD, USA), M. Schleef (Qiagen, Hilden, Germany), J. Reimann and R. Schirmbeck (University of Ulm, Germany), S.C. Watkins (University of Pittsburgh, PA, USA), and R.G. Whalen (CNRS URA-1115, College de France, Paris, France). We also wish to thank the other members of our laboratory for their ongoing contributions to this work: L. Comanita, M. McCluskie, L. St. Vincent, R. Weeratna and T. Wu.

References

1. Alberti A, Cavalletto D, Pontisso P, Chemello L, Tagariello G, Belussi F (1988) Antibody response to pre-S2 and hepatitis B virus induced liver damage. Lancet 25: 1421
2. Babinet C, Farza H, Morello D, Hadchouel M, Pourcel C (1985) Specific expression of hepatitis B surface antigen (HBsAg) in transgenic mice. Science 230: 1160
3. Buynak EB, Roehm RR, Tytell AA, Bertland AU, Lampson GP, Hilleman MR (1976) Development and chimpanzee testing of a vaccine against human hepatitis B. Proc Soc Exp Biol Med 151: 694
4. Coates RA, Halliday ML, Rankin JG, Stewart JD, Bristow NJ, Granero R, West DJ (1988) Immunogenicity and safety of a yeast-derived recombinant DNA hepatitis B vaccine in health care workers. In: Zuckerman AJ (ed) Viral hepatitis and liver disease. Liss, New York, pp 1038–1042
5. Centers for Disease Control (1987) Recommendations of the Immunization Practises Advisory Committee Update on hepatitis B prevention. MMWR 36: 353
6. Davis HL, Demeneix BA, Quantin B, Coulombe J, Whalen RG (1993) Plasmid DNA is superior to viral vectors for direct gene transfer in adult mouse skeletal muscle. Hum Gene Ther 4: 733
7. Davis HL, Michel M-L, Whalen RG (1993) DNA based immunization for hepatitis B induces continuous secretion of antigen and high levels of circulating antibody. Hum Mol Genet 2: 1847
8. Davis HL, Michel M-L, Mancini M, Schleef M, Whalen RG (1994) Direct gene transfer in muscle with plasmid DNA for the purpose of nucleic acid immunization. Vaccine 12: 1503
9. Davis HL, Schirmbeck R, Reimann J, Whalen RG (1995) DNA-mediated immunization in mice induces a potent MHC class-I restricted cytotoxic T lymphocyte response to the hepatitis B envelope protein. Hum Gene Ther 6: 1447
10. Davis HL, Mancini M, Michel M-L, Whalen RG (1996) DNA-mediated immunization to hepatitis B surface antigen: longevity of primary response and effect of boost. Vaccine 14: 910
11. Davis HL, McCluskie MJ, Gerin JL, Purcell RH (1996) DNA vaccine for hepatitis B: evidence for immunogenicity in chimpanzees and comparison with other vaccines. Proc Natl Acad Sci USA 93: 7213
12. Davis HL, Brazolot Millan CL, Watkins SC (1997) Immune-mediated destruction of transfected muscle fibers after direct gene transfer with antigen-expressing plasmid DNA. Gene Ther 4: 181
13. Ganem D, Varmus HE (1987) The molecular biology of the hepatitis B viruses. Annu Rev Biochem 56: 651
14. Gerety RJ (1988) Recombinant hepatitis B vaccines. In: Zuckerman AJ (ed) Viral hepatitis and liver disease. Liss, New York, pp 1017–1024
15. Gerin JL, Purcell RH, Lerner RA (1985) Use of synthetic peptides to identify protective epitopes of the heptitis B surface antigen. Vaccines 85. Cold Spring Harbor Laboratory Press, Cold Spring Harbor, pp 235–239
16. Gerlich WH, Bruss V (1993) Functions of hepatitis B virus proteins and molecular targets for protective immunity. In: Ellis RW (ed) Hepatitis B vaccines in clinical practise. Dekker, New York, pp 41–82
17. Guidotti LG, Ando K, Hobbs MV, Ishikawa T, Runkel L, Schreiber RD, Chisari FV (1994) Cytotoxic T lymphocytes inhibit hepatitis B virus gene expression by a noncytolytic mechanism in transgenic mice. Proc Natl Acad Sci USA 91: 3764
18. Hadler SC. Margolis HS (1993) Epidemiology of hepatitis B virus infection. In: Ellis RW (ed) Hepatitis B vaccines in clinical practise. Dekker, New York, pp 141–158
19. Hibberd PL, Rubin RH, Dienstag JL (1993) Needs unfulfilled by current hepatitis B vaccines. In: Ellis RW (ed) Hepatitis B vaccines in clinical practise. Dekker, New York, pp 323–336
20. Hilleman MR (1993) Plasma-derived hepatitis B vaccine: a breakthrough in preventive medicine. In: Ellis RW (ed) Hepatitis B vaccines in clinical practise. Dekker, New York, pp 17–40

21. Itoh Y, Takai E, Ohnuma H, Kitajima K, Tsuda F, Machida A, Mishiro S, Nakamura T, Miyakawa Y, Mayumi M (1986) A synthetic peptide vaccine involving the product of the pre-S(2) region of hepatitis B virus DNA: protective efficacy in chimpanzees. Proc Natl Acad Sci USA 83: 9174
22. Iwarson S, Tabor E, Thomas HC, Snoy P, Gerety RJ (1985) Protection against hepatitis B virus infection by immunization with hepatitis B core antigen. Gastroenterology 88: 763
23. Kane MA (1993) Global control of hepatitis B through universal infant immunization. In: Ellis RW (ed) Hepatitis B vaccines in clinical practise. Dekker, New York, pp 309–322
24. Krieg AM, Yi A-K, Matson S, Waldschmidt TJ, Bishop GA, Teasdale R, Koretzky GA, Klinman DM (1995) CpG motifs in bacterial DNA trigger direct B-cell activation. Nature 374: 546
25. Kruskall MS, Alper CA, Awdeh Z, Yunis EJ, Marcus-Bagley D (1992) The immune response to hepatitis B vaccine in humans: inheritance patterns in families. J Exp Med 175: 495
26. Lubeck MD, Davis AR, Chengalvala M, Natuk RJ, Morin JE, Molnar-Kimber K, Mason BB, Bhat BM, Mizutani S, Hung PP, Purcell RH (1989) Immunogenicity and efficacy testing in chimpanzees of an oral hepatitis B vaccine based on live recombinant adenovirus. Proc Natl Acad Sci USA 86: 6763
27. Mancini M, Hadchouel M, Tiollais P, Pourcel C, Michel M-L (1993) Induction of anti-hepatitis B surface antigen (HBsAg) antibodies in HBsAg producing transgenic mice: a possible way of circumventing "nonresponse" to HBsAg. J Med Virol 39: 67
28. Mancini M, Hadchouel M, Davis HL, Whalen RG, Tiollais P, Michel M-L (1996) DNA-mediated immunization breaks tolerance in a transgenic mouse model of hepatitis B surface antigen chronic carrier state. Proc Natl Acad Sci USA 93: 12496
29. Maugh TH (1980) Hepatitis B vaccine passes first major test. Science 210: 760
30. Maupas P, Goudeau A, Coursaget P, Drucker J (1976) Immunization against hepatitis B in man. Lancet 1: 1367
31. Michel M-L, Pontisso P, Sobczak E, Malpièce Y, Streeck RE, Tiollais P (1984) Synthesis in animal cells of hepatitis B surface antigen particles carrying a receptor for polymerized human serum albumin. Proc Natl Acad Sci USA 81: 7708
32. Michel M-L, Davis HL, Schleef M, Mancini M, Tiollais P, Whalen RG (1995) DNA-mediated immunization to the hepatitis B surface antigen in mice: aspects of the humoral response mimic hepatitis B viral infection in humans. Proc Natl Acad Sci USA 92: 5307
33. Milich DR (1988) T- and B-cell recognition of hepatitis B viral antigens. Immunol Today 9: 380
34. Moss B, Smith GL, Gerin JL, Purcell RH (1984) Live recombinant vaccinia virus protects chimpanzees against hepatitis B. Nature 311: 67
35. Murray K, Bruce SA, Hinnen A, Wingfield P, Erd PMCA van, Reus A de, Schellekens H (1984) Hepatitis B virus antigens made in microbial cells immunize against viral infection. EMBO J 3: 645
36. Neurath AR, Kent SBH, Strick N, Taylor P, Stevens CE (1985) Hepatitis B virus contains pre-S gene-encoded domains. Nature 315: 154
37. Neurath AR, Kent SBH, Parker K, Prince AM, Strick N, Brotman B, Sproul P (1986) Antibodies to a synthetic peptide from the preS 120–145 region of the hepatitis B virus envelope are virus-neutralizing. Vaccine 4: 35
38. Prince AM (1981) The use of chimpanzees in biomedical research. US Department of Health and Human Services: Trends in bioassay methodology in vivo, in vitro and mathematical approaches. NIH publication no. 82–2382. NIH, Bethesda, pp 81–98
39. Prince AM, Whalen RG, Brotman B (1997) Successful nucleic acid based immunization of newborn chimpanzees against HBV. Vaccine 15 : 916
40. Purcell RH, Gerin JL (1975) Hepatitis B subunit vaccine: a preliminary report of safety and efficacy tests in chimpanzees. Am J Med Sci 270: 395
41. Purcell RH, Gerin JL (1987) Hepatitis B vaccines past present and future: lessons for AIDS vaccine development. In: Robinson W, Koike K, Will H (eds) Hepadna viruses. Liss, New York, pp 465–479
42. Reesink-Brongers EE, Reesink HW, Brummelhuis HGJ, Schut BJT, Dees PJ, Lelie PN, Raap AK, Wilson-de Stürler LA, Aken WG van, Balner H, Eerd PMCA van, Schie TC van, Stitz LW, Steenis B van, Feltkamp-Vroom TM (1982) Preparation and evaluation of heat-inactivated HBsAg as a vaccine against hepatitis B. In: Szmuness W, Alter HJ, Maynard JE (eds) Viral Hepatitis 1981 International Symposium. The Franklin Institute Press, Philadelphia, pp 437–450
43. Ridge JP, Fuchs EJ, Matzinger P (1996) Neonatal tolerance revisited: turning on newborn T cells with dendritic cells. Science 271: 1723
44. Sato Y, Roman M, Tighe H, Lee D, Corr M, Nguyen M-D, Silverman GJ, Lotz M, Carson DA, Raz E (1996) Immunostimulatory DNA sequences necessary for effective intradermal gene immunization. Science 273: 353

45. Schirmbeck R, Melber K, Kuhröber A, Janowicz ZA, Reimann J (1994) Immunization with soluble hepatitis B virus surface protein elicits murine H-2 class I-restricted $CD8^+$ cytotoxic T lymphocyte responses in vivo. J Immunol 152: 1110
46. Stephenne J (1988) Recombinant versus plasma-derived hepatitis B vaccines: issues of safety immunogenicity and cost-effectiveness. Vaccine 6: 299
47. Tang D, DeVit M, Johnston SA (1992) Genetic immunization is a simple method for eliciting an immune response. Nature 356: 152
48. Thornton GB, Milich DR, Chisari F, Mitamura K, Kent SB, Neurath R, Purcell RH, Gerin JL (1987) Immune response in primates to the pre-S2 region of hepatitis B surface antigen: identification of a protective determinant. In: Chanock RM, Lerner RA, Brown F, Ginsberg H (eds) Vaccines 87. Cold Spring Harbor Laboratory Press, Cold Spring Harbor, pp 77–80
49. Tiollais P, Buendia M-A (1991) Hepatitis B virus. Sci Am 264: 48
50. Valenzuela P, Medina A, Rutter WJ, Ammerer G, Hall BD (1982) Synthesis and assembly of hepatitis B virus surface antigen particles in yeast. Nature 298: 347
51. Wolff JA, Malone RW, Williams P, Chong W, Ascadi G, Jani A, Felgner PL (1990) Direct gene transfer into mouse muscle *in vivo*. Science 247: 1465
52. Yano M, Tashiro A (1988) Clinical evaluation of recombinant yeast-derived hepatitis B vaccine. In Zuckerman AJ (ed) Viral hepatitis and liver disease. Liss, New York, pp 1050–1052

Gene vaccination for hepatitis C

Geneviève Inchauspé

INSERM U271, 151 Cours Albert-Thomas, F-69003 Lyon, France

Introduction

Hepatitis C virus (HCV) is a positive-strand RNA virus that codes for at least six different proteins (Fig. 1). Its worldwide prevalence ranges from 0.5% to 10% and it is currently believed that more than 70% of HCV-infected patients will evolve towards a chronic carrier state with the risk, in more than 40%, of developing cirrhosis associated with an enhanced change of evolution towards hepatocellular carcinomas (HCC) [32]. In France, HCV infections have become the prevalent cause of HCC and it is estimated that more than 30,000 cases of HCC directly related to HCV infection will be accounted for by the year 2010 [3]. Community acquired infection is still common causing a significant amount of morbidity as well as important economic burdens [26]. In addition, the current lack of efficient antiviral treatment makes the development of a vaccine desirable.

Several observations from clinical and experimental studies of humans and chimpanzees suggest that failure to mount an effective immune response against HCV is responsible for the high rate of chronicity characterizing infections by this agent. These studies have shown that (1) following a self-limited infection or during a chronic carrier state, re-infection with a heterologous or homologous inoculum can occur [10, 34], (2) infection by multiple genotypes, in particular in high-risk populations such as hemophiliacs or drug abusers, is possible [23], and (3) HCV exists in the infected host as a very complex population of mutant viruses of quasispecies [46]. The quasispecies distribution seems to fluctuate with duration of infection [19] and in response to antiviral treatment [9, 31], and may be responsible for the emergence of immune-escape mutants. Taken together these data suggest that the natural immunity fails to control the infection, although a certain degree of immunity appears to be mounted following primary infection. Indeed, Prince et al. [34] documented in the chimpanzee model that second episodes of hepatitis following challenge tend to be milder.

The development of a vaccine against HCV is obviously faced with multiple challenges. The identification of immunogenic antigens carrying neutralizing determinants has yet to be documented. Preliminary data suggest that the N-terminal part of the envelope glycoprotein E2, the so-called hypervariable region (HVR, [46]) could contain a neutralizing epitope [11, 18, 38]. This region contains several B cell as well as cytotoxic T lymphocyte (CTL) epitopes [18, 20, 24, 47], and specific antibodies directed at

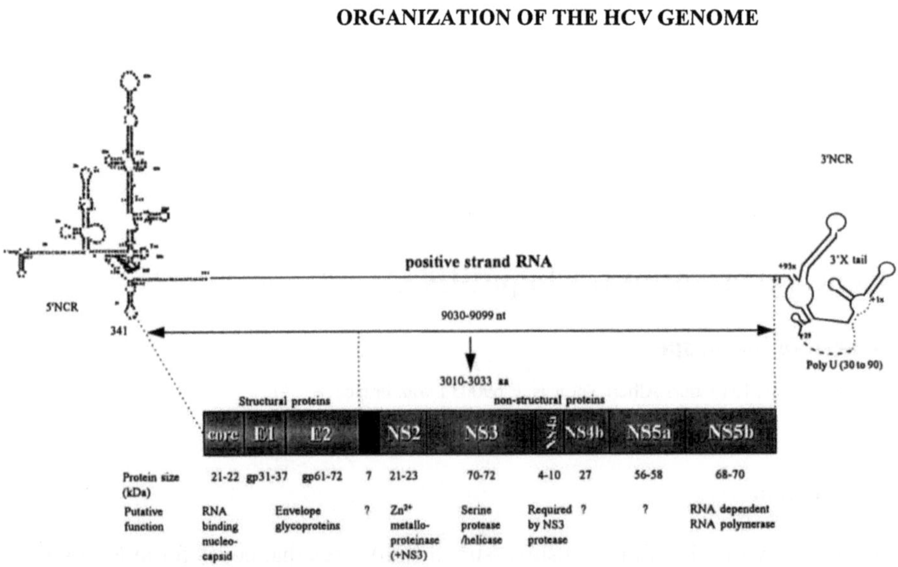

Fig. 1. Schematic representation of the hepatitis C virus (HCV) genome. Secondary structures found at the 5′ and 3′ non-coding regions *(NCR)* are indicated. Putative function of the different viral antigens (structural and non-structural) is indicated

this region were reported to block viral attachment to susceptible cells [49]. Due to the lack of a sensitive in vitro tissue culture assay for HCV, it has not yet been possible to test the neutralizing potential per se of such candidate antibodies, let alone their cross-neutralizing ability. Nonetheless, progress has been made in the development of substitute assays and a group has recently developed a specific cell-binding assay whereby the purified glycoprotein E2 is quantitatively absorbed onto susceptible cells [36]. Antibodies capable of neutralizing binding of E2 in this assay (neutralizing of binding antibodies or NOB antibodies) have been detected in up to 40% of chronically infected patients. In addition, protection of chimpanzees immunized with E1 and E2 was correlated not only with high anti-E2 antibody titers but also with high titers of NOB antibodies [36, 37].

Identification of components of the cellular immune machinery (such as $CD8^+$ CTL and $CD4^+$ T helper lymphocytes) capable of eliminating or facilitating the elimination of the virus are currently the focus of active investigations. Circulating blood lymphocytes as well as liver infiltrating lymphocytes have been successfully used to identify a number of CTL determinants (for review see [21]). These have been mapped to virtually all encoded HCV antigens. At present, no correlation has been established between CTL activity against any particular determinant or antigen and development or outcome of disease. A favorable response to interferon treatment appears nonetheless to be associated with enhanced CT1 activity. In earlier studies, an enhanced ($CD4^+$) proliferative response directed at the nucleocapsid (C) and the NS4 protein, had been found in association with self-limited or asymptomatic evolving infections [2, 12]. More recent studies have documented that $CD4^+$-type responses directed not only at these two antigens but also at the glycoproteins E1 and E2 and the non-structural proteins NS3 and NS5 were associated with control of infection and/or better response to antiviral treatments [12].

Both humoral and cellular immune responses are likely to be important for controlling HCV infection. Nucleic acid-based immunizations may thus be particularly fit for the generation of both types of responses. The goal of this chapter is to review the latest work reported in the field of gene immunization against HCV and discuss its potentialities for the development of both a preventive and therapeutic vaccine.

Plasmids encoding the viral nucleocapsid: direct injection and induced immune responses

HCV nucleocapsid (CAP) may represent a valuable component in the development of a vaccine as it is the most conserved viral antigen (about 95% homology at the amino acid level has been described between the different viral genotypes/subtypes). In addition, internal antigens such as nucleocapsids have been shown in various models (e.g., rabies virus, hepatitis B virus and influenza virus) to be associated with protective immune resonses, most likely via the generation of effective CTL [6, 16, 43]. Different

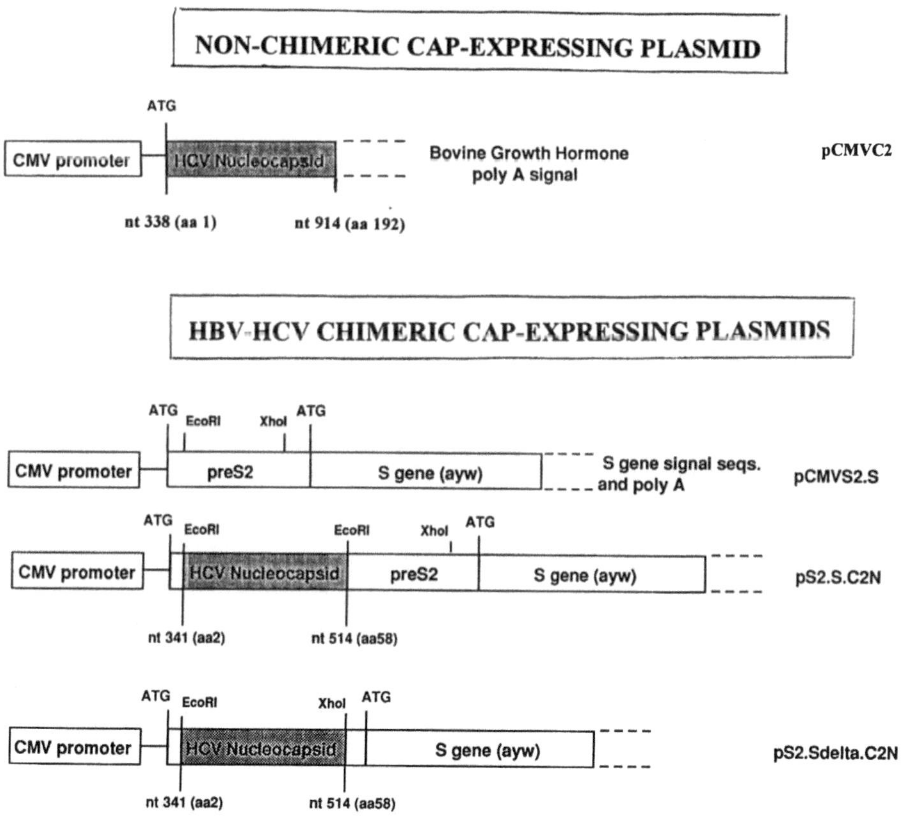

Fig. 2. Schematic representation of HCV nucleocapsid (CAP)-expressing plasmids: pCMVC2, a non-chimeric plasmid expressing the full-length CAP sequence directly under the control of the cytomegalovirus (CMV) promoter; and pS2.SC2N and pS2.Sdelta.C2N, HBV-HCV chimeric plasmids expressing the first 60 amino acids of CAP in fusion with the HBsAg sequences expressed in presence or absence of the preS2 sequence, respectively. Adapted from Major et al. [25]

strategies have been described for the design of HCV CAP-expressing plasmids. These have included the use of plasmids containing the full-length CAP sequence under the control of a cytomegalovirus (CMV) promoter [22, 25, 42] as well as plasmids containing truncated sequences of CAP expressed in fusion with the hepatitis B surface antigen (HBsAg, [15, 25]). HBsAg-derived hybrid proteins have been shown in different models to be particularly effective for the presentation of foreign epitopes in immunization experiments using particles produced in vitro [5, 27].

Figure 2 is an illustration of the different CAP-encoding plasmids used by Major et al. [25] and Inchauspé et al. [15] in recent studies. In vitro experiments demonstrated expression of both HCV and HBV antigens from these plasmids in the cytoplasms of transiently transfected cells. Secretion of HCV-CAP antigenic forms in the supernatants of transfected cells was only detected when CAP sequences were expressed as HBV-HCV fusion proteins [15]. Concentration of the secreted antigens in supernatants of these cells was nonetheless quite low (35 ng/ml at 96 h post transfection) and suggested that most of the expressed antigens remained as intracellular forms. The effect of the HBsAg preS2 sequence on the induction of antibodies following injection of the HVB-HCV chimeric plasmids was also evaluated, one speculation being that the immunodominant determinants present in this sequence could have a masking effect on the presentation of the CAP-HCV determinants. No effect was seen either on the seroconversion rates (100% by week 8 post immunization, p.i.) or on the titers of anti-CAP-induced antibodies (1 : 2500–3000 by week 18 p.i.), suggesting that the preS2 sequence neither favors nor inhibits the presentation of HCV-CAP determinants. Seroconversion rates and antibody titers were systematically found to be lower with plasmids expressing the HCV-CAP directly under the control of the CMV promoter (i.e., from a non-chimeric plasmid). Using both chimeric and non-chimeric CAP-expressing plasmids, comparative experiments were performed in three different haplotypes of mice, H-2^d, H-2^b and H-2^s [15]. While dramatic differences in seroconversion rates were observed between the different lines of mice for all immunogens, HBV-HCV chimeric plasmids were the most efficient at inducing anti-CAP antibodies independent of the haplotype of the mice. The fastest seroconversion rate to anti-CAP antibodies was observed in BALB/c mice (H-2^d). A detailed analysis of antigen-specific cytokine production in vitro by the splenic cells of plasmid-injected mice revealed the presence of numerous potential T helper epitopes, some of them being apparently unique to specific major histocompatibility complex backgrounds as described below.

Overall, induction of proliferative responses ($CD4^+$) following the direct injection of CAP-encoding plasmids was demonstrated in proliferation assays as well as in analysis of cytokine production in vitro following stimulation with purified CAP or specific synthetic peptides [15, 22]. Both interferon-γ (IFN-γ) and interleukin-2 (IL-2) could be detected (concentrations ranged from 30 to 1500 pg/ml), while IL-4 and IL-10 were not detectable or detectable at very low levels only (< 30 pg/ml). Such profiles were detected whether CAP was expressed as a fusion or a non-fusion with the HBsAg, and were comparable in different haplotypes of mice. In contrast, cultures of spleen from mice immunized with a highly purified CAP protein, in absence of adjuvant, gave rise to the production of IL-2, IL-4, IL-10 and IFN-γ ranging from 30 to 280 pg/ml. In these experiments, in vitro stimulation was performed using purified CAP as well as CAP-specific overlapping synthetic peptides. Putative T helper epitopes could be mapped and, overall, the same peptides had an identical effect on cells taken from DNA- or protein-injected animals, with the exception of one peptide [amino acids (aa) 79–103] that elicited a response in DNA- but not protein-immunized mice (see Fig. 2 of [15]).

In vitro and in vivo detection of specific ($CD8^+$) CTL was reported in different studies following intramuscular (IM) or intradermal (ID) injection of CAP-derived plasmids ([22, 42]) and O. Vidalin, personal communication). These studies illustrate the following points: (1) induction of CAP-specific CTL following DNA injection does not appear very efficient [maximal of 20% specific lysis for an effector to target (E : T) ratio of 1 : 100]. In comparison, for example, the CTL-specific lysis following one single injection of HBsAg-encoding plasmid DNA was typically found to be 80% for a E : T ratio of 1 : 20 (O. Vidalin, personal communication), (2) such a low level of detection is independent of the time of analysis p.i. and was found to be identical at 5 and 24 weeks p.i. (O. Vidalin, personal communication), and (3) in a mouse tumor-rejection model, CAP-specific CTL were nonetheless apparently capable of eliminating CAP-expressing tumors when compared to appropriate controls [42]. In this latter model, rejection of tumors was observed within a short period of follow-up post challenge (20 days) suggesting that CTL were efficiently primed in vivo. Up to three booster injections (using 100 μg DNA injection per mouse) were nonetheless necessary to achieve this rejection. Although somewhat artificial, this type of in vivo model may provide alternative ways to assess the induction of DNA-induced specific HCV CTL as small animal models are not available. We have observed that, using a synthetic peptide corresponding to a previously described murine CTL epitope [39], it is possible to detect up to 80% specific lysis following IM or ID injections of CAP-expressing plasmid DNA. Identification of additional putative CTL epitopes is in progress and should provide useful analytical tools.

We have recently performed comparative analysis of anti-CAP immune responses induced following IM or ID injection, using a Gene Gun, of CAP-expressing plasmids. Overall, anti-CAP seroconversion rates and antibody titers were found slightly higher following ID injections rather than IM but no differences could be observed at the level of CTL induction. Thus, changing the injection route of HCV CAP-plasmid DNA does not appear to enhance cellular immune responses to the antigen. Other strategies would have to be devised to achieve this goal, such as co-injection of cytokine-encoding plasmid DNA. Preliminary results obtained by Geissler et al. [13], who con-injected granulocyte-macrophage colony-stimulating factor-, IL-2- and IL-4-encoding plasmids with HCV CAP-plasmids showed that this approach could result in a two- to threefold increase in anti-CAP antibody titers or seroconversion rates, but did not apparently had no improving effect on the induced CTL.

Immune response following IM or ID injection of plasmids encoding the glycoprotein E2

Whether the participation of immune responses directed at HCV glycoproteins E1 and E2 can be exploited for the development of a vaccine is still not certain in view of accumulated data demonstrating that both antigenic domains, but particularly E2, are prone to mutational changes and appearance of immune escape mutants [14, 18, 45]. Nonetheless, the use of such antigens in a vaccine formulation should be evaluated as they seem to encode neutralizing determinants which remain to be identified. In fact, E2-specific determinants have not yet been analyzed. In particular identification of genotype- and/or subtype-conserved determinants has been limited in part because of difficulties in obtaining the corresponding purified antigens.

Recent studies have reported the successful induction of humoral responses following the direct injection of E2-encoding plasmids in mice [29, 30, 41]. These

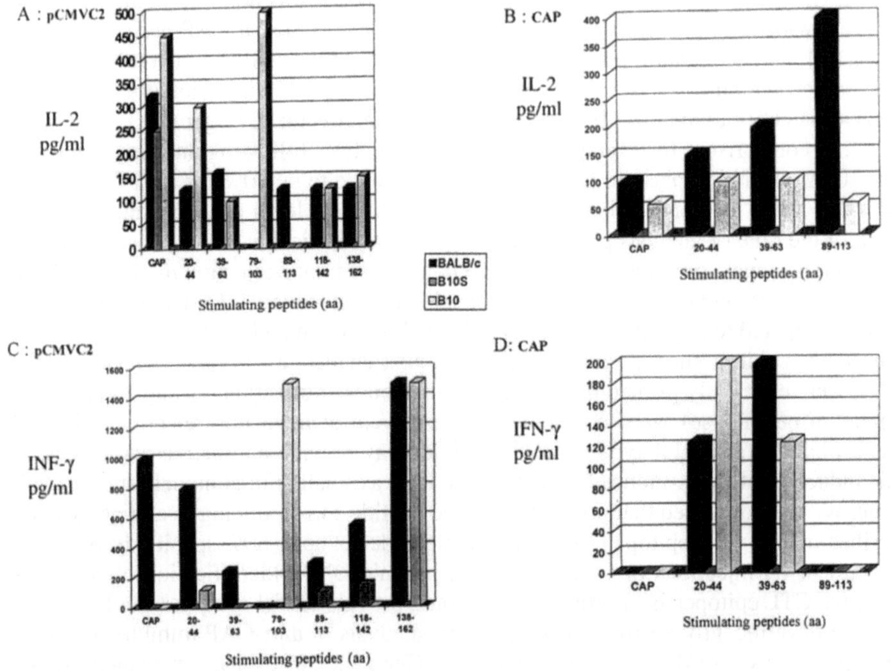

Fig. 3. Comparison of CAP-specific cytokine production by BALB/c, B10 and B10S splenic T cells following genetic or protein-based immunization. Groups of three mice were immunized with the pCMVC2 vector or purified CAP antigen. Splenic cells were cultured in the presence of the various indicated stimulating peptides used at three different concentrations (0.25, 2.5 and 6 mg/ml). Production of interleukin-2 (IL-2) following immunization with pCMVC2 (C) and CAP (D) were recorded and expressed in pg/ml. Results given are representative values from two separate experiments. Only those peptides that resulted in cytokine production are indicated. From Inchauspé et al. [15]

studies addressed issues related to the induction of anti-E2 humoral immune responses in terms of (1) evaluating the competency of DNA immunization for induction of high and stable anti-E2 antibody titers, (2) identifying E2 subtype- (variable or -conserved immunogenic regions, and (3) analyzing the capacity of E2-plasmid-induced antibodies to recognize a mature form of the protein as a predictor of neutralization.

In their study, Tedeschi et al. [41] used a plasmid expressing the near full-length HCV E2 sequence under the CMV promoter and were able to document seroconversion to anti-E2 antibodies as early as week 2 p.i. following IM injection of the DNA. The presence of plasmid DNA in the mice quadriceps was demonstrated up to 4 months p.i., confirming previous studies that have documented long-term persistence of the injected DNA in the injected tissues [4, 48]. The immuno-reactivity of the induced sera was assessed using a panoply of synthetic peptides and two linear epitopes were successfully mapped. Nakano et al. [30] have compared the induction of humoral immune responses generated after injection of a similar construct as well as a panoply of HBsAg-expressing plasmids carrying distinct, non-overlapping E2 putative antigenic domains (illustrated in Fig. 3). The latter insert sequences were cloned in fusion with the HBsAg sequences, in replacement of the pre-S2 sequence. None of these constructs appeared to secrete the expressed antigens efficiently. These were systemati-

Table 1. Anti-E2 antibody responses following IM or ID injection of plasmid DNA

Plasmids[a]	Injection Mode[b]	% Seroconversion[c]		Titers[c, d]		Isotypes
		Week 6	Week 18	Week 6	Week 18	
pS2.SE2C	IM	75	75	390 (390)	99 (90)	IGG2A
	ID	100	100	3 700 (1 862)	35 509 (13 337)	IG2a, 2b
pCIE2t	IM	75	75	1 288 (761)	31 590 (11 410)	IgG2a, 2b
	ID	100	100	3 637 (977)	> 43 700 (> 24 904)	IgG2a, 2b

[a] pS2.SE2C contains aa 504–556 expressed in fusion with the HBsAg, pCIE2t contains aa 384–674
[b] IM, intramuscular; ID, intradermal using a gene gun
[c] Measured post inoculation
[d] Numbers in bold represent maximal titers, numbers in parenthesis represent mean titers

cally located within the cytoplasms of transfected cells. All constructs were injected IM or ID into BALB/c mice to allow for a fine comparison of induced responses in correlation with the injection routes. Typical doses of 100 μg and 5 μg of gold-coated DNA/mouse, respectively, were injected IM and ID, and typically one booster injection was performed at 5 weeks p.i. Table 1 illustrates the results obtained for two of the injected plasmids: pCIE2t, expressing the near full-length coding region of E2 (aa 384–674) and pS2.SE2C expressing 60 aa of the central domain of E2 (aa 504–556) expressed in fusion with the HBsAg. Important differences were seen between the two injection modes for both plasmids in terms of seroconversion rates and antibody titers, while isotypes of induced antibodies were identical, IgG2a and IgG2b (IgG1 was never detected). As shown in Table 1, differences in antibody titers were particularly dramatic for the pS2.SE2C plasmid as ID-induced antibody titres were 100-fold higher than IM-induced ones at week 12 p.i. Because ID injections target plasmid DNA in a tissue, the epidermis, which is particularly rich in Langerhans cells (cells that play an important role in antigen presentation and immunocompetence of the skin [1, 40], it has been speculated that such an "environment" could explain why ID injections are generally more potent at inducing strong immune responses. In studies of Nakano et al. [29, 30], more intriguing was the observation that different determinants (linear epitopes) seem to be recognized depending on the injection mode of the plasmid DNA. Indeed, Western blot analysis and pepitide-based mapping revealed that, for both pS2.SE2C and pCIE2t induced sera, different epitopes were recognized by the induced antibodies, independent of their titers. In addition, cross-reactivity of the induced sera as tested against purified E2 proteins as well as synthetic peptides derived from two distinct viral subtypes was found to depend on the injection mode of the plasmids. These data suggest that not only quantitative but also qualitative differences in the induced immune responses can be observed that are linked to both the nature of the antigen expressed and the immunization route. It is interesting to note that similar observations have recently been described in the influenza model [33]. In this study, the authors report that the viral nucleoprotein-specific immunoglobulin subclass and cytokine responses elicited by DNA vaccination are dependent on the injection route of the DNA. While endpoint IgG titers were identical, muscle injection resulted in predominantly IgG2a responses and gene immunization yielded a preponderance of IgG1 antibodies. In addition, production of cytokines in vitro following specific recall T cell activation was quite different, as for example IL-4 production could never be detected

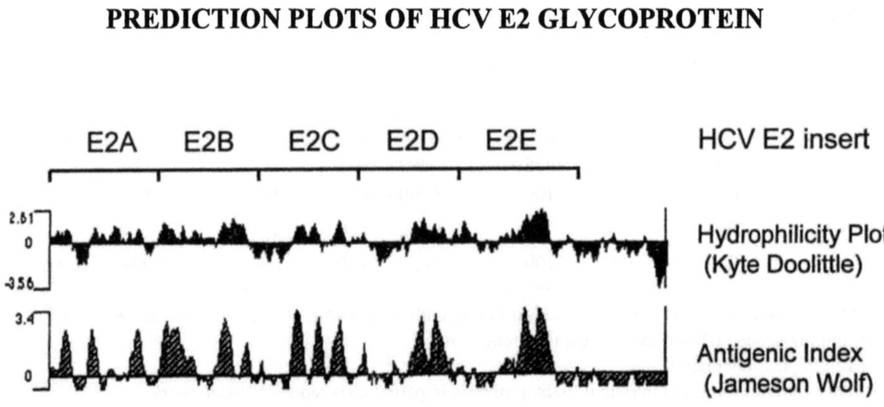

Fig. 4. Hydrophilic and antigenic predicted plots for HCV E2 glycoprotein. The map position of the different E2 insert sequences cloned in fusion with the HBsAg is indicated

following IM injection but increasing concentrations were observed following ID injection of the plasmids.

While it has been possible to document induction of humoral responses to the HCV-E2 protein following direct injection of plasmid DNA, induction of cellular responses remain to be documented. We have observed in preliminary experiments that IM injection of E2-encoding plasmids is indeed associated with the splenic production of IFN-γ but no IL-4, and that the levels of cytokines produced are low but constant over time, at least as observed between 3 and 24 weeks p.i. (I. Nakano, personal observation). A number of E2-specific CTL epitopes have been identified in chronically infected patients (for review see [21]), some of them mapping within rather conserved sequences of the antigen. Induction of such CTL could indeed be an important factor in the control of infection and vaccine strategies should also focus on designing E2 immunogens capable of inducing such responses.

Towards a nucleic acid-based vaccine against HCV?

As reviewed above, examples of studies focused on the evaluation of DNA-based immunization for the induction of immune responses specific for HCV antigens are still scarce. Work is ongoing in different laboratories, including ours, that focuses on additional genes encoding HCV antigens beside the viral nucleocapsid and the glycoprotein E2. These involve in particular the E1 glycoprotein potentially capable of inducing neutralizing antibodies, and the non-structural protein NS3 that has been shown to induce strong CTL. Experiments are also ongoing that use plasmids encoding the full-length HCV open reading frame (A. M. Prince, personal communication). Such experiments will provide complementary information to those obtained with strategies focused on expression of individual antigens. A genomic cDNA clone that is infectious in vivo has recently been reported [35] and should provide a very valuable tool for pursuing these studies. Among the many obstacles that face the development of an efficient HCV vaccine is the lack of appropriate analytical tools, including: (1) the lack of an in vitro replication assay, (2) the lack of a small susceptible animal model beside the chimpanzee, and (3) the lack of purified antigens, in particular the viral glycoproteins. HCV E1 and E2 antigens have been reported to associate and form two types of complex heterodimers, covalently and non-covalently linked, the latter presumably mimicking the native structure believed to exist on the surface of virions [7, 8]. Assessing the relevance of anti-envelope antibodies and their potential for neutralization, while awaiting for appropriate neutralization assays, should involve immunoprecipitation studies using such complexes as a potential marker for neutralizing capacity.

Finally, clinical studies have still to document what are the types of immune responses that are beneficial in the control and/or prevention of HCV infections. Such studies, as reviewed in the introduction of this chapter, seem to point towards the benefit of an early, strong and broad cellular response that appears to be asssociated either with spontaneous viral clearance or better outcome of antiviral treatments. Recent data, in addition, suggest that NOB antibodies may also be important for clearance of virus. Rosa et al. [37] have indeed documented, in long-term follow-up studies (up to 8 years), that spontaneous recovery from infection appears linked to the appearance of high anti-NOB antibody titers. Both fundamental and clinical studies are warranted for the design of the most efficient strategies for the development of a HCV vaccine, including a gene-based vaccine.

Acknowledgements. I would like to acknowledge the group at the INSERM U271 in Lyon who performed a number of experiments that were described in this chapter, Drs. G. Maertens, J. Dubuisson, and J. Haynes for their collaborative participation and fruitful discussion during the course of our studies and Dr. H. Lerat for his help with art work. Important financial contributions to our projects were from the ARC (Association pour la Recherche sur le Cancer) and the European Community through a BIOMED and a BIOTECH grant.

References

1. Bos JD, Kapsenberg ML (1993) The skin immune system: progress in cutaneous biology. Immunol Today 14 : 75
2. Botarelli P, Brunetto MR, Minutello MA, Calvo P, Unumaaz D, Weiner AJ, Choo QL, Shuster JR, Kuo G, Bonino F, Houghton M, Abrigiani S (1993) T lymphocyte response to hepatitis C virus in clinical courses of infection. Gastroenterology 104 : 580
3. Cahour A (1995) Les perspectives d'un vaccin contre l'hépatite C: quelle stratégie adopter? Méd Sci 11 : 81
4. Davis HL, Michel LM, Whalen RG (1993) DNA-based immunization induces continuous secretion of hepatitis B surface antigen and high levels of circulating antibody. Hum Mol Genet 3 : 1847
5. Delpeyroux F, Chenciner N, Lim A, Malpiece Y, Blondel B, Crainic R, Streeck RE (1986) A poliovirus neutralizing epitope expressed, on hybrid hepatitis B surface antigen particles. Science 233 : 472
6. Dietzschold B, Wang H, Rupprecht CE, Celis F, Tollis M, Ertl H, Heber-Katz E, Koprowski H (1987) Induction of protective immunity against rabies by immunization with rabies virus ribonucleoprotein. Proc Natl Acad Sci USA 84 : 9165
7. Dubuisson HJ, Hsu H, Cheung RC, Greenberg HB, Russell DC, Rice CM (1994) Formation and intracellular localization of hepatitis C virus envelope glycoprotein complexes expressed by recombinant vaccinia and Sindbis viruses. J Virol 68 : 6147
8. Dubuisson J, Rice CM (1996) Hepatitis C virus glycoprotein folding; disulfide bond formation and association with calnexi. J Virol 70 : 778
9. Enomoto N, Kuosaki M, Tanaka Y, Marumo F, Sato C (1994) Fluctuation of hepatitis C virus quasispecies in persistent infection and interferon treatment revealed by single-strand conformation polymorphism analysis. J Gen Virol 75 : 1361
10. Farci P, Alter HJ, Govindarajan S, Wong DC, Engle R, Lesniewski RR, Desai SM, Miller RH, Ogata N, Purcell RH (1992) Lack of protective immunity against reinfection with hepatitis C virus. Science 258 : 135
11. Farci P, Shimoda A, Wong D, Cabezon T, De Gionnis D, Srazzera A, Shimizu Y, Shapiro M, Alter HJ, Purcell RH (1996) Prevention of hepatitis C virus infection in chimpanzees by hyperimmune serum against the hypervariable region 1 of the envelope 2 protein. Proc Natl Acad Sci USA 93 : 15 394

12. Ferrari C, Valli A, Galati L, Penna A, Scaccaglia P, Giuberti T, Schienchi C, Missale G, Garcia Marin M, Fiaccadori F (1994) T cell response to structural and non-structural hepatitis C virus antigen in persistent and self-limited hepatitis C virus infection. Hepatology 19 : 286
13. Geissler M, Gesien A, Tokushige K, Wands JR (1997) Enhancement of cellular and humoral immune responses to hepatitis C virus (HCV) core protein using DNA based vaccines augmented with cytokine expressing plasmids. Abstracts of the Fourth International meeting on hepatitis C virus and related viruses, Kyoto, Japan, 6–10 March. Fujitsu Aprico, Tokyo, p 41
14. Higashi Y, Kakumi S, Yoshioka K, Wakita T, Mizokami M, Ohba K, Ito Y, Ishikawa TM, Nagai N (1993) Dynamics changes in the E2/NS1 region of hepatitis C virus in vivo. Virology 197 : 659
15. Inchauspé G, Vitviski L, Major ME, Jung G, Spengler U, Maisonnas M, Trépo C (1997) Plasmid DNA expressing a secreted or a nonsecreted form of hepatitis C virus nucleocapsid: comparative studies of antibody and T-helper responses following genetic immunization. DNA Cell Biol 16 : 185
16. Iwarson S, Tabor E, Thomas HC, Snoy P, Gerety RJ (1985) Protection against hepatitis B virus infection by immunization with hepatitis B core antigen. Gastroenterology 88 : 763
17. Kato N, Sekiya H, Ootsuyama Y, Nakasawa T, Hijikata M, Ohkoshi S, Shimotohno K (1993) Humoral immune response to the hypervariable region 1 of the putative envelope glycoprotein (gp70) of hepatitis C virus. J Virol 67 : 3923
18. Kato N, Ootsuyama Y, Sekiya H, Ohkoshi S, Nakazawa T, Hijikata M, Shimotohno K (1994) Genetic drift in hypervariable region I of the viral genome in persistent hepatitis C virus infection. J Virol 68 : 4776
19. Koizumi K, Enomoto N, Kurosaki M, Murakami T, Izumi N, Marumo F, Sato C (1995) Diversity of quasispecies in various diseases stages of chronic hepatitis C virus infection and its significance in interferon treatment. Hepatology 22 : 30
20. Kojima M, Osuga T, Tsuda F, Tanaka T, Okamoto H (1994) Influence of antibodies to the hypervariable region of E2/NS1 glycoprotein on the selective replication of hepatitis C virus in chimpanzees. Virology 204 : 665
21. Koshy R, Inchauspé G (1996) Evaluation of hepatitis C virus protein epitopes for vaccine development. Trends Biotechnol 14 : 365
22. Lagging LM, Meyer K, Hoft D, Houghton M, Belshe RB, Ray R (1995) Immune responses to plasmid DNA encoding the hepatitis C virus core protein. J Virol 69 : 5859
23. Lai ME, Mazzoleni AP, Argiolu F, De Virgilis S, Balestrieri A, Purcell RH, Cao A, Farci P (1994) Hepatitis C virus in multiple episodes of acute hepatitis in polytransfused thalassaemic children. Lancet 343 : 338
24. Leroux-Roels G, Alvadero Esquivel C, DeLeys R, Stuyver L, Elewaut A, Philippé J, Desombre L, Paradijs J, Maerteens G (1996) Lymphoproliferative responses to hepatitis C virus core, E1, E2 and NS3 in patients with chronic hepatitis C infection treated with interferon alfa. Hepatology 23 : 8
25. Major MM, Vivitski L, Mink MA, Schleef M, Whalen RG, Trépo C, Inchauspé G (1995) DNA-based immunization with chimeric vectors for the induction of immune responses against the hepatitis C virus nucleocapsid. J Virol 69 : 5798
26. Mast EE, Alter MJ (1993) Epidemiology of viral hepatitis: an overview. Semin Virol 4 : 273
27. Michel ML, Mancini M, Sobczak E, Favier V, Guetard D, Bahraoui EM (1988) Induction of anti-human immunodeficiency virus (HIV) neutralizing antibodies in rabbits immunized with recombinant HIV-hepatitis B surface antigen particles. Proc Natl Acad Sci USA 85 : 7957
28. Missale G, Bertoni R, Lamonaca V, Valli A, Massari M, Mori C, Rumi MG, Houghton M, Fiaccadori F, Ferrari C (1996) Different clinical behaviors of acute hepatitis C virus infection are associated with different vigor of the anti-viral-cell mediated immune responses. J Clin Invest 98 : 706
29. Nakano I, Maertens G, Major ME, Vitvitski L, Dubuisson J, Fournillier A, De Martynoff G, Trépo C, Inchauspé G (1997) Direct injection of HCV-E2 encoding plasmid DNA: induction of antibody responses and dependence on the immunization mode. Abstracts of the Fourth International Meeting on Hepatitis C virus and Related Viruses, Kyoto, Japan, 6–10 March. Fujitsu Aprico, Tokyo, p 79
30. Nakano I, Maertens G, Major ME, Vitvitski L, Dubuisson J, Fournillier A, De Martynoff G, Trépo C, Inchauspé G (1997) Immunization with plasmid DNA encoding hepatitis C virus envelope E2 antigenic domains induces antibodies whose immune reactivity is linked to the injection mode. J Virol 71 : 7101–7109
31. Okada SI, Akahane Y, Suzuki H, Okamoto H, Mishiro S (1992) The degree of variability in the amino-terminal region of the E2/NS1 protein of hepatitis C virus correlates with responsiveness to interferon therapy in viremic patients. Hepatology 16 : 619

32. Paterlini P, Driss F, Nalpas B, Pisi E, Franco D, Berthelot P (1993) Persistence of hepatitis B and hepatitis C genomes in primary liver cancers from HBsAg-negative patients: a study of a low-endemic area. Hepatology 17 : 20
33. Pertner TM, Roberts TR, Haynes JR (1996) Influenza virus nucleoprotein-specific immunoglobulin G subclass and cytokine responses elicited by DNA vaccination are dependent on the route of vector DNA delivery. J Virol 70 : 6119
34. Prince AM, Brotman B, Huima T, Pascual D, Jaffrey M, Inchauspé G (1992) Immunity in hepatitis C virus infection. J Infect Dis 165 : 438
35. Kolykhalov AA, Agapov EV, Blight KF, Mihalik K, Feinstone SM, Rice CM (1997) Transmission of hepatitis C by intrahepatic inoculation with transcribed RNA. Science 277 : 570–574
36. Rosa D, Campagnoli S, Moretto C, Cuenzi E, Cousens L, Chin M, Dong C, Weiner AJ, Lau JYN, Choo QL, Chien D, Pileri P, Houghton M, Abrignani S (1996) A quantitative test to estimate neutralizing antibodies to the hepatitis C virus: cytofluorimetric assessment of envelope glycoprotein 2 binding to target cells. Proc Natl Acad Sci USA 93 : 1759
37. Rosa D, Ishii K, Miyamura T, Houghton M, Abrigiani S (1977) High titers of envelope neutralizing antibodies correlate with both prevention of HCV infection and resolution of chronic hepatitis C. Abstracts of the Fourth International Meeting on Hepatitis C virus and Related Viruses, Kyoto, 6–10 March. Fujitsu Aprico, Tokyo, p 58
38. Sekiya H, Kato N, Ootsuyama Y, Nakazawa T, Yamauchi K, Shimotohno K (1994) Genetic alterations of the putative envelope proteins encoding region of the hepatitis C virus in the progression to relapsed phase from acute hepatitis: humoral immune response to hypervariable region 1. Int J Cancer 57 : 664
39. Shirai M, Okada H, Nishioka M, Akatsuka T, Wuchowski C, Houghten R, Pendleton CD, Feinstone SM, Berzofski JA (1994) An epitope in hepatitis C core region recognized by cytotoxic T cells in mice and humans. J Virol 68 : 3334
40. Stingl G, Tschachler E, Groh V, Wolff K, Hauser C (1989) The immune functions of epidermal cells. Immunol Sei 4 . 3
41. Tedeschi V, Akatsuka T, Wai-Kuo Shih J, Battegay M, Feistone SE (1997) A specific antibody response to HCV E2 elicited in mice by intramuscular inoculation of plasmid DNA containing coding sequences for E2. Hepatology 25 : 459
42. Tokushige K, Wakita T, Pachuk C, Moradpour D, Weiner DB, Zurawski VR, and Wands J (1996) Expression and immune response to hepatitis C virus core DNA based vaccine constructs. Hepatology 24 : 14
43. Ulmer JB, Donnelly JJ, Parker SE, Rhodes GH, Felgner PL, Dwarki VJ, Deck RR, DeWitt CM, Friedman A, Hawe LA, Leander KR, Martinez D, Perry HC, Shiver JW, Montgomery DL, Liu MA (1993) Heterologous protection against influenza by injection of DNA encoding a viral protein. Science 259 : 1745
44. Van Doorn LJ, Capriles I, Maertens G, DeLeys R, Murray, Kos T, Schellekens H, Hand II, Quint W (1995) Sequence evolution of the hypervariable region in the putative envelope region E2/NS1 of hepatitis C virus is correlated with specific humoral immune responses. J Virol 69 : 773
45. Weiner AJ, Brauer MJ, Rosemblatt J, Richman KH, Tung J, Crawford K, Bonino F, Saracco G, Choo QL, Houghton M, Han JH (1991) Variable and hypervariable domains are found in the regions of HCV corresponding to flavivirus envelope and NS1 proteins and the pestivirus envelope proteins. Virology 180 : 842
46. Weiner AJ, Geysens HM, Christopherson C, Hall EJ, Mason TJ, Saracco G, Bonino F, Crawford K, Marion CD, Crawford KA, Brunetto M, Barr PJ, Miyamura T, McHutchinson J, Houghton M (1992) Evidence of immune selection of hepatitis C virus (HCV) putative envelope glycoprotein variants: potential role in chronic HCV infections. Proc Natl Acad Sci USA 89 : 3468
47. Wolff JA, Ludtke JJ, Acsadi G, Williams P, Jani A (1992) Long-term persistence of plasmid DNA and foreign gene expression in mouse muscle. Hum Mol Genet 6 : 363
48. Zibert A, Schreier E, Roggendorf M (1995) Antibodies in human sera specific to hypervariable region 1 of hepatitis C virus can block viral attachment. Virology 208 : 653

Gene immunization for allergic disorders

Mark Roman[1], Hans L. Spiegelberg[3], David Broide[2], Eyal Raz[2]

[1] Dynavax Technologies Corporation, 3099 Science Park Road, San Diego, CA 92121, USA
[2] Department of Medicine, University of California San Diego, School of Medicine, La Jolla CA 92093, USA
[3] Department of Pediatrics, University of California San Diego, School of Medicine, La Jolla CA 92093, USA

Introduction

The allergic response

The allergic response is mediated by binding of allergens to specific IgE antibodies attached via IgE receptors to the surface of mast cells and basophils. The binding of allergens by surface IgE causes degranulation resulting in release of histamine and other mediators of inflammation including interleukin (IL)-4, and IL-5. This IgE-mediated response is called the immediate-phase (hypersensitivity) reaction [1], and occurs within seconds to minutes of allergen exposure. The late-phase response results from the secretion of proinflammatory mediators such as leukotrienes and platelet-activating factor [1], occurs 4–24 hours later and is characterized by the infiltration of eosinophils into the site of allergen exposure. These eosinophils are activated in response to immune complexes, Th2 and mast cell mediators, resulting in the release of toxic substances such as major basic protein (MBP) which causes tissue damage [2]. The release of proinflammatory mediators from both the immediate and late responses then lead to pulmonary allergic inflammation.

Immunotherapy versus pharmacological treatment for allergies

Immunotherapy for allergic disorders has been practiced since the beginning of the century and involves the subcutaneous injection of small, but gradually increasing amounts of allergen. However, the risk of inducing anaphylactic reactions by injection of soluble allergens and the general variability in efficacy with many allergens, has led to a decline in its practice over the last 15 years. Furthermore, the use of new pharmacological agents for allergic disorders allows for the control of allergic symptoms at a lower risk to benefit ratio than immunotherapy [3]. However, immunotherapy could regain status as a viable therapy for the treatment of allergies, if a safe and effective

Correspondence to: M. Roman

immunotherapeutic agent or modality were developed. The criteria for this therapy would be: (1) the therapeutic agent would not react with IgE bound to mast cells and trigger adverse or anaphylactic reactions; and (2) that the administration of these preparations would result in therapeutic improvement, i.e., a decrease in the severity of the allergic symptoms, reduced need of daily anti-allergic drugs such as β-agonists and corticosteroids, and reduction of medical attention.

Immunization with plasmid DNA (pDNA) which encodes allergens (antigens) may provide a novel method of immunotherapy for allergic disorders. Recent research in vaccine development has shown that gene vaccines do not induce local inflammation [4], do not induce IgE antibodies [5], and may actually down-regulate antigen-specific IgE synthesis and eosinophil abundance and infiltration in the lung [5, 6]. The role of DNA immunization as a modifier of allergic disorders is the subject of this review.

Induction of Th1 immune responses by gene immunization

Allergen-encoding pDNA injected (intradermally, i.d. or intramuscularly, i.m.) into mice induces long-lasting antigen-specific cellular and humoral immune responses with a Th1 phenotype [5, 7]. This response is characterized by the stimulation of the Th1 lymphocytes which secrete primarily interferon-γ (IFN-γ) and IL-2. IFN-γ plays a key role in Th1 responses by promoting the differentiation of naive T helper or Th0 cells to Th1 cells, thus increasing the abundance of antigen-specific Th1 cells capable of further secreting IFN-γ in response to specific antigen [8]. These IFN-γ-secreting Th1 cells then interact with their B cells, where they induce IgG2a antibody synthesis and inhibit IgE antibody secretion [9]. In addition, because Th1 and Th2-mediated responses are reciprocally regulated, the Th1 cytokine IFN-γ may inhibit the effects of the Th2 cytokines IL-4 and IL-5 [10], i.e., inhibiting Th0 cell differentiation to Th2 cells, IL-4-enhanced B cell secretion of IgE antibodies, and IL-5-stimulated proliferation of eosinophils. As a result of this negative regulation, the induction of Th1 responses may be beneficial to the treatment of allergies considered to result from enhanced Th2 responses to allergens [11, 12].

Gene immunization for allergic disorders

Gene versus protein immunization: the primary response

As mentioned, i.d. and i.m. gene injection of pDNA encoding antigens results in the induction of a Th1 immune response. In mice, the Th1 phenotype response is generally characterized by the induction of an IgG2a isotype and IFN-γ production [5], whereas a Th2 response (protein in alum immunization) mainly induces IgG1 and IgE antibodies, (Fig. 1) [13, 14] IL-4, IL-5 and IL-10 production. The immunization of mice with pDNA expressing the LacZ gene resulted in the induction of IgG2a antibodies [5], and the stimulation in vitro of their splenocytes with β-galactosidase (β-gal) resulted in the secretion of high levels of IFN-γ and low levels of IL-4 and IL-5, indicating a Th1 response (Table 1). In contrast, no IFN-γ but high levels of IL-4 and IL-5 were secreted from the splenocytes of β-gal protein in alum-immunized mice stimulated in vitro with antigen, indicating a Th2 response (Table 1) [5, 17].

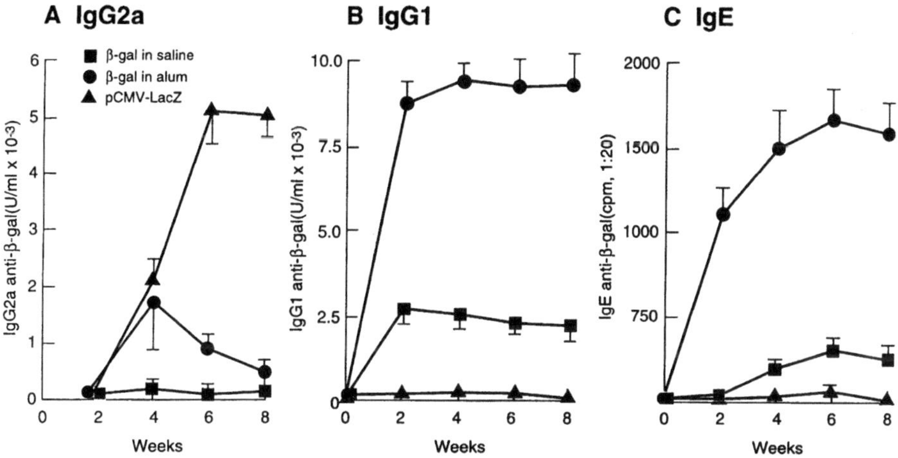

Fig. 1. Primary IgG subclass and IgE immune response of BALB/c mice after intradermal (i.d.) injection of 100 μg LacZ-pDNA (pCMV-LacZ) (▲), 10 μg β-galactosidase (β-gal) in saline (■) or 1 μg β-gal in alum (●)

Table 1. Lymphokine secretion by β-gal-activated CD4+ splenic T cells from pDNA and/or protein immunized mice[a]

Exp.	Priming	Boosting	IFN-γ pg/ml	IL-4 pg/ml	IL-5 Units/ml
A	None	None	< 10	< 2	< 2
B	LacZ-pDNA	None	741 ± 170	< 2	< 2
C	β-gal/saline	None	< 10	12 ± 2	15 ± 4
D	β-gal/alum	None	< 10	351 ± 24	642 ± 51
E	LacZ-pDNA	β-gal/alum	1050 ± 314	4 ± 2	46 ± 10
F	β-gal/saline	β-gal/alum	53 ± 48	126 ± 43	165 ± 54
G	β-gal/alum	LacZ-pDNA	730 ± 193	307 ± 128	183 ± 70

[a] LacZ-pDNA mice were injected with 100 μg pDNA (ampicillin resistance) encoding β-galactosidase (β-gal). β-gal/alum mice received 10 μg β-gal protein in alum. Cytokines were measured by enzyme-linked immunosorbent assay using Biosource kits or reagents.
Means ± SE of spleens from four mice per experiment (*β-gal* β-galactosidase, *pDNA* plasmid DNA, *IFN* interferon, *IL* interleukin)

Gene versus protein immunization: the secondary response

The results of protein or gene boosting of mice, which had previously been immunized with protein in alum or antigen-encoding pDNA, are shown in Fig. 2. When mice immunized with β-gal protein in alum were boosted with β-gal in alum, the levels of β-gal-specific IgG1 and IgE increased, as expected. In contrast, when LacZ-gene-immunized mice were boosted with β-gal in alum, further increases in specific IgG2a antibodies occurred without the induction of antigen-specific IgE antibodies [5]. However, if LacZ-pDNA-immunized mice were boosted with ovalbumin (OVA), IgE antibodies to OVA were induced demonstrating that the IgE antibody inhibition by pDNA immunization was antigen specific. Hsu et al. [15] recently reported that immunization of rats with pDNA encoding the house dust mite allergen Der p 5 inhibited subsequent IgE production, indicating a similar response to a human allergen [15].

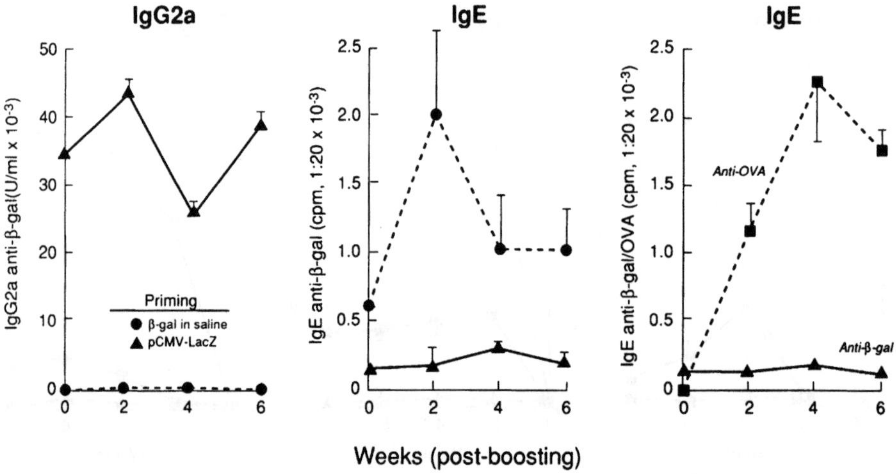

Fig. 2. IgG2a and IgE response of BALB/c mice primed with 100 μg LacZ-pDNA (pCMV-LacZ) and boosted with 1 μg β-gal in alum (▲). Control mice were primed with 10 μg β-gal in saline (●). For the antigen specificity control, mice primed with LacZ-pDNA were injected with 2 μg ovalbumin (OVA) in alum (■)

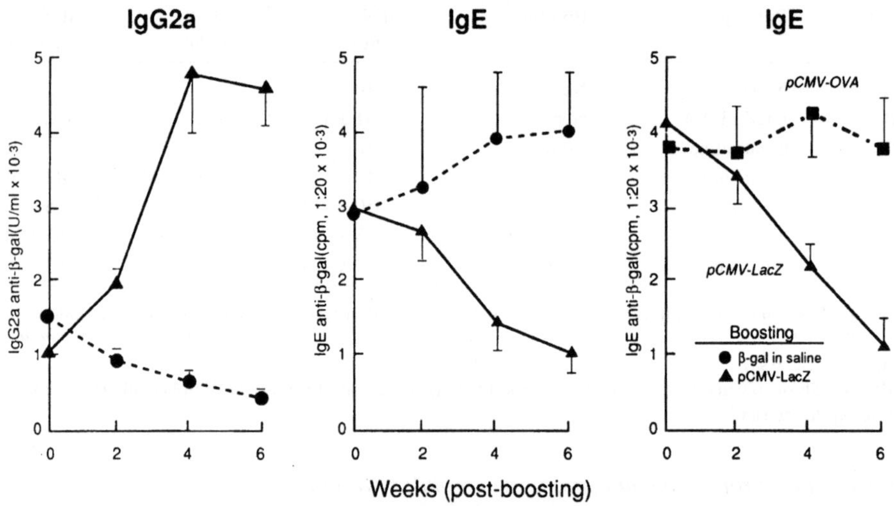

Fig. 3. IgG2a and IgE response of BALB/c mice primed with 1 μg β-gal in alum and boosted with 100 μg LacZ-pDNA (pCMV-LacZ) (▲). Control mice were primed with 1 μg β-gal in saline (●). For antigen specificity control, mice were boosted with OVA-pDNA (■)

Down-regulation of IgE antibodies by pDNA immunization

The prevention of IgE synthesis by pDNA immunization provoked us to investigate the use of pDNA immunization for the treatment of an animal model of a allergic disorder. If pDNA immunization could prevent subsequent formation of IgE, could it down-regulate an existing IgE response?

To mimic an allergic response, mice were primed with β-gal in alum to induce anti-β-gal IgE antibodies. Six weeks after priming, these mice were immunized with LacZ-pDNA, resulting in a 75% reduction of anti-β-gal IgE antibodies and in an increase in anti-β-gal IgG2a antibodies [5] (Fig. 3). The decrease in IgE antibody levels was antigen specific, as pDNA immunization with an OVA-encoding pDNA did not result in decreases in anti-β-gal IgE. Specific down-regulation of anti-Hev b 5 (latex allergen) IgE by gene immunization has been reported [16]. In this study a 23% decrease of the Hev 5 IgE antibody levels occurred 10 days after pDNA injection of rats previously induced to synthesize anti-Hev b 5 IgE. Taken together, these results demonstrate that genetic immunization can result in a decrease of antigen-specific IgE antibodies [5, 6]. A model of the presumed mechanism is illustrated in Fig. 4 and is discussed in the next section.

Potential mechanism of IgE Inhibition by pDNA immunization

It is difficult to know precisely what occurs in vivo as a result of gene vaccination. However, the analysis of the lymphokine secretion profiles of $CD4^+$ splenic T cells stimulated in vitro with antigen can give us some insight into what may be occurring in vivo. Splenocytes from LacZ-pDNA-immunized mice (either prior to or after β-gal in alum immunization) produced similar levels of IFN-γ after antigen stimulation in vitro (Table 1).

The IL-4 levels produced by these same groups were also similar, that is, the induction of IFN-γ secretion (in the LacZ-pDNA after β-gal in alum) did not inhibit IL-4 secretion. Therefore, it seems that the IFN-γ production by the newly induced Th1 cells appeared to be sufficient to cause the 75% decrease of the ongoing IgE antibody formation within the 6 week observation period, despite the influence of continued IL-4 production (Fig. 3). pDNA immunization results in prolonged antigen expression by the cells transfected in vivo [4]. Therefore, Th1 stimulation and recruitment may be a continual process that leads to increasing amounts of Th1-B cell interactions (Fig. 4). This would explain the progressive decrease of anti-β-gal IgE levels after injections of LacZ-pDNA. It remains to be shown whether a pre-existing Th2 response and IgE antibody formation can be completely eliminated over a longer period by multiple pDNA injections, can be replaced by a Th1 response, and to what extent the IgE-down-regulation will be therapeutic.

Gene immunization suppresses pulmonary eosinophilic inflammation

Immunization with allergen-encoding pDNA not only inhibits IgE antibody formation in mice and rats but also inhibits the allergic response in the lung after challenge with allergen inhalation [6]. Mice immunized with OVA-pDNA and challenged by OVA inhalation showed significantly reduced numbers of eosinophils in the bronchial airway lavage fluid (from 43% to 3.5%), in the lung tissue and also in the bone marrow (from 10.3% to 1.4%) as compared to control mice [6]. Taken together these findings indicate that immunization with pDNA encoding allergens suppresses not only IgE antibody formation (the hypersensitivity phase of the allergic reaction), but also inhibits the late-phase allergic reaction. The analysis of the lymphokine secretion profiles of $CD4^+$ splenic T cells stimulated in vitro with antigen (Table 1) showed that LacZ-

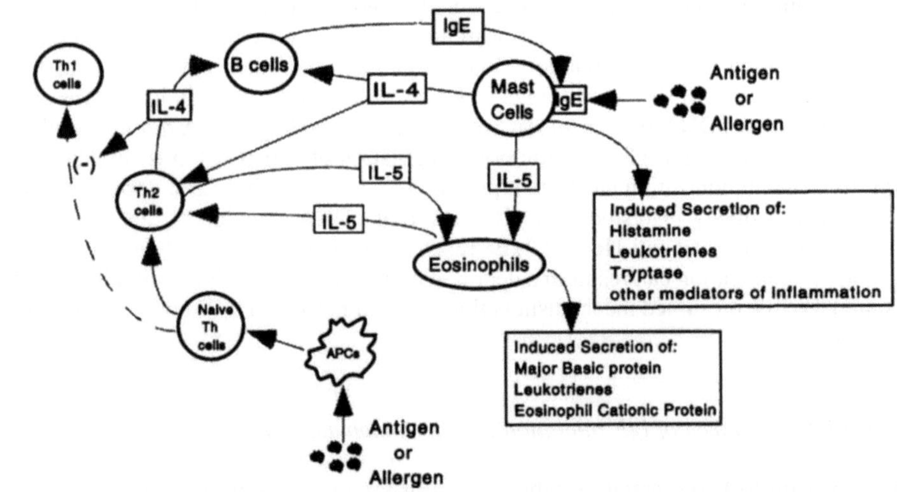

A Th 2 Response to Allergens Induces or Facilitates Allergic Inflammation

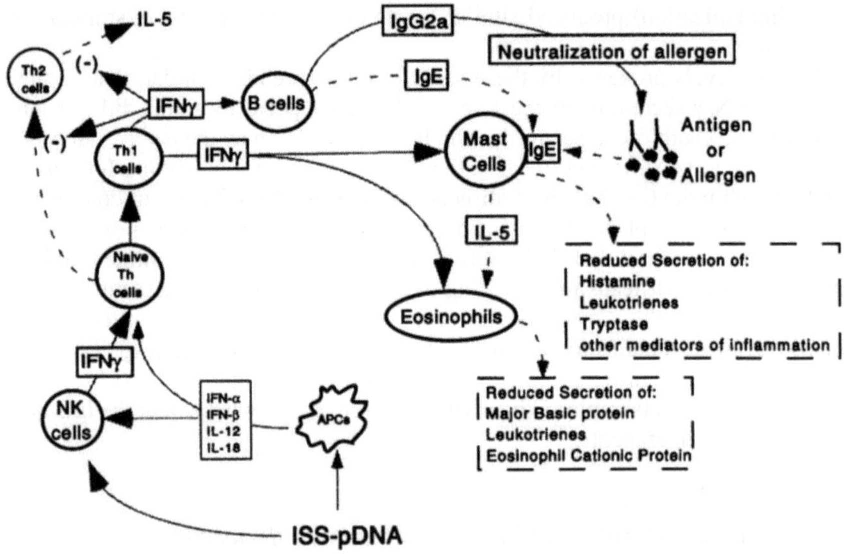

B Th 1 Response to Allergens Induced by Allergen Gene Vaccination Reduces Allergic Inflammation

pDNA immunization of β-gal protein-primed mice resulted in a decrease in IL-5 levels. Since IL-5 influences eosinophil differentiation and survival, it is probable that the observed decrease in eosinophil numbers mentioned above, was the result of IFN-γ inhibition of IL-5 secretion (Fig. 4).

◀ **Fig. 4.** How gene immunization may break the allergic cycle. Solid lines indicate enhanced responses, whereas dotted lines indicate inhibited responses. **A** Cellular interaction among theTh2 cells, mast cells and eosinophils generate the allergic response. The key cytokines interleukin (IL)-4 and IL-5 act to induce IgE production and eosinophil proliferation, respectively. The excessive production of IL-4 and IL-5 also influences naive Th cells to differentiate further into Th2 cells which further enhance the allergic response. Positive feedback of these factors leads to increases in allergic inflammation. **B** The induction of interferon-γ (IFN-γ) by allergen gene immunization may break the allergic cycle. Plasmid DNA contains the information for the allergen synthesis, and immunostimulatory sequences (ISS) which deliver an adjuvant effect with Th1-promoting properties. Antigen-presenting cells (APC) transfected in vivo secrete IFN-inducing cytokines, which enhances IFN-γ secretion from natural killer (NK) cells. Increased Th1 differentiation and subsequent IFN-γ secretion results in the inhibition of IL-5 secretion, decreased IgE secretion, and mast cell and eosinophil degranulation. Together, the induction of a allergen-specific Th1 response to the allergen inhibits the allergic reactions in various steps as shown above

Table 2. pDNA immunization inhibition of pulmonary eosinophilic inflammation[a]

Priming	Sensitization	Challenge	Blood	BM	BALF	Lung
1) Saline	+	+	5.0 ± 2.4	10.2 ± 1.8	39.5 ± 5.0	40.3 ± 15.8
2) OVA-pDNA	+	+	4.0 ± 0.8	3.1 ± 0.7	6.2 ± 1.8	12.0 ± 1.4
3) pUC19	+	+	8.1 + 0.7	8.4 ± 0.5	32.2 ± 7.2	38.5 ± 1.7
4) Naive	–	–	7.4 ± 2.0	3.7 ± 0.5	0 ± 0	0 ± 0

[a] Differential counts (%) of eosinophils in various tissues after ovalbumin (OVA) inhalation. OVA gene vaccines (50 μg OVA-pDNA administered i.d.) given prior to repeated OVA/alum administration (groups 2 and 3), inhibited the subsequent eosinophil infiltrate in the bone marrow (BM), in the bronchial airway lavage fluid (BALF) and in the lung tissue (Lung) after inhalation challenge with OVA (eight mice/group). Eosinophil cell counts were performed by a "blinded" investigator on slides coded with numbers. Five hundred white blood cells were counted in the BALF of each mouse and ten random light microscope fields of lung sections were analyzed for determination of the eosinophils in the lung tissue. Results are means ± S.E.

The adjuvanticity of DNA: the effect of immunostimulatory DNA sequences

The role of immunostimulatory sequences in pDNA immunization

While characterizing the immune responses induced by pDNA immunization, we found that the presence of specific DNA sequences were essential for the induction of a Th1 response [17]. Certain plasmids differing only in their antibiotic resistance gene, induced different levels of immune responses. Specifically, plasmids containing the kanamycin resistance (kanR) gene induced significantly lower anti-β-gal immune responses than the equivalent plasmid containing an ampicillin resistance (ampR) gene, even though the kanR construct produced higher levels of β-gal expression from cells transfected in vitro [17]. Consequently, it seemed that the ampR gene within the pDNA construct was having an adjuvant effect. It had previously been reported that palindromic single-stranded DNA sequences having the 5′-purine-purine-C-G-pyrimidine-pyrimidine-3′ (CpG motif) have an immunomodulatory effect [18, 19]. Screening of the ampR gene showed that it contained two 5′-AACGTT-3′ repeats, whereas the kanR gene used in our study contained no such sequences. The premise that the immunostimulatory sequences (ISS) were responsible for the differential outcome of the immune responses in vivo was confirmed when the insertion of one or two 14-bp double-stranded oligonucleotides containing the 5′-AACGTT-3′-ISS into the kanR gene-containing vector resulted in vectors which induced immune responses similar to the ampR vectors [17].

When pDNA expression vectors were compared for their ability to induce IgG2a antibodies and a cytotoxic T lymphocyte (CTL) response, ISS-deficient vectors were greatly reduced in their ability to induce either antibodies or CTL responses to the gene product [17]. Furthermore, when a non-antigen-encoding ISS-containing pDNA was co-injected (i.d.) with antigen-encoding pDNA, the adjuvant effect of the ISS-pDNA was observed (i.e., enhanced antibody and CTL responses to the gene product). The adjuvant effect was also observed when ISS-pDNA was co-injected with protein antigens. Indeed, the i.d. co-injection of ISS-containing plasmids (ampR gene-containing pUC19), or ISS-enriched KanR plasmids with protein antigens resulted in a Th1-like response to the protein antigens in mice, whereas the protein immunization alone or in alum resulted in a Th2-like immune response [20] (M. Roman, et al., Nature Medicine, in press). These experiments support the notion that the ISS act as an adjuvant which induces Th1-promoting cytokine secretion and suggest that the ISS play a major role in the induction of the Th1 response to encoded proteins observed in pDNA-vaccinated animals.

Cytokine induction by immunostimulatory DNA sequences

To investigate the potential mechanism of the adjuvant effect of ISS-containing DNA, we compared the cytokine response of murine and human cells to ISS-deficient DNA, ISS-containing DNA (oligonucleotides or plasmids), and methylated ISS-containing DNA (methylated at the cytosine of the CG) in vitro. The introduction of non-methylated ISS-containing DNA into human peripheral blood mononuclear cells (PBMC) resulted in the transcription of various cytokine genes including IFN-α, IFN-β, IFN-γ, IL-12, and IL-18, all of which are inducers of IFN-γ, while methylated or mutated (CG $\rightarrow$ GG) pDNA did not induce similar gene transcription [21] (M. Roman, et al., Nature Medicine, in press). Recently there has been much attention drawn to the induction of innate immune responses to ISS-containing DNA. In addition to the induction of IFN-α, IFN-β, IL-12, IFN-γ, and IL-18 mentioned above, ISS-containing DNA has been shown to activate natural killer (NK) cells to proliferate and secrete IFN-γ [22, 23], and to activate B cells to proliferate and to secrete IgM antibodies [24]. The innate responses to ISS-containing DNA occurs without the presence of antigen, yet this innate response contributes greatly to the antigen-dependent processes. This is apparent in the observed outcome of pDNA vaccination, in that ISS-containing DNA induces effective Th1 immune responses: (1) within antigen-encoding expression vectors, (2) when non-encoding ISS-containing DNA (adjuvant) is co-injected with antigen-encoding expression vectors, and (3) when non-encoding ISS-containing DNA (adjuvant) is co-injected with protein antigens.

The conclusion from these data is that, ISS-containing DNA exerts multiple influences on the innate and adaptive immune system, resulting in a Th1 bias, and a productive cellular immune response. Such ISS-containing DNA-induced responses are similar to those generated by viral infection or infection by certain pathogenic bacteria [4, 7, 17]. Therefore, the use of ISS-containing DNA can be exploited by current DNA-immunization techniques to yield Th1 responses which may be useful for the development of vaccines for allergies, infectious diseases, and cancer.

Conclusions

For immunotherapy to regain a major role as a treatment for allergic disorders, improvements in current allergen immunotherapy are needed to decrease treatment-associated risks when compared to the risks involved in current pharmacological management protocols [1]. The recent findings described in this review suggest that there is potential for the development of a novel form of immunotherapy, i.e., allergen gene vaccination, which would be safe and effective. Gene vaccination does not result in inflammation when injected i.d. and has been shown to down-regulate antigen-specific IgE antibodies in mice and rats, and in the reduction of late phase allergic responses. The presence of ISS-containing DNA in the vaccine formulation, whether within the pDNA expression vectors, or co-injected, is important in the induction of IFN-γ-mediated Th1 cell differentiation, IL-5 inhibition, and B cell isotype switching, which cumulatively may lead to the reduction of allergic responses (Fig. 4).

To date, all the in vivo experiments showing IgE inhibition have been performed in mice and rats. However, based on the combined observations that pDNA is also taken up by human skin cells transplanted onto nude mice [25], and that ISS-containing DNA induces Th1-promoting cytokines from human PBMC, it is possible that the anti-allergic responses observed in rodents will also occur in human. As for safety considerations, in vitro data indicate that the transfected cells secrete low levels of antigen which are unlikely to induce the anaphylactic reactions seen in vivo with classical immunotherapy. Furthermore, the allergens encoded by pDNA constructs can be designed to include a transmembrane domain and anchor, thereby preventing the secretion of allergen and possible induction of anaphylactic reactions.

Acknowledgements. Figures 1–3 are reproduced with the permission of Proc Natl Acad Sci USA (1996) 93: pages 5141–5145. This work was supported by US National Institutes of Health Grant AI 37305 and AI 40682.

References

1. Mygind N, Dahl R, Pederson S, Thestrup-Pederson K (1996) Essential allergy, 2nd edn. Blackwell Oxford
2. Frigas E, Motojima S, Gleich GJ (1991) The eosinophilic injury to the mucosa of the airways in the pathogenesis of bronchial asthma. Eur Respir J [Suppl] 13:123s
3. Adkinson NF, Eggleston PA, Eney D, Goldstein EO, Schuberth KC, Bacon JR, Hamilton RG, Weiss ME, Arshad H, Meinert CL, Tanascia J, Wheeler B (1997) A controlled trial of immunotherapy for asthma in allergic children. N Engl J Med 336:324
4. Raz E, Carson DA, Parker SE, Parr TB, Abai AM, Aichinger G, Gromkowski SH, Singh M, Lew D, Yankauckas MA, Baird S, Rhodes GH (1994) Intradermal gene immunization: the possible role of DNA uptake in the induction of cellular immunity to viruses. Proc Natl Acad Sci USA 91:9519
5. Raz E, Tighe H, Sato Y, Corr MP, Dudler JA, Roman M, Swain SL, Spiegelberg HL, Carson DA (1996) Preferential induction of a Th1 immune response and inhibition of specific IgE antibody formation by plasmid DNA immunization. Proc Natl Acad Sci USA 93:5141
6. Broide D, Orozco EM, Roman M, Carson DA, Raz E (1997) Intradermal gene vaccination down-regulates both arms of the allergic response. J Allergy Clin Immunol 99:S129
7. Ulmer JB, Donnelly JJ, Parker SE, Rhodes GH, Felgner PL, Dwarki VJ, Gromkowski SH, Randall-Deck RR, DeWitt CM, Friedman A, Hawe LA, Leander KR, Martinez D, Perry HC, Shiver JW, Montgomery DL, Liu MA (1993) Heterologous protection against influenza by injection of DNA encoding a viral protein. Science 259:1745
8. Mosmann TR, Coffman RL (1989) The Th1 and Th2 cells: differrent patterns of lymphokine secretion lead to different functional properties. Annu Rev Immunol 7:145–173

9. Coffman RL, Carty J (1985) A T cell activity that enhances polyclonal IgE production and its inhibition by interferon-γ. J Immunol 136:949
10. Snapper CM, Paul WE (1987) Interferon-γ and B cell stimulatory factor-1 reciprocally regulate Ig isotype production. Science 236:944
11. Parronchi P, Macchia D, Piccini MP, Biswas P, Simonelli C, Maggi E, Ricci M, Ansari AA, Romagnani S (1991) Allergen- and bacterial antigen-specific T-cell clones established from atopic donors show a different profile of cytokine production. Proc Natl Acad Sci USA 88:4538
12. Wierenga EA, Snock M, Groot C de, Chretien I, Bos JD, Jansen HM, Kapsenberg M (1990) Evidence for compartmentalization of functional subsets of $CD4^+$ T lymphocytes in atopic patients. J Immunol 144:4651–4656
13. Coutelier JP, Logt JTM van der, Heessen WA, Waarner G, van-Snick J (1987) IgG2a restriction of murine antibodies elicited by viral infections. J Exp Med 165:2373
14. Beck L, Spiegelberg HL (1989) The polyclonal and antigen-specific IgE and IgG subclass response of mice injected with ovalbumin in alum or complete Freund's adjuvant. Cell Immunol 123:1
15. Hsu CH, Chua KY, Tao MH, Lai YL, Wu HD, Huang SK, Hsieh KH (1996) Immunoprophylaxis of allergen-induced immunoglobulin E synthesis and airway hyper responsiveness in vivo by genetic immunization. Nature Med 2:540
16. Slater JE, Zhang YJ, Athur-Smith A, Colberg-Poley A (1997) A DNA vaccine inhibits IgE responses to the latex allergen Hev b 5 in mice. J Allergy Clin Immunol 99:S504
17. Sato Y, Roman M, Tighe H, Lee D, Corr MP, Nguyen MD, Silverman GJ, Lotz M, Carson DA, Raz E (1996) Immunostimulatory DNA sequences necessary for effective intradermal gene immunization. Science 273:352
18. Yamamoto S, Yamamoto T, Kataoka T, Kuramoto E, Yano O, Tokunaga T (1992) Unique palindromic sequences in sythetic oligonucleotides are required to induce IFN and IFN-mediated natural killer activity. J Immunol 148:4072–4076
19. Klinman DM, Yi AK, Beaucage SL, Conover J, Krieg AM (1996) CpG motifs present in bacterial DNA rapidly induce lymphocytes to secrete interleukin 6, interleukin 12, and interferon γ. Proc Natl Acad Sci USA 93:2879
20. Raz E, Roman M, Orozco EM, Carson DA (1997) Immunostimulatory DNA sequences (ISS) are a Th1 promoting adjuvant. J Allergy Clin Immunol 99:S365
21. Roman M, Orozco EM, Goodman J, Nguyen MD, Sato Y, Ronaghy A, Kornbluth RS, Richman DD, Carson DA, Raz E (1997) Immunostimulatory DNA sequences function as T helper-1-promoting adjuvants. Nat Med 3 : 849–854
22. Cowdery JS, Chace JH, Yi AK, Krieg AM (1996) Bacterial DNA induces NK cells to produce IFN-gamma in vivo and increases the toxicity of lipopolysaccharides. J Immunol 156:4570
23. Krieg AM, Yi AK, Matson S, Waldschmidt TJ, Bishop GA, Teasdale R, Koretzky GA, Klinman DM (1995) CpG motifs in bacterial DNA trigger direct B-cell activation. Nature 374:546
24. Liang H, Nishioka Y, Reich CF, Pisetsky DS, Lipsky PE (1996) Activation of human B cells by phosphorothioate oligodeoxynucleotides. J Clin Invest 98:1119
25. Hengge UR, Walker PS, Vogel JC (1996) Expression of naked DNA in human, pig, and mouse skin. J Clin Invest 97:2911

Immunization with DNA vaccines in early life: advantages and limitations as compared to conventional vaccines

Claire-Anne Siegrist, Paul-Henri Lambert

WHO Collaborating Center for Neonatal Vaccinology, Departments of Pathology and Pediatrics, University of Geneva, 1 rue Michel Servet, CH-1211 Geneva 4, Switzerland

The need for early life immunization

Neonatal or early infant immunizations are required to give protection from diseases caused by pathogens to which exposure occurs in early life. As an example, the median age of infants with a respiratory syncytial virus (RSV) infection severe enough to require hospitalization is below 3 months of age worldwide. A significant proportion of severe early infections are due either to encapsulated bacteria such as *Haemophilus influenzae, Streptococcus pneumoniae*, or *Neisseria meningitidis* or to intracellular agents such as viruses [RSV, measles virus (MV), rotavirus, herpes simplex viruses, cytomegalovirus], certain bacteria (*Listeria monocytogenes,* salmonella, mycobacteria) or other microorganisms (*Chlamydiae, Ureaplasma*). This enhanced susceptibility of newborns and infants to specific infectious diseases is due to limitations of both their innate and specific immune system.

Immune responses in early life differ from adult responses

The impaired function of monocytes/macrophages in newborns has been associated with reduced expression of major histocompatibility complex (MHC) class II and co-stimulatory molecules, decreased antigen-processing capacity and altered cytokine production. Although little is known about the development of human dendritic cells, their maturation appears to be slow and their function as antigen-presenting cells (APC) is rather poor at birth [10], thus probably contributing to the limitations of the induction of specific immune responses. Although natural killer (NK) cells are present in significant numbers at birth, their functional activity [reflected by interferon-γ (IFN-γ) production and NK cell-mediated lysis] also remains low for several weeks. It is not yet known precisely which part of these limitations reflects the intrinsic immaturity of infant NK cells or their impaired activation by cytokines or factors that prevail in the

Correspondence to: C.-A. Siegrist

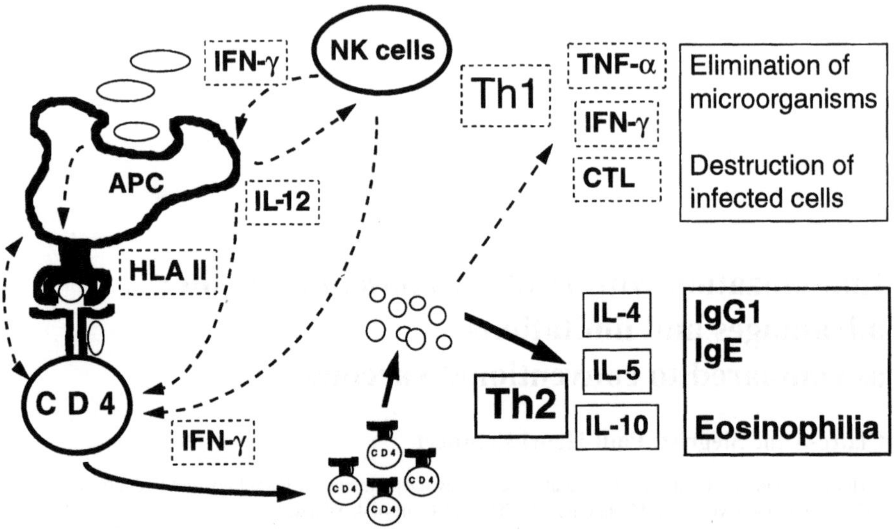

Fig. 1. Schematic representation of the preferential polarization of neonatal CD4 Th2 cell responses. Factors contributing to the preferential development of neonatal CD4 Th2 cell responses compared to adult responses have been identified at the level (i) of antigen-presenting cells (*APC*): decreased antigen processing, decreased expression of major histocompatibility complex class II and co-stimulatory molecules, decreased production of cytokines such as interleukin (IL)-12; (ii) of natural killer (NK) cells: decreased production of interferon-γ (IFN-γ) acting both on APC and CD4 T cells; (iii) of CD4 T cells themselves: hyporesponses to IL-12, hyperresponses to IL-4, decreased expression of CD40 ligand. These factors contribute to the preferential production of IL-4, IL-5 and IL-10, reflected by enhancement of IgG1and IgE antibodies and eosinophilia. In contrast, the low production of tumor necrosis factor-α (TNF-α), IFN-γ and weak generation of CD8 cytotoxic T lymphocytes (*CTL*) weakens the neonatal capacity to eliminate microorganisms and infected cells

microenvironment at the time of immune response triggering. As an example, reduced interleukin (IL)-12 production by activated mononuclear cells could be an important factor limiting NK cell activity since exogenous IL-12 was shown to enhance both IFN-γ and NK lytic activity of cord blood human NK cells up to adult levels [13]. Inversely, reduced IFN-γ production by NK cells probably affects the development of specific T cell responses, further contributing to the failure to generate the strong cellular responses required for clearance of intracellular microorganisms.

Antibody responses can be raised by newborns and infants in response to infectious agents or vaccines, although IgG responses are often slower and weaker than those elicited later in life. A lower avidity of vaccine-specific antibodies has also been reported, probably linked to poor T cell-driven affinity maturation of antibodies. This is best reflected by the additional doses of vaccines that must be given to fully immunize a 2-month-old infant compared to a 2-year-old toddler. Most importantly, responses to carbohydrate determinants such as those contained in bacterial capsules or in heavily glycosylated viral proteins can not be elicited in infants before 18–24 months of age. This does not relate to the capacity of B cells to recognize the antigen, and the basis for these impaired responses to carbohydrates – which explain infant susceptibility to encapsulated bacteria – remain largely unknown.

In vitro studies of neonatal T cells have indicated a low frequency of T cell precursors, poor responses to anti-CD2 and anti-CD3 stimulation in absence of anti-CD28 co-stimulation, poor B cell help in terms of both cytokine production and CD40 ligand expression by activated T cells, and low cytokine production (mainly IL-2 and IFN-γ). Recently, neonatal T cells have been shown to follow a preferential development into IL-4- and IL-5-producing effector cells [8, 28] and to respond to specific cytokines such as IL-12 not only by IFN-γ but also by IL-4 production [24].

Similar observations have been generated in vivo, in murine models of neonatal immunization with conventional vaccines. When the capacity of BALB/c mice at different stages of immunological maturation to respond to a selection of vaccine antigens and presentation systems was assessed, significant B and T cell responses to vaccine antigens (tetanus and MV peptides, tetanus toxoid, live viral attenuated MV, canarypox recombinant measles vector or BCG) were obtained already in the 1st week of life. However, these neonatal responses differed qualitatively from adult responses by a decreased IgG2a/IgG1 ratio of vaccine-specific antibodies, the secretion of significantly higher IL-5 and lower IFN-γ levels by vaccine-specific T cells and an impaired induction of cytotoxic T cell precursors [3]. This was interpreted as reflecting a biased pattern of Th2 versus Th1 responses induced upon early exposure to vaccines, and considered to reflect the situation occurring in human infants (Fig. 1). The polarization of T cells is believed to depend essentially on the APC capacity; antigen presentation by APC that do not express adequate levels of co-stimulators is indeed known to result in a selective Th2 activation [5]. Thus, the impaired development of Th1 neonatal responses to antigens, which directly contributes to their susceptibility to intracellular agents, could reflect defective neonatal APC-T cell interactions.

Which vaccines are required for immunization in early life?

The factors which limit infant responses to infectious agents also affect immune responses to vaccine antigens and result in an age-dependent immunogenicity of vaccines. Bacterial polysaccharide vaccines are not immunogenic before the age of 18–24 months, and although protein/conjugate vaccines can be offered already at a few weeks of age, their use in young infants requires the administration of additional vaccine doses to reach sufficient immunogenicity. Live viral or bacterial vaccines which are capable of inducing stronger cellular immune responses than subunit vaccines can often not be used in very early life; with a few exceptions, their early use is limited either by the persistence of antibodies of maternal origin or by safety concerns.

Thus, specific requirements have to be met by vaccines for them to be considered for immunization in early life. Candidate vaccines should induce protective vaccine responses against bacterial/viral pathogens to which infants are exposed early in life and represent a significant risk of either severe acute disease or persistent infections. These antibody/cellular responses should be inducible at a young age and confer protection before age of exposure to these specific microorganisms. Vaccine-induced immune responses should ideally be sufficiently sustained for long-term protection. In addition, novel vaccine candidates should avoid the induction of neonatal tolerance and induce infant vaccine responses in spite of the persistence of antibodies of maternal origin. Finally, specific vaccine safety issues associated with this early age of relative immunodeficiency have to be met. The purpose of this review is to evaluate how DNA vaccines compare to conventional vaccines for their potential use in early life, based on the experimental observations generated so far in murine models of immunization.

DNA s induce vaccine responses upon neonatal immunization

Optimal vaccine candidates for early life immunization should be more rapidly protective than has been achieved so far with conventional vaccines. This depends on both the earliest age at which immune responses can first be triggered and the kinetics of the development of such responses.

Experiments on neonatal DNA immunization have been initiated in mice, and are currently being extended to primates. The capacity of vaccines to induce specific responses at various stages of the immune maturation was assessed by immunizing mice intramuscularly prior to 3 weeks of age or as adults. Conventional and DNA vaccines were selected in view of their potential clinical significance to target potential infant pathogens such as measles {attenuated MV, immunodominant peptides of MV hemagglutinin (MV-HA), live recombinant canarypox (ALVAC-HA [26]) or DNA (MV-HA DNA [6]) vectors encoding MV-HA} and tetanus {tetanus toxoid (TT), immunodominant peptides of TT or DNA plasmid encoding its fragment C (TetC DNA [1])}.

Antibody responses

Characteristics of vaccine antibodies induced in both age groups by either conventional [3] or DNA [14] vaccines are summarized in Table 1. As a rule, conventional vaccines resulted in weaker primary antibody responses when used in early life than in adult mice, although antibody titers often reached similar antibody titers after administration of a booster immunization. In contrast, a single injection of DNA vaccines performed in adult or young mice resulted 4 weeks later in similar antibody titers in both age groups. These titers were in general lower than those raised in adult mice by a single dose of conventional vaccines. Administration of a second DNA immunization similarly boosted antibody levels (tenfold) in both age groups.

Analysis of vaccine-specific antibody isotypes induced by conventional vaccines revealed an age-dependent limitation of the induction of IgG2a vaccine-specific antibodies by neonatal immunization even in situations where similar titers of IgG1 responses were induced (Table 1) [3]. This was also true for live vaccines such as ALVAC-HA. In contrast, similar antibody patterns were induced by early or adult DNA immunization, characterized by a preferential IgG2a (MV-HA) or a mixed IgG1/IgG2a (TetC DNA) profile of vaccine-specific antibodies [14]. Thus, in contrast to conventional vaccines, the use of DNA vaccines was capable of inducing adult-like neonatal antibody responses, both quantitatively and qualitatively.

CD4 T cell responses

Comparison of CD4 T cell responses induced by adult/neonatal immunization with conventional vaccines revealed quantitatively similar T cell proliferation but significant qualitative differences (Table 2). The pattern of CD4 responses observed after immunization of 1- to 3-week-old mice with conventional vaccines consisted of a significantly higher production of IL-5 by antigen-specific T cells, as compared to cells from adult primed mice [3, 4]. This neonatal burst of IL-5 was mostly observed after neonatal immunization with alum-adsorbed subunit vaccines. It also occurred, however, upon immunization with live viral vaccines (live attenuated MV or ALVAC-HA),

Table 1. Vaccine-specific antibodies induced by conventional and DNA vaccines[a]

Vaccine types	Vaccines	Vaccine responses	Serum antibody titers (ELISA-log10)			
			Adult priming		Neonatal priming	
			IgG	IgG2a	IgG	IgG2a
Measles						
Peptide	MVH4972	Primary	2.2	< 1.6	1.7	< 1.6
	MVH4972	Secondary	3.8	1.8	1.9*	< 1.6
Atten. virus	MVSchwartz	Primary	5.5	4.0	4.7*	2.3*
	MVSchwartz	Secondary	6.8	4.2	6.8	2.3*
Avipox vect.	ALVAC-HA	Primary	5.4	4.2	4.3*	2.1*
	ALVAC-HA	Secondary	6.3	4.7	6.4	2.3*
DNA vacc.	MV-HA DNA	Primary	4.2	3.0	4.1	3.3
	MV-HA DNA	Secondary	5.1	3.3	5.2	3.6
Tetanus						
Peptide	TTP30	Primary	3.7	< 1.6	2.5*	< 1.6
	TTP30	Secondary	5.5	3.5	5.1	1.8*
Protein	TT	Primary	6.3	4.2	5.2*	2.9*
	TT	Secondary	7.2	5.0	6.6	3.4*
DNA vacc.	TetC DNA	Primary	4.3	3.9	4.2	3.6

[a] Antibody titers to measles virus hemagglutinin (MV-HA) or tetanus toxoid (TT) were measured by an enzyme-linked immunosorbent assay (ELISA) as described [3]. Analyses were performed in the serum after one or two immunizations of BALB/c mice primed either as adults or at 1 week of age with the following peptide (MVH4972: 100 μg in ALOH; TTP30: 100 μg in ALOH), protein (TT: 3 μg in ALOH), viral (MVSchwartz: 5×10^6 CCID50 in ALOH; ALVAC-HA: 5×10^7 pfu) or DNA (MV-HA DNA: 100 μg; TetC DNA: 100 μg) vaccines
* $P < 0.05$ between adult and neonatal responses, Wilcoxon rank test

which furthermore failed to induce in young mice adult levels of IFN-γ production by antigen-specific T cells.

These experiments, as well as those reported by others [9, 18, 19, 25], indicated that the impairment of neonatal cellular responses could derive from a preferential polarization of neonatal CD4 T cells towards a Th2 rather than a Th1 pattern, as reflected by the generation of antibodies of different isotypes (preferential IgG1 and IgE vs. IgG2a antibodies), by a low secretion of IFN-γ and by an excess of IL-5 production by antigen-specific CD4 T cells. Although the distinction between Th1/Th2 subsets is less stringent in humans, a tendency towards preferential Th2 development of neonatal responses has also been observed in a few studies involving human cells [8, 28]. It could account for the age-dependent clinical pattern of infectious diseases such as hepatitis, mononucleosis or toxoplasmosis in which symptoms are believed to be essentially immune mediated and which remain mostly asymptomatic in young children compared to adults. It would also explain the lower immunogenicity and higher frequency of complications following BCG immunization performed at birth rather than at a few months of age [11, 16]. Finally, it could be linked to the preferential induction of allergic reactions upon early exposure to environmental antigens.

The capacity of DNA vaccines to induce strong Th1 cellular responses in adult animals suggested that this novel antigen-presentation system could represent an inter-

Table 2. Antigen-specific cytokine production by T cells induced by conventional and DNA vaccines[a]

Vaccine types	Vaccines	Vaccine responses	Antibody-specifc cytokines			
			IFN-γ		IL-5	
			Adult	Neonatal	Adult	Neonatal
Measles						
Peptide	MVH4972	Primary	< 20	< 20	383	1310*
Atten. virus	MVSchwartz	Primary	230	100*	500	2150*
Avipox vect.	ALVAC-HA	Primary	150	52*	< 150	925*
DNA vacc.	MV-HA DNA	Primary	182	315	< 150	< 150
Tetanus						
Peptide	TTP30	Primary	< 20	< 20	< 150	800*
Protein	TT	Primary	< 20	< 20	< 150	1305*
DNA vacc.	TetC DNA	Primary	170	95	400	603

[a] Cytokine production by antigen-specific T cells was measured by ELISA as described [3] in the supernatant of splenocytes after in vitro restimulation with MV or TT. Analyses were performed after a single immunization of BALB/c mice primed either as adults or at 1 week of age with the following peptide (MVH4972: 100 μg in ALOH; TTP30: 100 μg in ALOH), protein (TT: 3 μg in ALOH), viral (MVSchwartz: 5×10^6 CCID50 in ALOH; ALVAC-HA: 5×10^7 pfu) or DNA (MV-HA DNA: 100 μg; TetC DNA: 100 μg) vaccines
* $P < 0.05$ between adult and neonatal responses, Wilcoxon rank test

esting vaccine strategy for neonatal immunization against intracellular agents. When CD4 T cell responses were assessed in mice immunized with DNA vaccines either as adults or at 1 week of age [14], similar levels of antigen-specific T cell proliferation were observed. Importantly, the cytokine profiles of in vitro-restimulated splenocytes were similar in both age groups (Table 2). Depending on the antigen, either a preferential secretion of IFN-γ (MV-HA) or mixed IFN-γ and IL-5 production (tetanus fragment C) was observed after DNA immunization. These patterns were directly associated with either the preferential IgG2a or the mixed IgG1/IgG2a profile of vaccine-specific antibodies, respectively. They demonstrate the induction of Th0/Th1 responses upon neonatal DNA immunization. This property of DNA vaccines to induce strong Th1 responses in early life appears quite unique: it is apparently only shared with low doses of live replicating viral agents ([19] and unpublished observations) and suggests the existence of specific requirements for complete activation of neonatal versus adult Th1 responses. Our working hypothesis is that activation of neonatal dendritic cells requires a prolonged exposure to antigen, a feature shared by both DNA and live replicating infectious agents or vaccines, to fully trigger NK cell and Th1 responses.

CD8 cytotoxic responses

Among conventional vaccines, only live viruses are capable of raising significant cytotoxic T lymphocyte (CTL) responses in immunologically mature animals or humans. However, these responses are weakly induced by neonatal immunization. As an example, adult-like murine CTL responses can not be induced before the age of 3 weeks even with live vaccines such as ALVAC-HA, which raise very strong CTL responses in adult animals: a greater than tenfold reduction of the frequency of CTL precursors

(CTLp) was observed upon immunization of 1- to 3-week-old versus adult-primed animals [3]. Although CTL can be induced in infants by infectious agents such as HIV or RSV, the limited generation of CTL responses in very early life is considered to participate in the impaired clearance of intracellular microorganisms. Furthermore, neonatal use of live vaccines is limited by both the relative physiological immunodeficiency and the presence of antibodies of maternal origin which limit the in vivo replication required by attenuated vaccines to reach sufficient immunogenicity.

DNA vaccines have emerged as potent inducers of CD8 cytotoxic responses in adult animals. This was found to be also the case upon neonatal DNA immunization. In contrast to the limited induction of neonatal CTL by ALVAC-HA, we observed the induction of adult-like CTL responses (assessed by similar frequency of CTLp in spleens) in BALB/c mice vaccinated either in the neonatal period or as adults with MV-HA DNA [14]. The same observation was made in C57BL/6 mice immunized either as adults or in the first weeks of life with a DNA plasmid encoding the nucleoprotein of another paramyxovirus, the Sendai virus [14]. Successful induction of CTL by DNA immunization was reported by Sarzotti et al. [20] in yet another mouse strain: 2-day-old NFS/N mice raised a protective CD8-mediated CTL response upon intramuscular immunization with a DNA plasmid encoding the full-length genome of a neuropathogenic retrovirus (Cas-Br-M murine leukemia virus). Thus, the generic property of DNA vaccines to induce strong CTL responses, which has been linked to the presence in bacterial DNA of specific unmethylated CpG motives capable of rapidly enhancing transcription of IL-6, IFN-α, IFN-γ and IL-12 in APC [2, 12, 21], is also effective in newborns. Through their adjuvant properties, DNA vaccines can fully activate neonatal dendritic cells, sharing only with live replicating agents the capacity to induce the adult-like neonatal CD8 responses required for clearance of intracellular microorganisms.

How rapidly do immune responses to neonatal DNA immunization develop?

In these murine models of neonatal immunization involving several mouse strains, plasmid vectors and antigens, a single DNA immunization performed in early life was capable of generating adult-like vaccine responses even in situations where conventional vaccines with the corresponding antigens failed to do so. However, the kinetics of vaccine response induced by DNA immunization was rather slow (2–6 weeks) in both adult and neonatally primed animals. This slow induction affected antibody responses, contrasting with the more rapid induction (1–2 weeks) of responses by corresponding conventional vaccines. Similarly, CTL induction was only detected in all mice at 8 weeks post DNA immunization [20], although occurring earlier (4–5 weeks) in some animals. This rather slow kinetic of DNA-induced vaccine responses appears as a generic property of DNA immunization which could represent a disadvantage for the induction of early infant protection. This is especially important in view of the difficulty in reverting neonatally induced Th2 responses towards Th1 responses. This could not be achieved either by Th1-driving adjuvants [4] or by DNA immunization [14] given at adult age after neonatal priming with conventional vaccines.

Does neonatal DNA immunization carry the risk of inducing tolerance rather than immunity?

Neonatal exposure to antigen under specific conditions has been shown in various rodent models to induce tolerance rather than immunity to the specific antigen. This was shown to depend on several factors such as the nature and dose of antigen and the timing of exposure, which usually has to occur within the first 24 h of life. Contradictory reports on the risk of inducing neonatal tolerance by DNA immunization have been generated to date. When newborn BALB/c mice were immunized once within their first 24 h of life with MV-HA DNA, we observed the induction of strong immune responses characterized by similar antibody titers, IFN-γ production and high frequency of CTLp as compared to 1-week-old or adult-primed mice. In another model, a single immunization of newborn C3H/He mice with a plasmid vector expressing the rabies virus glycoprotein was capable of raising significant antibody responses [29]. Neonatal priming was confirmed by booster administration, and antibody isotypes and cytokine production were reported as similar to those observed after adult immunization. In contrast to these results, a DNA vaccine encoding the circumsporozoite protein (CSP) of the *Plasmodium yoelii* malaria parasite was described as inducing long-lasting tolerance in 2-day- to 1-week-old mice who failed to raise immune responses upon adult boosting with DNA [15]. The mechanisms underlying this described tolerance induction are uncertain. They could be linked to unique properties of this CSP-DNA construct, which mainly induces Th2 rather than Th0/Th1 responses in adult mice [22] and whose immunogenicity clearly differs from the native CSP protein in terms of antigenic determinants [15]. Until further information is available, the induction of immune tolerance by DNA immunization of newborn mice with certain DNA plasmids can thus not be excluded. The importance of this specific observation might, however, not be directly relevant to human infant immunization, since the maturation of their immune system at birth is such that tolerance induction has not yet been induced by postnatal exposure to any antigen. Thus, neonatal DNA immunization appears worth assessing in conditions where induction of early immune responses are desired.

Can sustained vaccine responses be induced by neonatal DNA immunization?

Infant immunization against hepatitis B would be of little interest if protection waned before adolescence and its risk of exposure through sexual transmission. Waning of immunity in the absence of a booster is commonly observed with conventional vaccines such as inactivated or subunit vaccines, and there is little evidence yet that even live attenuated vaccines would provide life-long immunity in the absence of a repeat exposure to wild-type infectious agents. Interestingly, a single DNA immunization was shown in adult mice to induce long-lasting responses and life-long maintenance of memory cells to various antigens. Prolonged immune responses are similarly observed after neonatal DNA immunization [7, 27], and this could represent a significant advantage of DNA vaccines over conventional vaccines. However, experiments performed in non-human adult primates are now showing transient immune responses which suggest that this feature could be essentially a characteristic of rodent responses to DNA immunization. A weak and transient production of antibodies was also observed in a first study assessing DNA immunization of newborn chimpanzees against hepatitis B virus [17]. However, in spite of negative or very low antibody titers, the two animals were protected from a viral challenge performed at 33 weeks, suggesting the successful induction of cell-mediated responses.

Can vaccine responses be induced by neonatal DNA immunization in spite of the persistence of antibodies of maternal origin?

A number of infectious diseases can be either prevented or attenuated by the passive transfer of specific antibodies. Prevention of neonatal infections also relies on transplacental transfer of antibodies of maternal origin from mother to child. These antibodies progressively decline below the protective level, but nevertheless remain capable for a period of time of interfering with infant responses to immunization. The precise mechanisms responsible for the variable effects of maternal antibodies on infant responses have not yet been fully deciphered. It is known, however, that live attenuated vaccines have the greatest susceptibility to the inhibitory influence of maternal antibodies: by neutralizing part of the vaccine inoculum prior to viral entrance within host cells, antibodies interfere with the replication cycle in vivo that it requires to induce protective responses. This is of significant clinical importance for measles immunization in countries where vaccine coverage is not yet sufficient to limit the risk of contracting measles prior to the age at which maternal antibodies have sufficiently declined in most infants to allow successful immunization [23].

To assess the influence of MV specific maternal antibodies on neonatal responses to conventional or DNA vaccines expressing measles hemagglutinin, 2-week-old mice born of nonimmune mothers were passively transferred various concentrations of syngeneic immune serum raised by two immunizations with live attenuated measles vaccine. They were immunized 2 days later with either live attenuated measles vaccine, live recombinant ALVAC-HA or MV-HA DNA, and followed at regular intervals for determination of HA-specific antibodies. When immunization was performed in presence of HA-specific antibodies at titers corresponding to those observed in pups of immune mothers (> 4.5 $\log^{10}$), neither of the live vaccines nor DNA was capable of inducing HA-specific antibodies in the pups (manuscript in preparation). When concentrations of passively transferred antibodies were tenfold lower at time of immunization, both conventional and DNA vaccines were capable of inducing infant antibody responses. Thus, DNA vaccines could be reported either as capable or not of circumventing the inhibitory influence of maternal antibody, depending on the antibody titers present at time of immunization. This suggests that passive antibodies bind to a fraction of the antigen expressed by transfected muscle cells which is sufficient, or not, to prevent the induction of antibody responses. In this model of measles immunization, DNA vaccines, therefore, did not show any advantage over live conventional vaccines for infant immunization in the presence of passively transferred antibodies.

Does neonatal DNA immunization have to meet specific safety issues?

Ongoing human trials of DNA immunization suggest that these vaccines have no immediate or early side effects. However, nothing is known yet on the potential long-term consequences of such vaccines. The issues of prolonged antigen expression being potentially capable of triggering physiopathological immune responses and the questions of potential genomic integration will have to be specifically addressed in neonatal models of immunization, bearing in mind the ongoing maturation of the immune system and the high mitotic rates existing in infants.

Conclusion

DNA vaccines favorably compare to conventional vaccines in their unique capacity to induce, in murine models, adult-like antibody, Th1 and CTL responses at a time of yet significant immune immaturity. Immune responses to DNA vaccines are, however, significantly slower than the one induced by adjuvanted subunit or live vaccines. Although they persist for life in mice, preliminary data in non-human adult primates suggest that this could not be the case in higher mammals. The issue of potential tolerance induction will likely not emerge as a critical feature of human neonatal DNA immunization. However, DNA vaccines are unlikely to prove superior to conventional vaccines in their capacity to circumvent the inhibitory influence of maternal antibodies.

Thus, the greater perspectives for neonatal DNA immunization could be found in models where the induction of Th1 and CTL responses are of utmost importance. These are essentially infections with intracellular agents responsible for severe/persistent infections upon early exposure and for which no current efficient and safe conventional vaccine exists. Evaluating neonatal DNA immunization strategies against RSV or herpes viruses, tuberculosis or Chlamydiae therefore emerge as sound priorities.

Acknowledgements. Our work is supported by grants from the Swiss National Science Foundation, from W.H.O. Global Programme for Vaccines and Immunization, from Sandoz and from Pasteur-Mérieux Serums et Vaccins. C.A. Siegrist is supported by the Swiss National Science Foundation (SCORE A).

References

1. Anderson R, Gao SM, Papakonstantinopoulou A, Roberts M, Dougan G (1996) Immune response in mice following immunization with DNA encoding fragment C of tetanus toxin. Infect Immun 64:3168
2. Ballas ZK, Ramuaawn WL, Krieg AM (1996) Induction of NK activity in murine and human cells by CpG motifs in oligodeoxynucleotides and bacterial DNA. J Immunol 157:1840
3. Barrios C, Brawand P, Berney M, Brandt C, Lambert PH, Siegrist CA (1996) Neonatal and early life immune responses to various forms of vaccine antigens qualitatively differ from adult responses: predominance of a Th2-biased pattern which persists after adult boosting. Eur J Immunol 26: 1489
4. Barrios C, Brandt C, Berney M, Lambert PH, Siegrist CA (1996) Partial correction of the Th2/Th1 imbalance in neonatal murine responses to vaccine antignes through selective adjuvant effects. Eur J Immunol 26:2666
5. Burstein HJ, Shea CM, Abbas AK (1992) Aqueous antigens induce in vivo tolerance selectively in IL-2 and IFN-gamma producing Th1 cells. J Immunonol 148:3687
6. Cardoso AI, Blixenkrone-Moller M, Fayolle J, Liu M, Buckland R, Wild TF (1996) Immunization with plasmid DNA encoding for the measles virus hemagglutinin and nucleoprotein leads to humoral and cell-mediated immunity. Virology 225:293
7. Davis HL, Michel M, Whalen RG (1993) DNA-based immunization for hepatitis B induces continuous secretion of antigen and high levels of circulating antibody. Hum Mol Genet 2:1847
8. Demeure CE, Yang LP, Byun DG, Ishihara H, Vezzio N, Delespesse G (1995) Human naive CD4 T cells produce interleukin-4 at priming and acquire a Th2 phenotype upon repetitive stimulation in neutral conditions. Eur J Immunol 25:2722
9. Forsthuber T, Yip HC, Lehman PV (1996) Induction of TH1 and TH2 immunity in neonatal mice. Science 271:1728

10. Hunt DW, Huppertz HI, Jiang HJ, Petty RE (1994) Studies of human cord blood dendritic cells: evidence for functional immaturity. Blood 84:4333
11. Ildirim I, Sapan N, Cavusoglu B (1992) Comparison of BCG vaccination at birth and at third month of life. Arch Dis Child 67:80
12. Klinman DM, Yi AK, Beaucage SL, Conover J, Krieg AM (1996) CpG motifs present in bacterial DNA rapidly induce lymphocytes to secrete interleukin 6, interleukin 12 and interferon γ. Proc Natl Acad Sci USA 93:2879
13. Lee SM, Suen Y, Chang L, Bruner V, Quian J, Indes J, Knoppel E, Ven C van de, Cairo MS (1996) Decreased interleukin-12 (IL-12) from activated cord versus adult peripheral blood mononuclear cells and upregulation of interferon-gamma, natural killer and lymphokine-activated killer activity by IL-12 in cord blood. Blood 88:945
14. Martinez X, Brandt C, Saddallah F, Tougne C, Barrios C, Wild F, Dougan G, Lambert PH, Siegrist CA (1997) DNA immunization circumvents deficient induction of TH1 and CTL responses in neonates and during early life. Proc Natl Acad Sci USA (in press)
15. Mor G, Yamschchikov G, Sedegah M, Takeno M, Wang R, Houghten RA, Hoffman S, Klinman DM (1996) Induction of neonatal tolerance by plasmid DNA vaccination of mice. J Clin Invest 98:2700
16. Pabst HF, Godel JC, Spady DW, McKechnie J, Grace M (1989) Prospective trial of timing of BCG vaccination in Canadian Cree infants. Am Rev Respir Dis 140:1007
17. Prince AM, Whalen R, Brotman B (1997) Successful nucleic acid based immunization of newborn chimpanzees against hepatitis B virus. Vaccine (in press)
18. Ridge JP, Fuchs EJ, Matzinger P (1996) Neonatal tolerance revisited: turning on newborn T cells with dendritic cells. Science 271:1723
19. Sarzotti M, Robbins DS, Hoffman PM (1996) Induction of protective CTL responses in newborn mice by a murine retrovirus. Science 271:1726
20. Sarzotti M, Dean TA, Remington MP, Ly CD, Furth PA, Robbins DS (1997) Induction of CTL responses in newborn mice by DNA immunization. Vaccine (in press)
21. Sato Y, Roman M, Tighe H, Lee D, Corr M, Nguyen MD, Silverman GJ, Lotz M, Carson DA, Raz E (1996) Immunostimulatory DNA sequences necessary for effective intradermal gene immunization. Science 273:352
22. Sedegah M, Hedstrom R, Hobart P, Hoffman SL (1994) Protection against malaria by immunization with plasmid DNA encoding circumsporozoite protein. Proc Natl Acad Sci USA 90:4156
23. Shasby M, Shope T, Downs H, Herrmann KL, Polkowsky J (1977) Epidemic measles in a highly vaccinated population. N Engl J Med 296:585
24. Shu U, Demeure CE, Byun DG, Podlaski F, Stern AS, Delespesse G (1994) Interleukin 12 exerts a differential effect on the maturation of neonatal and adult human CD45RO- CD4 T cells. J Clin Invest 94: 1352
25. Singh RR, Hahn BH, Sercarz EE (1996) Neonatal peptide exposure can prime T cells and, upon subsequent immunization, induce their immune deviation: implications for antibody vs. T cell mediated autoimmunity. J Exp Med 183:1613
26. Taylor J, Pincus S, Tartaglia J, Richardson C, Alkhatib G, Briedis D, Appel M, Norton E, Paoletti E (1991) Vaccinia virus recombinants expressing either the measles virus fusion or hemagglutinin glycoprotein protect dogs against canine distemper virus challenge. J Virol 65:4263
27. Yakaucas MA, MorrowJE, Parker SE, Abai A, Rhodes GH, Dwarki VJ, Gromkowski SH (1993) Long-term anti-nucleoprotein cellular and humoral immunity is induced by intramuscular injection of plasmid DNA containing NP gene. DNA Cell Biol 12:771
28. Yang LP, Byun DG, Demeure CE, Vezzio N, Delespesse G (1996) Default development of cloned human naive CD4 T cells into interleukin-4- and interleukin-5-producing effector cells. Eur J Immunol 25:3517
29. Wang, Y, Xiang Z, Pasquini S, Ertl HCJ (1997) Immune response to neonatal genetic immunization. Virology 228:278

DNA vaccination by somatic transgene immunization

Maurizio Zanetti, Sidong Xiong and Mara Gerloni

The Department of Medicine and Cancer Center, University of California, San Diego, 9500 Gilman Drive, La Jolla CA 92093-0063, USA

New vaccines, old vaccinology

Possibly the most astonishing feature in vaccinology is the fact that vaccines have, and continue to be, developed on an empirical basis. The biotechnological revolution that took place in the eighties expanded the range of strategies and approaches for making novel vaccines, but while not establishing new principles for vaccinology [1] it acknowledged two factors: (a) effective and durable immunity can be achieved with suitable constituted non-infectious vaccines, and (b) the experience of infection is not required for inducing such an effect [2]. Although immunology as a science has made remarkable progress in elucidating the physiology and the molecular basis of the immune response, new vaccines are not developed at the pace needed.

Vaccines as strategy for the immunological control of pathogens need to focus on two objectives: prevent disease and be based on simple immunological principles. An ideal vaccine is one that elicits a durable immune response at both the T- and B-cell levels, against nonpolymorphic determinant(s) immunodominant in the largest possible assortment of MHC haplotypes [1] and essential for the survival of the pathogen. Forging vaccines molecules and programming the immune response along these principles is the task facing modern vaccinology.

DNA and immunogenicity

DNA itself is scarcely immunogenic. Although there exists clinical evidence for autoantibodies to double and single stranded DNA [3–5], inducing a response against DNA has proven extremely difficult [6]. Bacterial DNA has, however, properties that one may consider relevant to an immunogenic process. As early as 1965 it was noted that bacterial DNA could serve as adjuvant in immunization [7]. Subsequently, it was noted that mice immunized with *Escherichia coli* DNA complexed with methylated BSA in adjuvant produce significantly greater amounts of antibodies than mice immunized with calf thymus DNA [8, 9]. It is now recognized that bacterial DNA possesses immunostimulatory properties [10], is mitogenic for B cells and induces polyclonal antibody production [11], and enhances the lytic activity of natural killer cells with production of IFN-γ [10, 12]. These stimulatory properties are apparently linked to a six-base nucleotide motif consisting of an unmethylated CpG dinucleotide [13] expressed nearly twenty times more frequently in bacterial than in vertebrate DNA [14]. Noncoding, immunostimulatory sequences (ISS)-enriched plasmid DNA or ISS oligonucleotides stimulate immune responses to co-administered antigens [15] by activating IFN-γ -α and -β, and IL-12 and 18, all of which promote a Th1 response [15].

DNA vaccines

DNA vaccination is the latest revolution in modern vaccination [16]. Inoculation of functional genes into somatic cells of adult immunocompetent animals is a new and simple way to initiate an immune response in a way similar to immunity induced by natural infection (reviewed in [17]). Antibody production (B-cell immunity), and cell-mediated immunity of the helper or cytotoxic T cell-type have all been induced. Plasmid DNA containing antigen-coding sequences and regulatory elements for their expression, can be introduced in tissues by simple parenteral injection [18] or by particle bombardment [19].

As exemplified and discussed elsewhere in this volume the immunogenicity of plasmid DNA vaccines has been exploited to elicit immunity against viruses [20], bacteria [21, 22], parasites [23], tumor antigens [24], self antigens [25, 26] and allergens [27].

Issues in somatic transgenesis

The success of DNA vaccination is determined by a series of factors all of which depend on the efficiency of gene delivery and gene expression *in vivo*. Strategies have been developed for receptor-mediated gene delivery [28–30] to exploit specific structures on somatic cells and their mechanisms to internalize macromolecules. Targeted delivery of DNA needs to be gauged through the specificity of regulatory elements, *i.e.*, promoters and enhancers, which allow the transgene to be transcribed and translated in tissues. The efficiency of these processes constitutes the rate limiting factor for *in vivo* efficacy of DNA vaccination.

Our proposal: somatic transgene immunization

Our approach to immunization with plasmid DNA was developed keeping in mind factors that could affect the success of DNA immunization such as the efficiency of *in vivo* transfection including DNA uptake by host cells, the efficiency with which transfected cells utilize the DNA and synthesize the transgene product, and the ability of *in vivo* transfected cells to serve as antigen-presenting cells. The simple consideration that during immunity to natural infection pathogens activate lymphocytes in lymphoid organs made it clear that the most effective way to mimic natural infection would be to vaccinate using transgenes under the control of lymphoid tissue-specific regulatory elements. As an experimental system we considered the immunoglobulin heavy (H) chain gene under the control of B lymphocyte-specific promoter [31–34]. Studies *in vitro* existed to show that transfection of B cell lymphomas with rearranged Ig gene is followed by a prompt utilization of the transgene and by secretion of transgenic immunoglobulins (TgIg) [35]. A variety of rearranged functional Ig genes have also been introduced in the germline to create mice with homogeneous B-cell antigen receptor or secretion of Ig with identical chemical and immunologic characteristics (for review see [36]. It is obvious that DNA immunization with Ig genes, *e.g.*, heavy (H) chain genes under the control of their own tissue-specific promoter and enhancer elements, could be a way to target B lymphocytes specifically and to exploit the protein-synthesis machinery of these cells (a B cell can produce 10^3 molecules of antibody/second [37]) as well as their ability to present antigen [38]. We termed this approach somatic transgene immunization (STI) [39].

Germane to STI as a new method for vaccination is another concept developed in this laboratory: Antibody antigenization [40]. This refers to an antibody engineering approach for targeted modifications of the variable (V) regions of an antibody to create antibodies with new antigenic and immunogenic characteristics. The method allows for the expression of peptide from foreign antigens with characteristics suited for immunogencity at the B and T cell level.

B cell immunity is dictated by the shape of antigens since the B cell receptor for antigen recognizes the conformation of antigenic determinants. The primary paradigm of an antigen:antibody interaction is that the three-dimensional structure of the six hypervariable (HV) loops of an antibody recognize and bind a specific antigenic surface determined by the three-dimensional structure of the antigen. This interaction occurs over large sterically and electrostatically complementary areas, *i.e.*, charged side chains interact with side chains of opposite charge, and proton donors and acceptors are involved in hydrogen bonds. Consequently, the ability to induce immunity relies on the ability of the immunogen to reproduce the topochemical characteristics of antigens, a prerequisite essential to generate biologicallly-active antibodies for protection. Heterologous peptides conformationally-constrained within an antibody HV loop have sufficient structure stability to interact with somatic receptors in a discriminating way. Numerous demonstrations from this [41–43] and other laboratories [44–48] support the view that that antigenized antibodies are effective antigens and elicit antibody responses focused on selected, biologically-relevant epitopes.

Activation of T cells requires that antigen be presented in the form of small peptides in the context of MHC molecules at the cell surface. Long peptides are trimmed into small peptides intracellularly. For this to happen it is necessary that peptide sequences of relevance for the MHC molecules be cut with some precision on both extremities. Studies on antigenized antibodies show that peptides in the HV loops are trimmed and presented in MHC class I [49–51] and class II [44, 52] molecules for effective recognition by specific T cells and activation of responsive T cells. As to class II MHC presentation, quantitative experiments showed that a T cell epitope borne on antigenized antibody is presented 100 to 1000 times more efficiently than free synthetic peptide [44]. T cell peptides engineered on antibody V regions are easily generated within the cell degradative machinery. Neither the position relative to the N terminus nor flanking residues influence this process. In short, HV loops are cleavable sites and, as such, antigenized V regions deliver T cell peptides to the B cell synthesizing the antigenized antibody or, if secreted, to conventional antigen-presenting cells (monocyte/macrophage or dendritic cells).

The above considerations predict that endogenously-synthesized antigenized antibodies serve simultaneously as a source of exogenous B- and T-cell epitopes: conformationally-constrained B-cell peptides are expressed with controlled geometry and spatial and T-cell peptides are easily processed from the H chain scaffold and presented in the MHC molecules.

To summarize, STI allows for programmable induction of immunity (antibodies against selected immunodominant epitopes and activation of T cells) and, as it will be discussed below, the establishment of durable immunologic memory. Unlike conventional DNA vaccines STI targets the lymphoid tissue in a way that expression of the transgene, release of vaccine molecules, and the cellular events that follow, are clearly identified. While mimicking the replicating nature of infection STI is rationally designed to fully integrate the immune system into the vaccination process.

Immunologic characteristics of STI

A single intra-spleen inoculation of adult mice with plasmid DNA containing a chimeric (mouse/human) Ig H chain gene is followed within a week by secretion of transgenic Ig and production of IgM anti-Ig antibodies. Transgenic H chains are invariably detected in the circulation in amounts ranging between 15 and 30 ng/ml [39], and are associated with endogenous κ light chains. Transgenic Ig (TgIg) and anti-Ig antibodies have superimposable kinetics of serum appearance. Both develop around day 5–7 and peak on day 18–21. Whereas anti-Ig antibodies remain detectable almost indefinitely, TgIg become undetectable after 3–4 weeks. We speculate this to be due to saturation by anti-Ig antibodies. Upon booster injection with the corresponding Ig a typical secondary immune response with IgG1 and IgG2b antibodies is seen [39]. Therefore, a single inoculation of an Ig H chain gene targeted to spleen lymphocytes is sufficient to initiate immunity and establish immunologic memory. STI general characteristics are listed in Table I.

Table 1. General Characteristics of Somatic Transgene Immunization

- Single inoculation of DNA
- Detection of TgIg in serum (15–30 μg/ml)
- Induction of lifelong antibodies against TgIg (mainly IgM)
- Activation of specific T cell immunity
- Establishment of durable immunologic memory
- 100% efficiency

Induction of antibodies specific for a B-cell epitope of an exogenous antigen

To verify whether STI could be used to induce antigen-specific immunity we used a transgene coding for three repeats of the amino acid sequence *Asn-Ala-Asn-Pro* (NANP), the immunodominant B-cell epitope of *Plasmodium falciparum* malaria sporozoites [53]. Antibodies against this epitope develop in people living in endemic areas for malaria [Zavala, 1985 #145], in volunteers vaccinated with irradiated sporozoites [54, 55], and are protective against experimental sporozoite challenge in human volunteers [56, 57]. Our earlier studies demonstrated that immunization with an antibody antigenized with three NANP repeats induced NANP-specific antibodies in mice and rabbits [41]. Following the induction of STI, antibodies against the NANP peptide appeared around day 14, reached a plateau by day 28, and persisted for as long as two years [58].

Establishment of immunologic memory

Long-lasting humoral immunity after DNA inoculation has already been documented by others [59, 60], although in many reports multiple DNA injections seem to be required [23, 61, 62]. Somatic transgene immunizationStudies with STI were designed to verify whetherestablish whether a single intra-spleen inoculation of plasmid DNA g1NANP was sufficient to induce immunologic memory. We used again the NANP epitope as a model system.

In a first round of experiments, wTo this end, we analyzed the secondary response following a booster immunization 45 days after DNA inoculation. The booster injection consisted in either 50 μg of the corresponding antigenized antibody in incomplete Freunds' adjuvant or in a single injection of 10^5 malaria parasite sporozoites. Mice primed with DNA had greater booster responses to sporozoites than mice primed with the antigenized antibody in complete Freunds' adjuvant (CFA) . These sera also reacted strongly with the surface of air-dried sporozoites by immunofluoresence assay confirming that the DNA-immunized mice had been primed with a B-cellB cell epitope with a conformation that iwas substantially similar to that present on the surface of the target pathogen. After booster, we observed a sharp rise in the IgG1 response and a minor but significant rise in IgG2a and IgG2b antibodies. In a second round of experiments immunologic memory was tested 30 and 104 weeks after the DNA inoculum, respectively [58]. The anamnestic response against the NANP epitope was measured 2 and 5 weeks after booster. A strong memory response was noted in both goups. When compared with mice boosted after 6 weeks only, it became evident that memory responses became stronger with time. In mice boosted on week 30, circulating antibodies persisted at a high titer for an additional 17 months.

That a single inoculation of appropriately formulated plasmid DNA establishes persistent immunologic memory is reminiscent of the earlier observation that immunologic memory that follows a single dose of a suitably potent vaccine increases over time and persists thereafter [63]. STI triggers and subsequently maintains, a state of durable immunity and, possibly irreversible, immunologic memory without the periodic need for reinforcement. Therefore, STI may be applicable to those pathogens or conditions which require memory-dependent immunity [2].

Studies on T cell immunity

a. Induction of Th cells

Experiments had already shown that antigenized antibodies carrying Th cell peptides in one of their HV loops are cleaved from the H chain polypeptide and presented in class II MCH molecules [44, 52]. Whether or not the same phenomenon could be generated *in vivo* during STI was demonstrated in a series of experiments in which the transgene coded for a bona fide Th cell determinant also from the circumsporozoite protein of *P. falciparum*. In these experiments (Gerloni et al., in preparation) T cell proliferation and IL-2 production were reproducibly measured starting from day 7 after DNA inoculation. Of interest, neither IL-4 nor IFN-γ were detected indicating that STI immunizes without imprinting modifications in the cytokine balance. Put in lay terms STI does not precondition the immune response. This opens to future possibilities of immunomodulation via cytokine-mediated amplification and cross-regulation during priming.

Th cell activation distally from the site of DNA inoculation was also studied. We were interested to verify whether T cells in lymphnodes would also proliferate to the Th cell determinant included in the transgene. This question was more than academic since we knew that cells harboring the transgene do not migrate to other lymphoid organs as soluble TgIg molecules. Proliferation in lymphnodes was marked on day 7 and day 14, and decreased by day 21 (Table II) (Gerloni et al., in preparation). Compared with a simultaneous test performed on spleen cells, it appeared that the magnitude of the proliferative response by lymphnode cells was delayed over that of spleen cells, a fact arguing in favor of the possibility that the proliferative response in the lymphnodes follows the levels of TgIg which peak around day 15 and spread to other lymphoid organs through the bloodstream.

Table 2. T Cell Proliferation in Mice Vaccinated Via STI

	DAY 7 (No. = 6)		DAY 14 (No. = 6)		DAY 21 (No. = 3)	
	B Cell Epitope	T Cell Epitope	B Cell Epitope	T Cell Epitope	B Cell Epitope	T Cell Epitope
Lymphnodes	1.2* ± 0.3 (1 – 1.5)**	4.4 ± 1.7 (2.2 – 6.8)	1.2 ± 0.2 (< 1 – 1.5)	9.3 ± 6.7 (3.9 – 19.8)	< 1 (< 1)	1.5 ± 0.2 (1.2 – 1.7)
Spleen	1.1 ± 0.2 (< 1 – 1.3)	10.9 ± 6.9 (2.6 – 20)	1.1 ± 0.3 (< 1 – 1.6)	7.8 ± 3.7 (3.9 – 12.5)	1.2 ± 0.1 (1.1 – 1.3)	2.2 ± 0.2 (1.9 – 2.4)

* Values refer to stimulation indexes (SI) expressed as mean ±SD. The number of mice examined at each time point is indicated in parenthesis. Results include assays performed on different dates. Tests were done in triplicate.

** Values in parenthesis indicate the range of SI values in each group. B cell epitope = (NANP)3; T cell epitope = NANPNVDPNANP [52]

b. Linked association between B- and T-cell epitopes on the same antigenized V region enhances immunogencity

It is well known that the antibody response to protein antigens requires the cooperation between B cells and T helper (Th) cells [64] with optimal conditions occurring when B and Th cells are specific for different determinants on the same molecule (associative recognition). Many synthetic peptide vaccines [65–68] or recombinant subunit vaccines [69, 70] have been built on this principle.

To optimize the immunogenic potential of STI, we engineered an antigenized antibody gene coding for a B and Th cell epitope from the malaria sporozoite circumsporozoite antigen, one in HV3 and the other in HV2, and tested the immune response. *In vitro* secretion of TgIg was within a normal range (1.6 – 3.3 10^3 molecules/cell/day). Inoculation *in vivo* of plasmid DNA coding for the two epitopes yilded an antibody response against the B cell epitope higher than in mice inoculated with plasmid DNA coding for the B cell epitope alone [52].

c. In vivo activation of cytotoxic T lymphocytes (CTL)

Proof that STI induces CTL *in vivo* was obtained using as a model system an Ig H chain gene engineered in CDR3 to code for a class I MHC (D^b)-restricted CTL epitope, ASNENMETM of the influenza virus nucleoprotein (NP) [71]. *In vitro* studies showed that B lymphoma cells harboring this transgene present the virus peptide to a specific T cell clone [50]. *In vivo* experiments showed that C57BL6 mice inoculated with the same transgene develop specific CTL during priming with a specific lytic activity as high as 40% (Langlade et al., in preparation). Initial studies also show that STI-induced CTL are protective against lethal challange with live virus.

Studies on the transgene *in vivo*

a. The transgene is harbored in B cells

We formally demonstrated that B lymphocytes are the target cell population *in vivo* [72]. Starting from the second week after plasmid DNA inoculation, splenic B and T lymphocytes were isolated to a high degree of purity (97–99%) by FACS sorting (Figure 1). Genomic DNA was extracted from the two cell populations and amplified

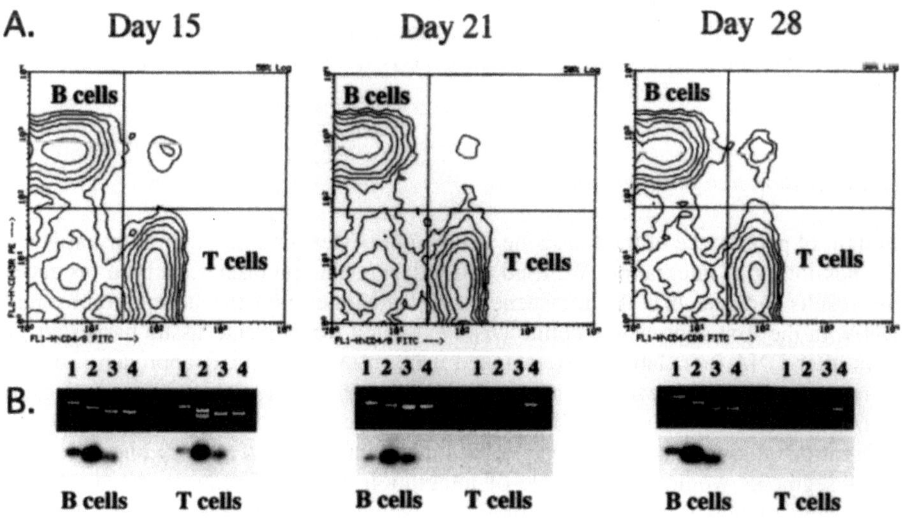

Fig. 1. Isolation of splenic B and T lymphocytes and detection of the transgene H chain in the purified lymphocyte populations. B and T lymphocytes from the spleen of DNA-inoculated mice were sorted and purified on a fluorescence-activated cell sorter (FACS) at the times indicated. The lanes are as follows: 1 – fragment amplified with the primers pCL/pCD (VDJ); 2 – fragment amplified with the primers pSE/pNAD [$(NANP)_3$]; 3 – fragment amplified with the primers pNEL/pNED (NESTED); 4 – fragment amplified with the primers pbA1/pbA2 (β-actin). From ref. [72]

by PCR. At the 15 day time point distinct amplification products were readily detectable in both B and T lymphocytes (left panel). However, at both the 21 and 28 day time points, specific amplification was observed only in B cells (middle and right panels). Southern blot hybridization confirmed the specificity of the amplification products. This analysis suggests, therefore, that B lymphocytes in the spleen are the target cell population. As to the mechanism of uptake of plasmid DNA by B cells little is known. It is possible that binding and internalization may occur either through surface Ig specific for DNA [73, 74] or through a non-Ig DNA receptor [75].

b. Life span and tissue distribution

PCR and Southern blot hybridization were used to monitor the kinetics of the transgene *in vivo* [72]. Genomic DNA extracted from the spleen of inoculated mice was analyzed at various times after inoculation. Amplification of the transgene VDJ region was visible up to 12 weeks after a single DNA inoculation. No amplification was seen at subsequent time points (16, 24, 36 and 52 weeks). Southern blot analysis using a probe specific for the NANP-coding region further confirmed the PCR results. Thus, after inoculation the transgene H chain persists *in vivo* for a period of 3 months. We also determined the tissue distribution of the transgene *in vivo*. We analyzed genomic DNA extracted from various lymphoid (*i.e.*, spleen, lymphnodes and bone-marrow) and non-lymphoid (*i.e.*, liver, kidney, lung and muscle) tissues explanted at different times, and analyzed for specific amplification of the transgene VDJ by PCR. An amplification product was readily visible in genomic DNA of the spleen. No specific amplification occurred in any of the other tissues. This did not vary at any of the time points analyzed. No amplification of the transgene was possible from peripheral blood lymphocytes. Collectively, these results suggest that in all likelihood the destiny of spleen B lymphocytes harboring the transgene is to remain localized in the tissue in which they were transfected.

c. Integration into host genomic DNA

In light of persistence of the transgene in B lymphocytes for 3 months we investigated the possibility of integration. We used two independent approaches. In both instances the results indicate that the transgene likely integrates into the host chromosomal DNA. In the first approach genomic DNA extracted from splenic tissue harvested 17 days after DNA inoculation was analyzed using a multiplex PCR approach [76–78] using seven pairs of specific primers to amplify seven different fragments of plasmid DNA. Primers were designed to facilitate the detection of fragmented plasmid and integration break-points in the plasmid, reasoning that failure to amplify one or several DNA segments would be indicative of integration. In experiments repeated under a wide range of $MgCl_2$ molar concentrations as well as different annealing temperatures two fragments consistently failed to amplify [39]. In the second approach genomic DNA from splenic tissue was first digested with Xba I and subsequently ligated and amplified [72]. In this instance we reasoned that a pattern of multiple molecular size products would suggest integration of the transgene whereas a single band of m.w. ~ 15 kb would suggest persistence of the transgene in episomal form. Both genomic DNA extracted from the spleen 4 and 12 weeks after plasmid DNA inoculation gave rise to amplified products of multiple molecular sizes. No such a pattern was observed in the genomic DNA extracted 36 weeks after inoculation, consistent with the kinetics of transgene detection. A non-integrated (episomal) form of the transgene cold not be detected.

d. The transgene does not mutate in vivo

Because the antigenic and the immunogenic potential of a transgene-encoded H chain must rely on the fact that no sense somatic mutation will affect the nucleotide sequence of the transgene while harbored *in vivo,* it became essential to verify whether V regions coding for heterologous epitopes accumulate somatic mutations. Hypermutation is of frequent occurrence in the V region of Ig, in particular in the complementarity-determining regions (CDR), a fact in agreement with the notion that hypermutation takes place during antigen selection and affinity maturation of the antibody response [79]. No evidence of hypermutation was found in the VDJ region of the transgene even after 3 months *in vivo* (Table III) indicating that *in vivo* persistence for months does not cause accumulations of mutations in the transgene [39, 72]. This result is consistent with the prediction that in the absence of a transmembrane domain in the transgene no antigen-driven somatic mutation would take place.

Table 3. Lack of Transgene Mutations In PCR-Generated Spleen Genomic DNA Clones

Time (Weeks)	No. of Clones Sequenced	No. of Clones Mutated	No. of Nucleotides Mutated	Rate of Mutation* (%)
2	6	1/6	1**	2.9×10^{-4}
4	3	0/3	0	–
12	3	0/3	0	–

* Number of mutations/total number of base pairs sequenced.
** A silent (C → T) mutation in FR3. From ref. [72].

Conclusions

The data presented constitute, in our opinion, convincing evidence that STI is a new, rational system for vaccination. The method to express exogenous peptides in antigenic and immunogenic form is simple and different from existing ones. Unlike vaccines produced by synthetic approaches antigenized antibodies *(i)* express epitopes with intrinsic tri-dimensional conformation for B cell immunogenicity, *(ii)* provide B cells with a continuous source of antigenic peptides for presentation in MHC molecules; and *(iii)* target antigen-presenting cells via the Fc receptor hence maximizing antigen presentation by class II MHC molecules. That STI's immunogenic molecules (TgIg) are manufactured *in vivo* by B lymphocytes as part of a self-determined event allows STI to induce immunity through mimicking of the replicating nature of pathogens, free from their infectious threat, and program immune cells to manufacture large quantities of vaccine molecules, without harming the immune system in the process. Table IV lists relevant immunological differences between conventional DNA vaccines and STI.

STI's conceptual simplicity makes it possible to undertake new directions of study and application. For instance, it may be possible to have a detailed account of the interplay of various cells during priming as well as during the establishment of immunologic memory. Answering questions such as number of B cells transfected *in vivo* and effects on B- and T-cell responses, and the exact role of dendritic cells in the immunogenic process *in vivo*, may be key to enhance the efficacy of vaccination and tailor it to needs on an *ad hoc basis*. Immunity through STI is programmable *in vitro* by assorting different epitopes and relies on simple immunological criteria for the induction of all three major types of adaptive immunity, generation of antibodies and activation of Th and cytotoxic T cell responses. Unlike other antigens TgIg can cross the placenta and carry foreign antigen epitopes from the mother to the offspring, hence rendering T-cell immunity transmissible. Finally, using DNA conveniently chimerized with a cytokine it will be possible to amplify the effect of vaccination and/or program the immune response toward predetermined immunological characterisitics as we have already shown using a DNA/GM-CSF chimeric transgene [80].

Table 4. Differences Between STI and Conventional DNA Vaccines

Conventional DNA Vaccines	STI Vaccines
• Mimic conventional immunization	• Conceptually new
• Directed against a pathogen or a molecule recognized as central to a pathogenic process	• Genetically engineered to assemble epitopes which may or may not belong to the same molecule or pathogen, and permit to attack a pathogenic event
• No specific *in vivo* cell targeting	• Target B cells as vaccine minifactories
• No demonstrable synthesis of transgenic vaccine molecules in bodily fluids	• Active endogenous synthesis of vaccine molecules that are secreted in the circulation. Vaccine molecules redistribute throughout organism (spreading of immunity)
• Induce antibodies after several inoculations	• Induce antibodies after one inoculation
• Unknown involvement of antigen presenting cells	• B cells serve as primary antigen presenting cells. Suitable genetic engineering of the vaccine allows for selective recruitment of dendritic cells. Vaccine molecules are constitutively able to target antigen presenting cells via Fc receptors
• No proof of induction of long term immunologic memory	• Induction of long term immunologic memory
• DNA may include epitopes with potentially adverse effects on the immune response (e.g., antigen competition, suppression, immune deviation etc.)	• Epitopes are selected ad hoc to maximize the immunization process
• Shown to induce tolerance to pathogens	• Does not induce tolerance
• Vaccine products do not cross the placenta	• Vaccine molecules cross the placenta

Acknowledgements. This work was supported by NIH grants AI36467 to M.Z.. M.Z. is Faculty Member of the Biomedical Sciences Graduate Program.

References

1. Zanetti M, E Sercarz, and J Salk (1987) The immunology of new generation vaccines. Immunol. Today 8:18
2. Salk J, and M Zanetti (1989) Next step in the evolution of vaccinology. In Progress in Vaccinology, GP Ta;war Ed., Springer-Verlag, New York. p 451
3. Tan EM, PH Schur, RI Carr, and HG Kunkel (1966) Deoxybonucleic acid (DNA) and antibodies to DNA in the serum of patients with systemic lupus erythematosus. J Clin Invest 45:1732
4. Koffler D, RI Carr, V Agnello, T Fiezi, and HG Kunkel (1969) Antibodies to polynucleotides: distribution in human serums. Science 166:1648
5. Pincus T, PH Schur, JA Rose, JL Decker, and N Talal (1969) Measurement of serum DNA-binding activity in systemic lupus erythematosus. N Engl J Med 281:70
6. Madaio MP, S Hodder, RS Schwartz, and BD Stollar (1984) Responsiveness of autoimmune and normal mice to nucleic acid antigens. J Immunol 132:872
7. Braun W, and M Nakano (1965) Influence of oligodeoxyribonucleotides on early events in antibody formation. Proc. Soc. Exp. Biol. Med. 119:701
8. Gilkeson GS, JP Grudier, and DS Pisetsky (1989) The antibody response of normal mice to immunization with single-stranded DNA of various species origin. Clin Immunol Immunopathol 51:362
9. Gilkeson GS, JP Grudier, DG Karounos, and DS Pisetsky (1989) Induction of anti-double stranded DNA antibodies in normal mice by immunization with bacterial DNA J Immunol 142:1482
10. Tokunaga T, H Yamamoto, S Shimada, H Abe, T Fukuda, Y Fujisawa, Y Furutani, O Yano, T Kataoka, T Sudo, and a. l. et (1984) Antitumor activity of deoxyribonucleic acid fraction from Mycobacterium bovis BCG. I. Isolation, physicochemical characterization, and antitumor activity. J Natl Cancer Inst 72: 955
11. Messina JP, GS Gilkeson, and DS Pisetsky (1993) The influence of DNA structure on the *in vitro* stimulation of murine lymphocytes by natural and synthetic polynucleotide antigens. Cell Immunol 147:148
12. Yamamoto S, T Yamamoto, S Shimada, E Kuramoto, O Yano, T Kataoka, and T Tokunaga (1992) DNA from bacteria, but not from vertebrates, induces interferons, activates natural killer cells and inhibits tumor growth. Microbiol Immunol 36:983
13. Krieg AM, AK Yi, S Matson, TJ Waldschmidt, GA Bishop, R Teasdale, GA Koretzky, and DM Klinman (1995) CpG motifs in bacterial DNA trigger direct B-cell activation. Nature 374:546
14. Cardon LR, C Burge, DA Clayton, and S Karlin (1994) Pervasive CpG suppression in animal mitochondrial genomes. Proc Natl Acad Sci U SA 91.3799
15. Roman M, OE Martin, JS Goodman, MD Nguyen, Y Sato, A Ronaghy, RS Kornbluth, DD Richman, DA Carson, and E Raz (1997) Immunostimulatory DNA sequences function as T helper-1-promoting adjuvants [see comments]. Nat Med 3:849
16. Cohen J (1993) Naked DNA Points Way to Vaccines. Science 259:1691
17. Ulmer JB, JC Sadoff, and MA Liu (1996) DNA vaccines. Curr Opin Immunol 8:53
18. Wang B, K Ugen, V Srikantan, M Agadjanyan, K Dang, Y Refaeli, A Sato, J Boyer, W Williams, and D Weiner (1993) Gene inoculation generates immune responses against human immunodeficiency virus type 1) Proc. Natl. Acad. Sci. USA 90:4156
19. Tang D, M DeVit, and SA Johnston (1992) Genetic immunization is a simple method for eliciting an immune response. Nature 356:152
20. Ulmer JB, JJ Donnelly, SE Parker, GH Rhodes, PL Felgner, VJ Dwarki, SH Gromkowski, RR Deck, CM Dewitt, A Friedman, LA Hawe, KR Leander, D Martinez, HC Perry, JW Shiver, DL Montgomery, and MA Liu (1993) Heterologous protection against influenza by injection of DNA encoding a viral protein. Science 259:1745
21. Huygen K, J Content, O Denis, DL Montgomery, AM Yawman, RR Deck, CM DeWitt, IM Orme, S Baldwin, C D'Souza, A Drowart, E Lozes, P Vandenbussche, J-P Van Vooren, MA Liu, and JB Ulmer (1996) Immunogenicity and protective efficacy of a tuberculosis DNA vaccine. Nat. Med. 2:893
22. Tascon RE, MJ Colston, S Ragno, E Stavropoulos, D Gregory, and DB Lowrie (1996) Vaccination against tuberculosis by DNA injection. Nat. Med. 2:888
23. Sedegah M, R Hedstrom, P Hobart, and SL Hoffman (1994) Protection against malaria by immunization with plasmid DNA encoding circumsporozoite protein. Proc. Natl. Acad. Sci. USA 91:9866
24. Conry RM, AF LoBuglio, J Kantor, J Schlom, F Loechel, SE Moore, LA Sumerel, DL Barlow, S Abrams, and DT Curiel (1994) Immune response to a carcinoembryonic antigen polynucleotide vaccine. Cancer Res 54:1164

25. Gilkeson GS, P Ruiz, AM Pippen, AL Alexander, JB Lefkowith, and DS Pisetsky (1996) Modulation of renal disease in autoimmune NZB/NZW mice by immunization with bacterial DNA J Exp Med 183: 1389
26. Waisman A, PJ Ruiz, DL Hirschberg, A Gelman, JR Oksenberg, S Brocke, F Mor, IR Cohen, and L Steinman (1996) Suppressive vaccination with DNA encoding a variable region gene of the T-cell receptor prevents autoimmune encephalomyelitis and activates Th2 immunity. Nat. Med. 2:899
27. Raz E, H Tighe, Y Sato, M Corr, JA Dudler, M Roman, SL Swain, HL Spiegelberg, and DA Carson (1996) Preferential induction of a Th1 immune response and inhibition of specific IgE antibody formation by plasmid DNA immunization. Proc Natl Acad Sci U SA 93:514
28. Wu CH, JM Wilson, and GY Wu (1989) Targeting genes: delivery and persistent expression of a foreign gene driven by mammalian regulatory elements *in vivo*. J Biol Chem 264:16985
29. Ferkol T, JC Perales, F Mularo, and RW Hanson (1996) Receptor-mediated gene transfer into macrophages. Proc Natl Acad Sci USA 93:101
30. Ferkol T, JC Perales, E Eckman, CS Kaetzel, RW Hanson, and PB Davis (1995) Gene transfer into the airway epithelium of animals by targeting the polymeric immunoglobulin receptor. J Clin Invest 95:493
31. Gillies SD, SL Morrison, VT Oi, and S Tonegawa (1983) A tissue-specific transcription enhancer element is located in the major intron of a rearranged immunoglobulin heavy chain gene. Cell 33:717
32. Banerji J, L Olson, and W Schaffner (1983) A lymphocyte-specific cellular enhancer is located downstream of the joining region in immunoglobulin heavy chain genes. Cell 33:729
33. Mason JO, GT Williams, and MS Neuberger (1985) Transcription cell type specificity is conferred by an immunoglobulin VH gene promoter that includes a functional consensus sequence. Cell 41:479
34. Grosschedl R, and D Baltimore (1985) Cell-type specificity of immunoglobulin gene expression is regulated by at least three DNA sequence elements. Cell 41:885
35. Morrison S (1985) Transfectomas provide novel chimeric antibodies. Science 229:1202
36. Storb U (1987) Transgenic mice with immunoglobulin genes. Annu Rev Immunol 5:151
37. Langman RE, and M Cohn (1987) The E-T (elephant-tadpole) paradox necessitates the concept of a unit of B-cell function: the protecton. Mol. Immunol. 24:675
38. Lanzavecchia A (1985) Antigen specific interaction between T and B cells. Nature 314:537
39. Gerloni M, R Billetta, S Xiong, and M Zanetti (1997) Somatic transgene immunization with DNA encoding an immunoglobulin heavy chain. DNA and Cell Biology 16:611
40. Zanetti M (1992) Antigenized antibodies. Nature 355:466
41. Billetta R, RM Hollingdale, and M Zanetti (1991) Immunogenicity of an engineered internal image antibody. Proc. Natl. Acad. Sci. USA 88:4713
42. Lanza P, R Billetta, S Antonenko, and M Zanetti (1993) Active immunity against the CD4 receptor using an antibody antigenized with residues 41–55 of the first extracellular domain. Proc. Natl. Acad. Sci. USA 90:11683
43. Rossi F, R Billetta, Z Ruggeri, and M Zanetti (1995) Engineered idiotypes. Immunochemical analysis of antigenized antibodies expressing a conformationally constrained Arg-Gly-Asp motif. Mol Immunol 32:341
44. Zaghouani H, R Steinman, R Nonacs, H Shah, W Gerhard, and C Bona (1993) Presentation of a viral T cell epitope expressed in the CDR3 region of a self immunoglobulin molecule. Science 259:224
45. Zaghouani H, SA Anderson, KE Sperber, C Daian, RC Kennedy, L Mayer, and CA Bona (1995) Induction of antibodies to the human immunodeficiency virus type 1 by immunization of baboons with immunoglobulin molecules carrying the principal neutralizing determinant of the envelope protein. Proc Natl Acad Sci U SA 92:631
46. Cook J, and BH Barber (1995) Recombinant antibodies containing an engineered B-cell epitope capable of eliciting conformation-specific antibody responses. Vaccine 13:1770
47. Corthesy B, M Kaufmann, A Phalipon, M Peitsch, MR Neutra, and JP Kraehenbuhl (1996) A pathogen-specific epitope inserted into recombinant secretory immunoglobulin A is immunogenic by the oral route. J Biol Chem 271:33670
48. Cook J, and BH Barber (1997) Recombinant antibodies with conformationally constrained HIV type 1 epitope inserts elicit glycoprotein 160-specific antibody responses *in vivo*. Aids Res Hum Retroviruses 13:449
49. Zanetti M, F Rossi, P Lanza, G Filaci, RH Lee, and R Billetta (1992) Theoretical and pratical aspects of antigenized antibodies. Immunol. Rev. 130:125
50. Billetta R, G Filaci, and M Zanetti (1995) Major histocompatibility complex class I-restricted presentation of influenza virus nucleoprotein peptide by B lymphoma cells harboring an antibody gene antigenized with the virus peptide. Eur J Immunol 25:776

51. Zaghouani H, M Krystal, H Kuzu, T Moran, H Shah, Y Kuzu, J Schulman, and C Bona (1992) Cells expressing an H chain Ig gene carrying a viral T cell epitope are lysed by specific cytolytic T cells. 148: 3604
52. Xiong S, M Gerloni, and M Zanetti (1997) Engineering vaccines with heterologous B and T cell epitopes using immunoglobulin genes. Nature Biotech. 15:882
53. Zavala F, JP Tam, MR Hollingdale, AH Cochrane, I Quakyi, RS Nussenzweig, and V Nussenzweig (1985) Rationale for Development of a Synthetic Vaccine Against Plasmodium falciparum Malaria. Science 228:1436
54. Clyde DF, VC McCarthy, RM Miller, and RB Hornick (1973) Specificity of protectionof man immunized against sporozoite-induced falciparum malaria. Am. J. Med. Sci. 266:398
55. Egan JE, SL Hoffman, JD Haynes, JC Sadoff, I Schneider, GE Grau, MR Hollingdale, WR Ballou, and DM Gordon (1993) Humoral immune responses in volunteers immunized with irradiated Plasmodium falciparum sporozoites. Am J Trop Med Hyg 49:166
56. Edelman R, SL Hoffman, JR Davis, M Beier, MB Sztein, G Losonsky, DA Herrington, HA Eddy, MR Hollingdale, DM Gordon, and al. et (1993) Long-term persistence of sterile immunity in a volunteer immunized with X-irradiated Plasmodium falciparum sporozoites. J Infect Dis 168:1066
57. Stoute JA, M Slaoui, DG Heppner, P Momin, KE Kester, P Desmons, BT Wellde, N Garcon, U Krzych, M Marchand, WR Ballou, and JD Cohen (1997) A preliminary evaluation of a recombinant circumsporozoite protein vaccine against Plasmodium falciparum malaria. RTS, S Malaria Vaccine Evaluation Group [see comments]. N Engl J Med 336:86
58. GerloniM, S Xiong, and M Zanetti (1997) Durable immunity and immunologic memory to a parasite antigen induced by somatic transgene immunization. Vaccine 16
59. Raz E, DA Carson, SE Parker, TB Parr, AM Abai, G Aichinger, SH Gromkowski, M Singh, D Lew, MA Yankauckas, SM Baird, and GH Rhodes (1994) Intradermal gene immunization: the possible role of DNA uptake in the induction of cellular immunity to viruses. Proc. Natl. Acad. Sci. USA 91:9519
60. Davis HL, M Mancini, M Michel, and R Whalen (1996) DNA-based immunization to hepatitis B surface antigen: longevity of primary and effect of boost. Vaccine 14:910
61. Xiang ZQ, SSpitalnik, M Tran, WH Wunner, J Cheng, and HC Ertl (1994) Vaccination with a plasmid vector carrying the rabies virus glycoprotein gene induces protective immunity against rabies virus. Virology 199:132
62. Anderson R, X-M Gao, A Papakonstantinopoulou, M Roberts, and G Dougan (1996) Immune response in mice following immunization with DNA encoding fragment C of tetanus toxin. Infect. Imm. 64:3168
63. Salk J (1984) One-dose immunization against paralytic poliomyelitis using a noninfectious vaccine. Rev Infect Dis:S444
64. Mitchison NA (1971) The carrier effect in the secondary response to hapten-protein conjugates. II. Cellular cooperation. Eur J Immunol 1:18
65. Herrington DA, DF Clyde, G Losonsky, M Cortesia, JR Murphy, J Davis, S Baqar, AM Felix, EP Heimer, and D Gillessen (1987) Safety and immunogenicity in man of a synthetic peptide malaria vaccine against Plasmodium falciparum sporozoites. Nature 328:257
66. Tam JP, and YA Lu (1989) Vaccine engineering: enhancement of immunogenicity of synthetic peptide vaccines related to hepatitis in chemically defined models consisting of T- and B-cell epitopes. Proc Natl Acad Sci U SA 86:9084
67. Tam JP, P Clavijo, YA Lu, V Nussenzweig, R Nussenzweig, and F Zavala (1990) Incorporation of T and B epitopes of the circumsporozoite protein in a chemically defined synthetic vaccine against malaria. J Exp Med 171:299
68. Munesinghe DY, P Clavijo, MC Calle, RS Nussenzweig, and E Nardin (1991) Immunogenicity of multiple antigen peptides (MAP) containing T and B cell epitopes of the repeat region of the P. falciparum circumsporozoite protein. Eur J Immunol 21:3015
69. Ballou WR, SL Hoffman, JA Sherwood, MR Hollingdale, FA Neva, WT Hockmeyer, DM Gordon, I Schneider, RA Wirtz, and JF Young (1987) Safety and efficacy of a recombinant DNA Plasmodium falciparum sporozoite vaccine. Lancet 1:1277
70. Herrington DA, GA Losonsky, G Smith, F Volvovitz, M Cochran, K Jackson, SL Hoffman, DM Gordon, MM Levine, and R Edelman (1992) Safety and immunogenicity in volunteers of a recombinant Plasmodium falciparum circumsporozoite protein malaria vaccine produced in Lepidopteran cells. Vaccine 10:841
71. Rotzschke O, K Falk, K Deres, H Schild, M Norda, J Metzger, G Jung, and H-G Rammensee (1990) Isolation and analysis of naturally processed viral peptides as recognized by cytotoxic T cells. Nature 348:252

72. Xiong S, M Gerloni, and M Zanetti (1997) *in vivo* role of B lymphocytes in somatic transgene immunization. Proc. Natl. Acad. Sci. USA 94:6352
73. Holmberg D, AA Freitas, D Portnoi, F Jacquemart, S Avrameas, and A Coutinho (1986) Antibody repertoires of normal BALB/c mice: B lymphocyte populations defined by state of activation. Immunol. Rev. 93:147
74. Glotz D, M Sollazzo, S Riley, and M Zanetti (1988) Isotype, VH genes, and antigen-binding analysis of hybridomas from newborn BALB/c mice. J. Immunol. 141:383
75. Bennett RM, GT Gabor, and MM Merritt (1985) DNA binding to human leukocytes. Evidence for a receptor-mediated association, internalization, and degradtion of DNA J. Clin. Invest. 76:2182
76. Donaldson YK, MJ Arends, E Duvall, and CC Bird (1993) A PCR approach to discriminate between integrated and episomal HPV DNA in small clinical specimens. Mol Cell Probes 7:285
77. Chen CM, MP Shyu, LC Au, HW Chu, WT Cheng, and KB Choo (1994) Analysis of deletion of the integrated human papillomavirus 16 sequence in cervical cancer: a rapid multiplex polymerase chain reaction approach. J Med Virol 44:206
78. Daniel B, G Mukherjee, L Seshadri, E Vallikad, and S Krishna (1995) Changes in the physical state and expression of human papillomavirus type 16 in the progression of cervical intraepithelial neoplasia lesions analysed by PCR. J Gen Virol:2589
79. Griffiths GM, C Berek, M Kaartinen, and C Milstein (1984) Somatic mutation and the maturation of immune response to 2-phenyl oxazolone. Nature 312:271
80. Gerloni M, D Lo, and M Zanetti (1998) DNA immunization in relB-deficient mice discloses a role for dendritic cells in IgG1→IgM switch *in vivo*. Eur. J. Immunol. In press, (1998

DNA vaccines: safety and efficacy issues

Dennis M. Klinman, Mitsuhiro Takeno, Motohide Ichino, Mili Gu, Galina Yamshchikov, Gil Mor, Jacqueline Conover

Section of Retroviral Immunology, Division of Viral Products,
Center for Biologics Research and Evaluation, Food and Drug Administration,
Bldg 29A Rm 3 D 10 HFM 454, Bethesda, MD 20892, USA

Summary. DNA technology has been harnessed to produce a variety of plasmid-based vaccines designed to prevent viral, bacterial and parasitic infections. The rapid adoption and implementation of this novel vaccine strategy carries with it important safety and efficacy concerns. This review will focus on whether DNA vaccines (1) are likely to induce systemic or organ-specific autoimmune disease, (2) have the potential to induce tolerance rather than immunity, and (3) are as effective in individuals with depressed immune function as they are in healthy adults.

Overview

Infectious organisms are a major source of morbidity and mortality worldwide. Preventing these infections is a public health priority and the primary goal of vaccine research. The development of new vaccines has been revolutionized by the finding that antigen-encoding DNA plasmids can be used to induce cellular and humoral immune responses against immunogenic determinants on viruses, parasites and bacteria [5, 43, 52, 54, 55]. These vaccines successfully prevent infection in a variety of animal models.

DNA vaccines consist of an antigen-encoding gene whose expression is regulated by a strong mammalian promoter located on a plasmid backbone of bacterial DNA [54, 56]. When injected intramuscularly (i.m.) or intradermally, DNA vaccines are transcribed, translated, and the protein they encode expressed in the context of self major histocompatibility complex (MHC) [29, 54, 56].

While the immunogenicity of DNA vaccines has been established in species ranging from mouse to man, the long-term safety and efficacy of these products is less well characterized. A number of concerns associated with the use of DNA vaccines have been raised, including the possibility that they may: (1) integrate into the host genome, thereby increasing the risk of malignancy (by activating oncogenes or inactivating tumor suppressor genes), (2) induce responses against self antigens thereby triggering

Correspondence to: D. M. Klinman

the development of autoimmune disease, (3) induce a local inflammatory response against cells producing the vaccine-encoded antigen (such as muscle or skin cells), (4) induce tolerance rather than immunity, and/or (5) stimulate the production of cytokines that alter the host's ability to resist other infectious agents. Compounding these concerns is the relative dearth of information concerning the mechanisms involved in plasmid uptake, persistence, processing and presentation in vivo. This article will focus on findings from our laboratory relevant to several of these issues.

Can DNA vaccines induce anti-DNA autoantibody production and/or promote the development of autoimmune disease?

Introduction

DNA vaccines can induce strong, protective antibody and cytotoxic responses. Contributing to the immunogenicity of DNA vaccines are elements of bacterial origin in their plasmid backbone [22, 24, 37]. These elements have intrinsic immunostimulatory properties that by promoting immune activation may contribute to the development of autoimmune disease. For example, bacterial (but not mammalian) DNA can stimulate normal mice to produce IgG anti-DNA autoantibodies and develop glomerulonephritis [10, 11, 36, 48]. Bacterial DNA can also accelerate autoantibody production by lupus-prone mice [10, 11]. Both the hypergammaglobulinemia and increased cytokine production triggered by bacterial DNA have been associated with the development of systemic autoimmune disease [17, 19, 28].

Many of these effects are linked to differences in the structure of bacterial versus mammalian DNA. In particular, unmethylated CpG dinucleotides are nearly 20 times more common in bacterial than mammalian DNA due to a combination of 'CpG suppression' and CpG methylation [4, 38]. We and others have shown that unmethylated CpG motifs present in bacterial DNA induce polyclonal T, B and natural killer (NK) cell activation, resulting in the release of immunomodulatory cytokines such as interleukin (IL)-6, interferon-γ (IFN-γ), IL-12 and tumor necrosis factor-α (TNF-α), as well as the polyclonal activation of IgM-secreting lymphocytes [13, 22, 24]. Recent work demonstrates that these CpG motifs are present in the plasmid backbone of DNA vaccines, where they facilitate the development of antigen-specific immune responses [23, 41]. These same motifs may contribute to the activation of anti-DNA-secreting B cells and/or the development of autoimmune disease.

DNA vaccination activates anti-DNA-secreting B cells

We examined whether DNA vaccines could induce or accelerate the development of systemic or organ-specific autoimmune responses. Normal BALB/c mice were immunized and boosted multiple times with each of three different plasmid (p)DNA vaccines. Sensitive and specific ELIspot assays were used to monitor the production of antigen-specific and anti-self responses in these mice [18, 21].

All three plasmids behaved similarly. Adult BALB/c mice immunized with 40 μg of the pCSP DNA vaccine (encoding the circumsporozoite protein of malaria) stimulated a 100-fold increase in the number of cells producing IgG anti-CSP antibodies ($P < 0.01$) and a 1,000-fold increase in serum anti-CSP titer (Table 1). Multiple im-

Table 1. Effect of immunization on antigen-specific B cell activation

Immunogen	Age (months)	Number of IgG secreting cells/106 spleen cells[a]				Serum Anti-DNA[b]
		DNA	Myosin	CSP	OVA	
I. BALB/c mice						
None	3	4 ± 2	1 ± 1	1 ± 1	1 ± 1	1.0 ± 0.2
pCSP	3	14 ± 4	1 ± 0	108 + 14	1 + 0	1.5 ± 0.2
1012 plasmid	3	15 ± 5	1 ± 0	1 ± 0	2 + 1	1.6 ± 0.3
Ovalbumin/IFA	3	3 ± 1	1 ± 1	1 ± 1	68 ± 14	1.0 ± 0.1
CS.1/IFA	3	4 ± 2	ND	49 ± 7	1 ± 1	1.0 ± 0.2
II. NZB/W mice						
None	3	46 ± 9	16 ± 5	1 ± 1	ND	4.3 ± 1.2
None	5.5	142 ± 38	35 ± 14	2 ± 1	ND	38 ± 11
pCSP	5.5	158 ± 42	31 ± 11	38 + 14	ND	34 ± 9
1012 plasmid	5.5	165 ± 56	29 ± 9	2 ± 1	ND	41 ± 12

ND, Not done; pCSP, plasmid circumsporozoite protein of *Plasmodium yoelii* (PyCSP); CS.1, recombinant purified CSP; IFA, incomplete Freund's adjuvant; OVA, ovalbumin

[a] BALB/c and NZB/W mice were immunized and boosted with 40–50 µg of plasmid DNA, or 50 µg of ovalbumin in an equal volume of IFA. The number of splenic B cells secreting IgG antibodies reactive with each antigen was determined by ELIspot assay 1 week post boost. Data represent the average ±SD of 6–12 mice/group

[b] A 1:50–1:500 dilution of serum from immunized mice was analyzed by ELISA for IgG ant-DNA antibodies

munizations with this DNA vaccine had no effect on the number of B cells or serum antibody levels reactive with the muscle cell autoantigen myosin or the control antigen ovalbumin (Table 1).

Whereas primary immunization did not activate B cells to secrete IgG antibodies reactive with mammalian DNA, booster immunizations elicited up to a threefold rise in the number of spleen cells producing IgG anti-DNA autoantibodies ($P = 0.004$, Table 1). This was accompanied by a modest but reproducible increase in serum IgG anti-DNA antibody levels (35–60%) in BALB/c mice immunized and boosted with either the pCSP vaccine or the 1012 vector from which pCSP was constructed (Table 1). Mice immunized with conventional protein antigens (such as ovalbumin) produced IgG antibodies against the corresponding target antigen but not against mammalian DNA (Table 1).

Effect of pDNA vaccination on B cell activation in lupus-prone mice

(NZB × NZW)F_1 mice develop life-threatening renal disease associated with the spontaneous overproduction of pathogenic IgG anti-DNA autoantibodies [6, 26, 50]. The number of B cells secreting these autoantibodies increases over time, a process accelerated by the administration of bacterial DNA [11]. As seen in Table 1, the number of B cells spontaneously secreting IgG anti-DNA autoantibodies increased over time in both control and vaccine-treated NZB/W mice. Vaccination did not significantly increase the production of autoantibodies reactive with DNA or myosin (Table 1).

Table 2. Effect of immunization on the development of autoimmunity

Treatment	Serum[a]		Kidney Histology[b]	Survival[c] (Days)
	BUN (mg/100 ml)	Cr (mg/100 ml)		
A. BALB/c mice				
Saline	22 ± 2	0.1 ± 0.1	0.5 ± 0.3	> 460
pCSP X 4	21 ± 8	0.1 ± 0.1	0.4 ± 0.2	> 460
B. B/W mice				
Saline	74 ± 38	0.3 ± 0.2	16 ± 7	260
pCSP X 4	83 ± 34	0.3 ± 0.2	18 ± 9	280

[a] Mice were primed and boosted 4 times with 50 µg of pCSP
[b] Sera were analyzed for blood urea nitrogen (BUN) and creatinine (Cr) levels
[c] Kidneys from these mice were formalin fixed and analyzed histologically for pathological changes associated with the development of immune-mediated glomerulonephritis. This analysis is based on a 39 point scale that evaluates interstitial and glomerular inflammation, tubular atrophy/fibrosis and case formation. The difference in kidney histology between saline treated and 1012/PyCSP DNA vaccine-treated mice was not statistically significant between treated and control mice of the same strain. Data provided are the mean ± SD of 6 mice/group
[d] The survival of mice primed and boosted 4 times with 50 µg of pCSP was monitored. Data represent the lifespan reached by one-half of all mice in each group (n = 30/group)

Absence of clinical sequelae following DNA vaccination

Cohorts of 30 BALB/c and 30 B/W mice were immunized four times with the pCSP DNA vaccine and monitored for the appearance of glomerulonephritis, myositis, and death. BALB/c mice remained healthy (no myositis, no proteinuria) throughout the 16 month observation period [33]. Three mice from this group were boosted a final time (at 20 months) and were killed 2 weeks later. Tissues from these animals were examined histologically for evidence of autoimmune disease. Kidneys from vaccinated mice showed no evidence of glomerulonephritis or immune complex deposition, and their muscle beds showed no increase in Ig- or cytokine-secreting cells when compared to excipient-treated controls (legend, Table 2).

Immunized and saline-treated B/W mice developed signs and symptoms of active autoimmune disease as they grew older. The age of onset and severity of proteinuria, and the lifespan of vaccinated versus control B/W mice, were similar (Table 2). Kidneys from a separate group of B/W mice immunized four times and killed at 9 months of age showed histological evidence of glomerulonephritis associated with IgG immune complex deposition. The degree of renal damage in saline-treated versus DNA-vaccinated animals was similar (Table 2).

Overview

These studies examined whether repeated DNA vaccination of normal or lupus-prone mice resulted in the activation of autoantibody-secreting B cells or the induction/acceleration of autoimmune disease. Our goal was to unmask autoimmunity by (1) studying lupus-prone B/W mice at high risk for the development of DNA-induced autoimmunity, and (2) monitoring autoantibody-secreting cells using extremely sensitive ELIspot assays [18, 21]. Our results showed that a threefold increase in the number of B cells secreting IgG antibodies against mammalian DNA was induced when mice were repeatedly immunized with pDNA vaccines (Table 1), whereas serum anti-DNA antibody titers rose 35–60%. Conventional protein immunogens did not increase anti-DNA antibody production, indicating that the observed effect was DNA vaccine specific.

Despite the increase in IgG anti-DNA autoantibody production induced by pDNA vaccination, no effect on the onset or severity of autoimmune disease was observed in multiply-vaccinated normal or lupus-prone mice. We believe this absence of clinical sequelae reflects the fairly short-lived and modest effect of vaccination on systemic autoantibody production. For example, mice with active lupus have nearly 40-fold higher serum anti-DNA antibody titers than normal mice vaccinated four times with a DNA vaccine. While the possibility remains that a subset of DNA vaccines (particularly those encoding determinants cross-reactive with self antigens) may stimulate an autoimmune response, our findings suggest that the level of autoantibody production elicited by these DNA vaccines is insufficient to induce active autoimmunity. More problematic may be the preferential production of type 1 cytokines (IFN-γ, IL-12) induced by immunization with bacterial DNA and plasmid vaccines [23]. Ongoing studies suggest that the overproduction of type 1 cytokines may promote or aggravate the development of organ-specific autoimmune syndromes. Additional research to assess the safety of DNA vaccines in the general population is needed.

Studies of neonatal tolerance induced by a DNA vaccine

Introduction

Most investigators study the immunogenicity of DNA vaccines in healthy adult animals [5, 39, 43, 51, 54]. Yet most vaccines intended for human use are administered to individuals with reduced immune function (e.g., infants, children, the elderly, and the immunosuppressed). We have, therefore, examined the safety and immunogenicity of DNA vaccines in these populations.

The integrity of the immune system is reduced in newborns and the elderly. For example, newborns exposed to foreign antigens are at risk of developing tolerance rather than immunity due to the functional immaturity of their lymphocytes and antigen-presenting cells [47]. A number of factors influence the development of neonatal tolerance including the type, concentration and method by which the antigen is introduced, and the age of the host [30, 40, 46]. Evidence suggests that recognition of foreign determinants is acquired at distinct stages of maturation, ranging from early gestation until days or weeks after birth [16, 20, 30, 46, 49]. Since the protein encoded by a DNA vaccine is produced endogenously and expressed in the context of self MHC, the potential exists for the neonatal immune system to recognize it as 'self', resulting in the development of tolerance rather than immunity. Our studies examined the effect of administering the pCSP DNA vaccine to newborns, since this vaccine induces a protective antibody and cytotoxic T lymphocyte (CTL) response in adult BALB/c mice [43].

Table 3. Induction of neonatal tolerance by the pCSP DNA vaccine

Age of vaccine recipient			Serum antibody levels[a]	Cytokine production[b]		CTL activity[c]
2 days	2 months	6 months		IL-4	IFN-γ	
	Vector		< 0.1	1.0	1.1	4 ± 2
	pCSP		0.5 ± 0.2	4.5	0.9	ND
	pCSP	pCSP	1.1 ± 0.4	1.4	7.4	34 ± 10
pCSP			< 0.1	0.9	1.0	3 ± 3
pCSP	pCSP		< 0.1	1.0	1.1	ND
pCSP	pCSP	pCSP	< 0.1	0.9	1.1	6 ± 2
Vector	pCSP		0.4 ± 0.1	ND	ND	ND

CTL, Cytotoxic T lymphocytes

BALB/c mice were injected in both quadriceps muscles with either pCSP or the plasmid vector from which it was derived. Immune responses were studied 3 weeks after the initial immunization and 1 week after subsequent immunizations

[a] A 1:100 dilution of serum was assayed by ELISA for IgG antibodies reactive with CS.1 protein. Data represent the mean absorbance (A) ± SD from 5 mice/group

[b] Cytokine ELIspot assays were used to detect IL-4 and IFN-γ-secreting cells in the spleen [44, 45]. Results reflect the fold increase in number of spleen cells actively secreting cytokine in vivo when compared to age-matched controls

[c] Spleen cells were stimulated *in vitro* for 5 days with a synthetic CTL peptide from PyCSP and then assayed for cytolytic activity. Results reflect the percent specific cytolysis of peptide-pulsed MHC-matched P815 cells less non-specific lysis of negative controls

Induction of humoral tolerance by the pCSP DNA vaccine

Two-day-old BALB/c mice were injected i.m. with 10 μg pCSP. Whereas vaccination stimulated 2-month-old mice to produce anti-CSP antibodies, no serum antibody response was detected in newborn animals (Table 3). This finding suggested that newborns either did not recognize the CSP, or that they were tolerized by the vaccine-encoded antigen. To discriminate between these alternatives, mice were injected with pCSP at 2 days of age and then re-immunized as adults. Mice injected as neonates were unresponsive to subsequent pCSP immunization (Table 3). This lack of reactivity was directly associated with pCSP vaccination, since (1) neonatal mice treated with 1012 vector (lacking the CSP-encoding gene) were not tolerized to the CSP, and (2) the same vaccine administered to adult mice was highly immunogenic (Table 3). Thus, the pCSP DNA vaccine induced tolerance rather than immunity in neonatal BALB/c mice.

Effect of pCSP on cytokine production

The pattern of cytokines elicited by the pCSP DNA vaccine was also examined. Priming adult BALB/c mice with pCSP stimulated the production of the type 2 cytokines IL-4 and IL-6 (Table 3 and [32]), while secondary immunization preferentially induced the secretion of the type 1 cytokine IFN-γ (see [32]). In contrast, no cytokine production was detected when neonatally tolerized mice were immunized or boosted with pCSP (Table 3). These findings suggest that classical neonatal tolerance (characterized by the absence of antibody or cytokine production) was elicited against epitopes expressed by the pCSP-encoded antigen.

An antigen re-stimulation assay was used to determine whether memory T cells were present in tolerized mice. Initial experiments examined the response of spleen cells from adult BALB/c mice immunized with pCSP. When spleen cells from vaccinated adults were cultured in vitro with an immunogenic peptide from CSP, IL-4 and IFN-γ production was induced. In contrast, splenocytes from neonatally tolerized mice did not respond to in vitro stimulation with full-length CSP or the immunostimulatory peptide (data not shown). These findings support the conclusion that pCSP is a toleragen rather than an immunogen in neonatal mice.

Effect of pCSP DNA vaccination on cytotoxic T cell responses

A final series of experiments examined the capacity of neonatally tolerized mice to generate antigen-specific CTL. We found that mice immunized and boosted as adults with pCSP mounted a strong cytotoxic response against peptide-pulsed MHC-matched targets (data not shown). Unpulsed targets and peptide-pulsed targets expressing the wrong MHC type were not lysed. In contrast, spleen cells from mice tolerized as newborns and immunized as adults with pCSP were unable to generate CTL against MHC-matched peptide-pulsed targets, despite in vitro re-stimulation with an optimally immunogenic CTL peptide (Table 3).

Overview

Long-lasting neonatal tolerance (persisting for more than 9 months) resulted from the administration of pCSP to newborn BALB/c mice. Tolerized mice were unable to mount antibody, cytokine or CTL responses when re-immunized with pCSP as adults. The induction of tolerance was critically dependent on both the age at which the vaccine was administered and the presence of the PyCSP-encoding gene. Tolerance was only induced when pCSP was administered to mice under 8 days of age. However, tolerance induction was not MHC restricted since newborn C57B*L*/6 (H-2^h) as well as BALB/c (H-2^d) mice could be tolerized by neonatal administration of pCSP. These findings suggest that tolerance rather than immunity may result when the neonatal immune system is confronted with an antigen produced endogenously and expressed in the context of self MHC following DNA vaccination.

However, not all DNA vaccines induce neonatal tolerance. Studies in our laboratory and elsewhere indicate that antigen-encoding plasmids may elicit active immune responses in neonatal mice. Establishing the factors responsible for the development of tolerance rather than immunity should improve our ability to design efficacious vaccines.

Decreased immunogenicity and efficacy of DNA vaccination in aged mice

Introduction

The elderly as well as the young are at heightened risk from infectious diseases [3]. Increased age is associated with a decline in cell-mediated and humoral immune responsiveness [31, 53]. Numerous factors have been identified that might contribute to this

Table 4. DNA vaccination of aged mice: reduced immunogenicity and efficacy

	Age of vaccine recipient		
	Untreated	2 months	> 26 months
1° IgG anti-CSP response[a]	0.32 ± 0.03	1.31 ± 0.24	0.42 ± 0.06
2° IgG anti-CSP response[a]	0.35 ± 0.04	2.17 ± 0.38	0.70 ± 0.15
CTL activity[b]	< 6	13 ± 3	39 ± 8
Protective efficacy[c]	0	80	40

BALB/c mice were injected in both quadriceps muscles with either pCSP or the plasmid vector from which it was derived. Immune responses were studied 3 weeks after immunization and 1 week post boost

[a] A 1:100 dilution of serum was assayed by ELISA for IgG antibodies reactive with the CS.1 protein. Data represent the mean A ± SD from 4 mice/group

[b] Spleen cells were stimulated in vitro for 5 days with a synthetic CTL peptide from the CS protein and then assayed for cytolytic activity. Results reflect the percent specific cytolysis of peptide-pulsed MHC-matched P815 cells minus lysis of negative controls at a 30:1 effector:target ratio. The difference between young and aged mice was statistically significant ($P < 0.03$)

[c] Boosted mice were challenged i.v. with 12 ID_{50} of live malaria sporozoites. Data represent the percent of animals protected from infection

age-related reduction in immunity, including thymic involution, loss of T effector cell precursors, diminished antigen-presenting cell activity, and changes in the number, frequency and activation state of type 1 and type 2 cytokine-secreting cells [2, 7–9, 14, 15, 25, 27, 31, 42, 53].

Vaccines used by the elderly must compensate for this decline in immune function since impaired vaccine responses are associated with increased mortality and morbidity in this population [35]. Having observed that the immunogenicity of the pCSP vaccine was reduced in newborns, we examined its efficacy in aged mice.

Antibody and CTL responses of aged mice vaccinated with pCSP

Young (2-month-old) and aged (> 26-month-old) BALB/c mice were immunized and boosted twice i.m. with 50 µg pCSP. Primary immunization elicited a strong IgG anti-CSP response in young adults but virtually no IgG anti-CSP antibodies in aged mice ($P < 0.01$, Table 4). The number of B cells secreting IgG anti-CSP antibodies increased 30-fold over background in young animals, but less than 2-fold in aged mice ($P < 0.001$, data not shown). Repeated pCSP vaccination stimulated an IgG anti-CSP antibody response in these aged animals, although their serum antibody levels remained significantly below those of similarly treated young mice ($P < 0.02$, Table 4).

Cells from these pCSP vaccinated animals were re-stimulated with antigen in vitro, and then monitored for cytotoxicity against peptide-pulsed targets. As seen in Table 4, CTL activity in cells from young mice was approximately 3-fold higher than from aged animals ($P < 0.03$, Table 4).

Protective efficacy of pCSP vaccination

Young and aged BALB/c mice were challenged intravenously with graded numbers of live malaria sporozoites. Both populations of unvaccinated mice were equally susceptible to sporozoite infection (ID_{50} of 8 and 9 sporozoites/animal, respectively). Mice primed and boosted with pCSP were then challenged with 100 viable malaria sporozoites. This dose induced fulminant infection in virtually all unimmunized BALB/c mice. Among vaccinated young mice, 12/15 (80%) were protected from sporozoite challenge. By comparison, only 4/10 (40%) of vaccinated aged mice were protected ($P = 0.078$).

Overview

These findings demonstrate that pCSP vaccination elicits significantly lower IgG anti-CSP antibody production, reduced CTL activity, and provides less protection against sporozoite challenge in aged than young adult animals. Coupled with the findings presented above, these results indicate that the effectiveness of DNA vaccines may be reduced in populations with diminished immune function (such as the elderly, the young, and the immunosuppressed/immunodeficient).

Both the primary and secondary immune response of aged mice to pCSP vaccination resulted in a disproportionate decrease in the ratio of cells secreting type 1 versus type 2 cytokines when compared to similarly treated young mice (data not shown). This change may underlie the reduced CTL activity of pCSP-immunized elderly mice since an IL-4-dominated primary response can impede the generation of type 1-dependent CTL. This finding is consistent with evidence that the ratio of type 1 : type 2 cytokine-secreting cells, rather than the absolute number of such cells, determines the nature of an immune response [12, 34].

Although both cytokine and antibody production were significantly reduced in pCSP immunized aged mice, their secretion increased significantly when these animals were repeatedly boosted with the same DNA vaccine. These findings suggest that age-related defects in immune responsiveness may be overcome, underscoring the need for additional research designed to improve the immunogenicity of DNA vaccines, especially in populations with diminished immune function.

Conclusion

DNA vaccines moved very rapidly from laboratory phenomena into clinical trials. This rapid transition was sustained by our ability to harness the tools of molecular biology to design antigen-encoding plasmids to induce immune responses against pathogens for which no conventional vaccine was available.

However, enthusiasm for this new technology must be tempered by an appreciation of its potential risks. The long-term sequelae of DNA vaccination have received little attention, despite the capacity of these plasmids to persist in vivo for many months or years. As multi-component DNA vaccines and DNA vaccines encoding both cytokines and antigens become more common, the possibility for detrimental side-effects will increase. Since many of the DNA vaccines currently undergoing clinical testing would (if licensed) be administered to millions of children and/or adults, even adverse events occurring at low frequency (< 1 per 1,000) would effect many thousands of otherwise healthy individuals.

The findings reviewed above demonstrate that important safety and efficacy issues relevant to DNA vaccines persist. We found DNA plasmids were unlikely to induce or accelerate the development of systemic autoimmune disease, despite their capacity to activate small numbers of IgG anti-DNA-secreting B cells. However, certain DNA vaccines (and the immunostimulatory CpG motifs they contain) may facilitate the development of certain organ-specific autoimmune diseases. We remain concerned that DNA vaccines may induce tolerance rather than immunity in some populations, and may be ineffective in others. Only adequate pre-clinical studies coupled with large-scale human trials will establish the risk of this new vaccine approach. To aid in this effort, the Food and Drug Administration has published a "Points to Consider" document that provides valuable suggestions for the evaluation of the safety, potency and immunogenicity of candidate DNA vaccines [1].

Acknowlegements. This work was supported in part by a grant from the National Vaccine Program. The authors appreciate the reagents and support provided by Drs. Steve Hoffman, Ion Norman and Peter Hobart. The ascertations herein are the private ones of the authors and are not to be construed as official or as reflecting the views of the FDA.

References

1. Points to consider on Plasmid DNA Vaccines for Preventive Infectious Disease Indications (1996) Obtain from: Office of Communication, Training and Manufacturers Assistance (HFM-10) Center for Biologics Evaluation and Research, FDA, Bethesda
2. Bloom ET, Kubota LF, Kawakami K (1988) Age-related decline in the lethal hit but not the binding stage of cytotoxic T cell activity in mice. Cell Immunol 114:440
3. Broody JA, Brock DB (1985) In: Finch CE, Schneider FL (eds) Handbook of the biology of aging, 2nd edn. Epidemiologic and statistical characteristics of this United States elderly population. Van Nostrand Reinhold, New York, pp 3–20
4. Cardon LR, Burge C, Clayton DA, Karlin S (1994) Pervasive CpG suppression in animal mitochondrial genomes. Proc Natl Acad Sci USA 91:3799
5. Cox GJ, Zamb TJ, Babiuk LA (1993) Bovine herpesvirus 1: immune responses in mice and cattle injected with plasmid DNA. J Virol 67:5664
6. Ebling FM, Hahn BH (1980) Restricted subpopulations of DNA antibodies in kidneys of mice with systemic lupus. Arthritis Rheum 23:392
7. Effros RB, Walford RL (1983) Diminished T cell response to influenza virus in aged mice. Immunology 49:387
8. Effros RB, Walford RL (1984) The effect of age on the antigen-presenting mechanism in limiting dilution precursor cell frequency analysis. Cell Immunol 88:531
9. Ernst DN, Hobbs MV, Torbett BE, Glasebrook AL, Rehse MA, Bottomly K, Hayakawa K, Hardy RR, Weigle WO (1990) Differences in the expression profiles of CD45 membrane antigens and in the patterns of lymphokine secretion by splenic CD4+ T cells from young and aged mice. J Immunol 145:1295
10. Gilkeson GS, Riuz P, Howell D, Lefkowith JB, Pisetsky DS (1993) Induction of immune-mediated glomerulonephritis in normal mice immunized with bacterial DNA. Clin Immunol Immunopathol 68: 283
11. Gilkeson GS, Pippen AM, Pisetsky DS (1995) Induction of cross-reactive anti-dsDNA antibodies in pre-autoimmune NZB/NZW mice by immunization with bacterial DNA. J Clin Invest 95:1398
12. Hagiwara E, Gourley M, Lee S, Klinman DM (1996) Disease severity in patients with systemic lupus erythematosus correlates with an increased ratio of IL-10: IFN-gamma secreting cells in the peripheral blood. Arthritis Rheum 39:379
13. Halpern MD, Kurlander RJ, Pisetsky DS (1996) Bacterial DNA induces murine interferon-gamma production by stimulation of IL-12 and tumor necrosis factor-alpha. Cell Immunol 167:72
14. Hobbs MV, Weigle WO, Ernst DN (1994) IL-10 production by splenic CD4+ cells and cell subsets from young and old mice. Cell Immunol 154:264
15. Horvath JA, Mostowski HS, Okumura K, Bloom ET (1992) Pore-forming protein in individual CTL. The effect of senescence provides a probe for understanding the lytic mechanism. Eur J Immunol 22:2649

16. Klinman NR (1972) The mechanism of antigenic stimulation of primary and secondary clonal precursor cells. J Exp Med 136:241
17. Klinman DM (1990) Polyclonal B cell activation in lupus-prone mice precedes and predicts the development of autoimmune disease. J Clin Invest 86:1249
18. Klinman DM (1992) Analysis of B lymphocytes cross-reactivity at the single cell level. J Immunol Methods 152:217
19. Klinman DM, Steinberg AD (1987) Systemic autoimmune disease arises from polyclonal B cell activation. J Exp Med 165:1755
20. Klinman NR, Sigal NH, Metcalf ES, Pierce SK, Gearhart PJ (1976) The interplay of evolution and environment in B-Cell diversification. Cold Spr Harbor Symp Quant Biol 41:165
21. Klinman DM, Shirai A, Ishigatsubo Y, Conover J, Steinberg AD (1991) Quantitation of IgG and IgM secreting B cells in the peripheral blood of patients with systemic lupus erythematosus. Arthritis Rheum 34:1404
22. Klinman DM, Yi A, Beaucage SL, Conover J, Krieg AM (1996) CpG motifs expressed by bacterial DNA rapidly induce lymphocytes to secrete IL-6, IL-12 and IFN-γ. Proc Natl Acad Sci USA 93:2879
23. Klinman DM, Yamshchikov G, Ishigatsubo Y (1997) Contribution of CpG motifs to the immunogenicity of DNA vaccines. J Immunol 158 : 3635
24. Krieg AM, Yi A, Matson S, Waldschmidt TJ, Bishop GA, Teasdale R, Koretzky GA, Klinman DM (1995) CpG motifs in bacterial DNA trigger direct B-cell activation. Nature 374:546
25. Kubo M, Cinader B (1990) Polymorphism of age-related changes in interleukin production: differential changes of T helper subpopulations, synthesizing IL-2, IL-3, and IL-4. Eur J Immunol 20:1289
26. Lambert PH, Dixon FJ (1968) Pathogenesis of the glomerulonephritis of NZB/W mice. J Exp Med 127:507
27. Lehtonen L, Eskola J, Vainio O, Lehtonen A (1990) Changes in lymphocyte subsets and immune competence in very advanced age. J Gerontol 45:M108
28. Linker-Israeli M, Deans R, Wallace D, Prehn J, Ozeri-Chen T, Klinenberg J (1991) Elevated levels of endogenous IL-6 in systemic lupus erythematosus. J Immunol 147:117
29. Manthorpe M, Cornefert JF, Hartikka J, Felgner J, Rundell A, Margalith M, Dwarki V (1993) Gene therapy by intramuscular injection of plasmid DNA: studies on firefly luciferase gene expression in mice. Hum Gene Ther 4:419
30. Marodon G, Rocha B (1995) Activation and 'deletion' of self-reactive mature and immature T cells during ontogeny of Mls-1a: implications for neonatal tolerance induction. Int Immunol 6:1899
31. Miller RA (1989) The cell biology of aging: immunologic models. J Gerontol 44:B4
32. Mor G, Klinman DM, Shapiro S, Hagiwara E, Sedegah M, Norman JA, Hoffman SL, Steinberg AD (1995) Complexity of the cytokine and antibody response elicited by immunizing mice with *Plasmodium yoelii* circumsporozoite protein plasmid DNA. J Immunol 155:2039
33. Mor G, Singla M, Steinberg AD, Hoffman SL, Okuda K, Klinman DM (1997) Do DNA vaccines induce autoimmune disease? Hum Gene Ther 8:293
34. Oshima T, Delespesse G (1997) T cell derived IL-4 and dendritic cell-derived IL-12 regulate the lymphokine-producing phenotype of alloantigen primed naive human CD4 T cells. J Immunol 158:629
35. Paganelli R, Scala E, Quinti I, Ansotegui IJ (1994) Humoral immunity in aging. Aging Clin Exp Res 6:143
36. Pincus T, Schur PH, Rose JA, Decker JL, Talal N (1970) Measurement of serum anti-DNA binding activity in systemic lupus erythematosus. N Engl J Med 281:701
37. Pisetsky DS, Reich C, Crowley SD, Halpern MD (1995) Immunological properties of bacterial DNA. Ann NY Acad Sci 772:152
38. Razin A, Friedman J (1981) DNA methylation and its possible biological roles. Prog Nucleic Acid Res Mol Biol 25:33
39. Robinson HL, Feltquate DM, Morin MJ, Haynes JR, Webster RG (1995) DNA vaccines: a new approach to immunization. Int J Immunopharmacol 17 : 79
40. Sarzotti M, Robbins DS, Hoffman PM (1996) Induction of protective CTL responses in newborn mice by a murine retrovirus. Science 271:1726
41. Sato Y, Roman M, Tighe H, Lee D, Corr M, Nguyen M, Carson DA, Raz E (1996) Non-coding bacterial DNA sequences necessary for effective intradermal gene immunization. Science 273 : 352
42. Scollary RGE, Butcher EC, Weissman IL (1980) Thymus cell migration. Quantitative aspects of cellular traffic from the thymus to the periphery in mice. Eur J Immunol 10:210
43. Sedegah M, Hedstrom R, Hobart P, Hoffman SL (1994) Protection against malaria by immunization with plasmid DNA encoding circumsporozoite protein. Proc Natl Acad Sci USA 91:9866

44. Shirai A, Holmes K, Klinman DM (1993) Detection and quantitation of cells secreting IL-6 under physiological conditions in BALB/c mice. J Immunol 150:793
45. Shirai A, Sierra V, Kelly CI, Klinman DM (1994) Individual cells simultaneously produce both IL-4 and IL-6 under physiologic conditions in vivo. Cytokine 6:329
46. Silverstein AM (1997) Ontogeny of the immune response: a perspective. In: Cooper MD (ed) Development of Host Defenses. Raven Press, New York, pp 1–10
47. Silverstein AM, Segal S (1975) The ontogeny of antigen-specific T cells. J Exp Med 142:802
48. Steinberg AD, Krieg AM, Gourley MF, Klinman DM (1990) Theoretical and experimental approaches to generalized autoimmunity. Immunol Rev 118:129
49. Sterzl J, Silverstein AM. (1967) Developmental aspects of immunity. Adv Immunol 6:337
50. Steward MW, Hay FC (1976) Changes in immunoglobulin class and subclass of anti-DNA antibodies to DNA and RNA. II. Sequential switch from IgM to IgG in NZB/W F1 mice. Clin Exp Immunol 26:363
51. Tang D, DeVit M, Johnston SA (1992) Genetic immunization is a simple method for eliciting an immune response. Nature 356:152
52. Tascon RE, Colston MJ, Ragno S, Stavropoulos E, Gregory D, Lowrie DB (1996) Vaccination against tuberculosis by DNA injection. Nature Med 2:888
53. Thoman ML, Weigle WO (1989) The cellular and subcellular bases of immunosenescence. Adv Immunol 46:221
54. Ulmer JB, Donnelly JJ, Parker SE, Rhodes GH, Felgner PL, Dwarki VJ, Gromkoski SH, Deck RR, DeWitt CM, Friedman A (1993) Heterologous protection against influenza by injection of DNA encoding a viral protein [see comments]. Science 259:1745
55. Wang B, Ugen KE, Srikantan V, Agadjanyan MG, Dang K, Refaeli Y, Sato A, Boyer J, Williams WV, Weiner DB (1993) Gene inoculation generates immune responses against human immunodeficiency virus type 1. Proc Natl Acad Sci USA 90:4156
56. Wolff JA, Malone RW, Williams P, Chong W, Ascadi G, Jani A, Felgner PL (1990) Direct gene transfer into mouse muscle in vivo. Science 247:1465

Genetic vaccines – a revolution in vaccinology?

Z. Q. Xiang, S. Pasquini, Z. He, H. Deng, Y. Wang, M. A. Blaszczyk-Thurin, H. C. J. Ertl

The Wistar Institute, 3601 Spruce Street, Philadelphia, PA 19104, USA

Introduction

Vaccination is the most efficacious medical treatment to prevent human morbidity and mortality due to infectious agents. Although viral vaccines have been used since the 17th century, to date vaccines to only about 25 different human pathogens are available. Traditionally, vaccines were generated by inactivation or attenuation of pathogens, using infectious agents that afflict a different species and are comparatively nonvirulent in humans or by modifications of toxins. Considering the multitude of existing and newly emergent infectious agents, novel approaches for vaccine development are needed. Subunit vaccines based on purified proteins or another pathogen have been explored extensively [1, 18, 28, 45, 64, 69] and led to an improved hepatitis B virus vaccine [39] and a recombinant vaccine for immunization of wild live animals to rabies virus [64]. A novel type of subunit vaccine based on plasmid vectors expressing antigens under the control of a suitable promoter has been under intensive investigation for the last 5 years. Such constructs, termed DNA vaccines, polynucleotide vaccines or genetic vaccines, were initially tested for their suitability as gene therapy vehicles. It was shown during these studies that circular vector DNA, upon intramuscular inoculation into mice, is taken up by muscle cells surrounding the inoculation site causing prolonged expression of the transgene [65, 66]. Uptake of DNA by muscle cells did not require precipitation of DNA, formation of liposomes, or any of the other techniques that are needed for successful transfection of cell lines in vitro. Shortly after these initial studies, another group using a vector expressing human growth hormone demonstrated stimulation of an antibody response to the transgene product [59]; thus starting the era of DNA vaccines.

The first report of induction of a B cell response upon genetic immunization of mice using the human growth factor as the antigen [59] has been confirmed with a variety of other antigens such as: the hemagglutinin of influenza virus [24], the envelope and the Nef protein of human immunodeficiency virus (HIV) 1 [3, 61], the glycoprotein (G protein) of rabies virus [67], the glycoprotein B of herpes simplex virus [38], the core protein of hepatitis C virus [32], the hepatitis B virus surface antigen [13], the

Correspondence to: H. C. J. Ertl

glycoproteins D and B of herpes simplex virus type 2 [40], rotavirus [27], lymphocytic choriomeningitis virus [74], murine cytomegalovirus (CMV) [25], the nucleoprotein of measles virus [20], the large T antigen of Simian virus 39 [53], the circumsporozoite protein of *Plasmodium yoelii* [54], the major surface protein of *Leishmania major* [70], the OspA antigen of *Borrelia burgdorferi* [37], *Toxoplasma gondii* [2], the hsp65 antigen of *Mycobacterium tuberculosis* [35], and others (reviewed in [29]). Regardless of the antigen or the technical approach of genetic immunization, the reports were rather similar in describing stimulation of antibodies and cytolytic T cells and, where the appropriate animal model was available, induction of protection to challenge with the pathogen. The initial studies conducted in mice were rapidly and successfully expanded to other species such as ferrets [63], rabbits [24], primates [7, 14], chickens [49] and cattle [10]. In addition to targeting infectious diseases, genetic vaccines were also shown to provide immunity to tumor antigens such as idiotopes expressed on B cell lymphomas [57], or sequences derived from a mutated oncoprotein present in a chemically induced tumor cell line [8].

Characteristics of vectors used for genetic immunization

Different expression vectors have been used successfully for the construction of genetic vaccines. Most of these vectors carried viral promoters that caused constitutive expression of antigen in a large variety of cell types. The early promoter of CMV has been used most frequently. We directly compared the immune response to the rabies virus G protein using vectors driving expression of the protein under the control of the simian virus (SV) 40 promoter or the CMV promoter [68]. The plasmids were identical but for the regulatory element. In our experiments the vector containing the SV40 promoter, which in most cell types induces only ~ 5% of the expression levels achieved with the more potent CMV promoter, induced a slightly superior immune response, especially with regard to long-term persistence of antibody titers. We were also able to induce a good immune response using the major histocompatibility (MHC) class I promoter that drives expression in most cells. In contrast, another vector utilizing the MHC class II promoter that is only functional in a small fraction of cells such as macrophages, dendric cells or B lymphocytes induced a rather low response to the rabies virus antigen. The rabies virus G protein of the ERA strain used for our experiments is toxic upon overexpression, and might thus be exceptional. In most systems strong promoters seem to result in more efficacious genetic vaccines, although other characteristics of the vector, such as size or form (circular versus linear), most likely affect DNA uptake and thus overall levels of antigen expression as well.

Bacterial DNA, such as the sequences of a mammalian expression vector backbone, contains unmethylated CpG sequences that have immunomodulatory functions [9, 31]. CpG sequences carried by oligonucleotides or bacterial DNA were shown to cause activation of B cells and of macrophages, resulting in the production of interferon (IFN)-γ [30, 71], which induces interleukin (IL)-12, a cytokine known to activate natural killer cells, to drive immune responses towards the Th1 pathway. There is some evidence that CpG sequences present in genetic vaccines have an adjuvant effect that is crucial for initiation of the immune response [52]. Upon intramuscular inoculation, genetic vaccines induce an immune response that is predominantly (but not exclusively) of the Th1 type [67]. Again CpG sequences present in the vector backbone might, by causing release of IL-12, be instrumental in the preferential induction of antibodies of the IgG2a isotypes and T helper cells secreting IL-2 and IFN-γ. "Classical" CpG sequences are present in the ampicillin resistance gene but not in the kanamycin resistance gene. Although most genetic vaccines that have been used to date rely on ampicillin as a selective marker, some of the high expression vectors utilize the kanamycin resistance gene. Whether deletion of some CpG sequences by, for example, replacing the ampicillin resistance gene with the kanamycin resistance gene, or alternatively addition of CpG sequences into the vector backbone, negatively or positively affect the efficacy of genetic vaccines remains to be investigated.

Delivery of genetic vaccines

In the first publication on genetic immunization, vector DNA was coated to gold beads and shot directly into the cells of the epidermis using a gene gun [59]. In subsequent experiments, vector DNA was applied by a syringe into muscle [60, 67]. Some investigators found that a hypertonic solution such as sucrose increased the response [12], others used reagents such as cardiotoxin [13] or buvocain [61], which cause muscle damage, to increase DNA uptake by regenerating muscle cells. We used saline or distilled water [67] and also tried sucrose solutions and did not find one diluent clearly superior to the other. Vector DNA was also shown to induce an immune response upon intradermal [47], subcutaneous or intranasal [24] application. In general, gene gun delivery of DNA coated to gold beads seems to be the most efficient way of application [4]; it forces the DNA-coated beads directly into the skin cells, thus circumventing uptake of DNA through cell membranes which is presumably rather inefficient. Nanogram amounts of DNA applied by particle bombardment result in an immune response, while in most experimental systems 20–100 times more DNA is needed to elicit a maximal response upon intramuscular inoculation. One group reported that gene gun delivery of DNA to the skin results in a Th2-type response [23], while the vectors injected intramuscularly induce a preferential Th1 response, suggesting that antigen presentation of vector encoded antigen by cells present in the skin might differ qualitatively from that in muscle tissue. Nevertheless, other groups reported induction of a Th1-like response, i.e., antibodies of the IgG2a isotype and cytolytic T cells, upon gene gun delivery of vector DNA [4, 44], suggesting that the finding of a preferential Th2 induction upon particle bombardment should currently not be generalized. In collaboration with Drs. S. A. Johnston and M. Barry, we tested the above-mentioned vector expressing the rabies virus G protein under the control of the SV40 promoter (termed pSG5rab.gp) for induction of an antibody response upon inoculation with a gene gun. Although this vector induces a potent antibody response upon intramuscular, subcutaneous, intradermal or even intratracheal application if used at 50 μg/mouse, delivery of 1 μg/mouse (the maximal amount that can easily be applied to gold beads) failed to cause seroconversion in any of the mice tested, indicating that gene gun application of low doses of plasmid might not be suitable for every construct (unpublished data).

Ease of delivery is a trait that is demanded of vaccines designed for mass vaccination. Oral or intranasal routes are preferable to the more cumbersome systemic routes. Delivery of DNA by gene gun is time consuming even for experimental purposes; it requires coating of the DNA to gold beads, loading of the gun, careful cleaning of the skin, or even shaving or using depilatory agents which, for some of the lesser obedient species such as mice or high-spirited canines, warrants sedation. Also, the gene gun is

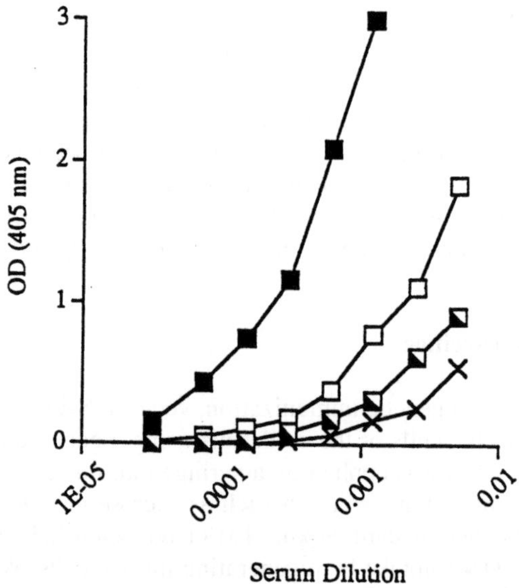

Fig. 1. Induction of antibodies to rabies virus upon application of the pSG5rab.gp vector systemically or to mucosal membranes of the airways: Groups of C3H/He mice were inoculated with pSG5rab.gp either intramuscularly (■), intranasally (◪) or intratracheally (□). Serum antibody titers were determined 8 weeks later by an ELISA, Normal mouse serum (×)

a rather expensive and sophisticated instrument and requires a helium tank to supply velocity. For mass vaccinations, especially under field conditions or in developing countries, this approach is clearly not suitable. Several groups including ours have demonstrated that DNA applied to the mucosal membranes of the airways results in an immune response [24]. In our system, again using the pSG5rab.gp vector, we found that both intranasal, as well as intratracheal inoculation, caused seroconversion. The response was clearly superior upon intratracheal inoculation, which targets the lower airways, than upon intranasal inoculation which goes towards the upper airways, Nevertheless, even upon intratracheal inoculation the response was lower than upon intramuscular injection (see Fig. 1). Using cationic lipids or other types of liposomes, as well as spray devises that form droplets which can readily reach the lower airways upon intranasal application, should improve the efficacy of this route of delivery.

Nature of the antigen

A number of antigens derived from viruses, bacteria, protozoa, parasites and cancer cells have been used successfully in genetic vaccines. Some of these antigens were surface proteins, such as the rabies virus glycoprotein, the gp120 of HIV or the influenza virus hemagglutinin. Others were retained within the transfected cells, such as the influenza virus nucleoprotein, and a third category was secreted, such as the circumsporoite antigen of *Plasmodium*. All of these antigens induced an immune response that was qualitatively similar. Assuming that secretion of an immunogenic protein might facilitate presentation by professional antigen-presenting cells (APCs), we compared the immune response to the full-length rabies virus G protein which is firmly anchored into the cell membrane to a truncated, secreted form, using the pSG5 vector for delivery [68]. Both forms induced a comparable T cell response, while the B cell response was clearly superior upon application of the vector expressing the full-length protein. Most of the B cell epitopes of the rabies virus G protein are conformation dependent, which is most likely the reason why the altered protein showed a loss in immunogenicity. Our assumption that a secreted protein would facilitate antigen presentation, and thus stimulation of T helper cells was shown to be incorrect.

The immune response to genetic immunization

Inoculation of mice (or other species) with a genetic vaccine results in stimulation of antibodies, T helper cells and cytolytic T cells. Bone marrow-derived cells are assumed to serve as APCs [15] either upon direct transfection or upon reprocessing of antigen provided by other cells such as muscle cells. The kinetics of the immune response clearly differ from that seen upon immunization with a traditional antigen: the immune response in most systems, including ours based on the rabies virus G protein, comes up slowly [68]. Again using the rabies virus system as an example, mice develop measurable antibody titers upon vaccination with a recombinant vaccine, such as an E1-deleted adenovirus expressing the rabies virus G protein, within a week. After genetic immunization, applying the pSG5rab.gp vector intramuscularly, antibodies cannot be detected in most experiments until 2 or 3 weeks after immunization. They reach plateau levels after about 10–12 weeks and stay at these levels for at least a year [68]. Antibody titers in mice immunized once with a recombinant vaccine, or inactivated rabies virus, come up rapidly and then decline after a few weeks and no longer provide protection to challenge given after a year. The long-lasting immune response, that at least in mice provides protection for life [11, 16, 72], is surprizing considering the small amount of antigen that is expressed after genetic immunization. Life-long immunity is generally only provided by natural infections. Even attenuated pathogens that have limited replication capacity fail to achieve protective immunity for more than a few years. It is assumed that the antigenic load achieved by a virulent agent induces a sufficiently large pool of memory T and B lymphocytes to provide long-lasting protection to rechallenge. There is some, albeit disputed, evidence that at least B cell memory requires persistence of antigen [26]. This can be provided by antigen-antibody complexes deposited in the form of immunocomplexes on follicular dendritic cells of lymph nodes [56]. Once antibody titers decline, these complexes are thought to be released, thus maintaining a response. In addition to the antigenic load that is highest upon natural infections, the duration of antigen expression might also affect the magnitude and the kinetic of the immune response. We have shown that a replication-defective E1-deleted adenoviral recombinant expressing the rabies virus G protein stimulates, upon inoculation of 10^3 plaque-forming units (pfu), an antibody response that is higher comparable to that induced by 10^6 pfu of a replication competent vaccinia virus recombinant expressing the same antigen [69]. Vaccinia viruses kill infected cells within 24–48 h, the E1-deleted adenovirus, on the other hand, is non cytopathic; immunoincompetent mice inoculated with E1-deleted adenoviral recombinant viruses carrying a reporter gene were shown to express the transgene for at least 6 months [73]. In immunocompetent mice the transgene product can be detected for about 10 days until $CD8^+$ T cells eliminate the infected cells [73]. Persistent expression of antigen by the replication defective adenovirus might provide a better stimulus compared

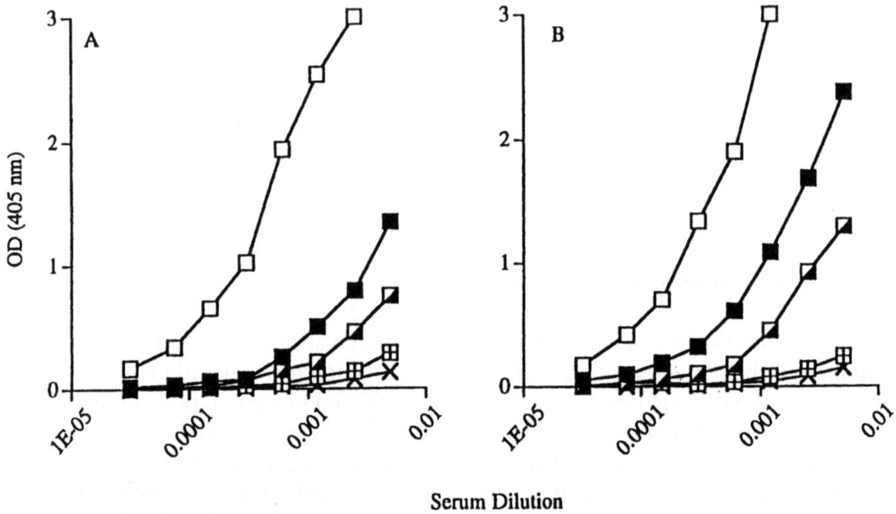

Fig. 2 A, B. Genetic immunization primes the immune system to booster immunizations. Groups of C3H/He mice were inoculated subcutaneously with 10^6 pfu of a vaccinia rabies virus recombinant (◪) or 10^6 pfu of an adenoviral recombinant expressing the rabies virus G protein (□), or 50 μg of pSG5rab.gp (■) or pSG5lacZ (⊞) (control construct expressing β-galactosidase). Mice were bled 8 weeks later and serum antibody titers were determined (**A**). Mice were boosted with 10^4 pfu of the adenoviral recombinant and bled 5 days later to determine serum antibody titers (**B**). Normal mouse serum (×)

to a larger dose of antigen, such as that provided by the vaccinia virus recombinant, present for a much shorter period of time. Vector DNA sequences, as well as vector-encoded antigen, can be demonstrated upon genetic immunization in transfected cells for several weeks [66]. Persistent native antigen in presence of an ongoing B cell response could favor formation of antigen-antibody complexes on follicular dendritic cells, which might then maintain a long-lasting immune response.

Booster immunization with the genetic vaccine (at least within the first 10 weeks after priming with a vector) seems to have little influence on the magnitude of the response, while a follow-up immunization with a conventional vaccine on the other hand has a clear booster effect (Fig. 2). Although, in the majority of systems, the immune response to DNA immunization is exceptionally long lasting, in some cases a rapid decline of antibody titers could be observed. One example was a genetic vaccine to the gp120 of HIV-1 that resulted in a transient antibody response that could not be sustained by booster inoculations [36]. Whether this reflects tolerization to this protein remains to be investigated.

Genetic vaccines can overcome genetic unresponsiveness

T cell-mediated immune responses are under Ir gene control [5]. MHC class I and II molecules of genetically distinct haplotypes have different sequences forming pockets in their peptide binding groove, which determines the profile of immunodominant T cell epitopes present on a given antigen. For example, we tested the responsiveness of rabies virus-immune T helper cell derived from mice of the H-2^k or H-2^b haplotype, using overlapping synthetic peptides delineated from the rabies virus nuceloprotein

[19]. T cells from mice of the H-2^k haplotype responded vigorously to a single peptide (called 31D) that corresponded to amino acids 404–418 of the protein. In contrast, mice of the H-2^b haplotype secreted cytokine in response to two peptides termed 3D and 30D, which corresponded to amino acids 21–35 and 394–408 of the nucleoprotein. Other proteins can induce a T cell-mediated immune response in some mouse strains but are completely immunologically silent in others. Again, responsiveness is linked to the MHC haplotype. For example, the nominal phosphoprotein of rabies virus induces a potent $CD8^+$ cytolytic T cell response in H-2^k mice, but can not be recognized by $CD8^+$ T cells derived from rabies virus immune H-2^d mice [34].

The ability of T cells to respond to a given epitope or protein not only depends on the presence of anchoring sequences for MHC binding, but also on the T cell repertoire. T cells that recognize epitopes that closely resemble self determinants are either deleted in the thymus, or are tolerized in the periphery [43]. Overexpression of a protein, even a self protein, can reveal so-called hidden (or cryptic) epitopes [33, 55]. These are epitopes that, as opposed to immunodominant epitopes, normally fail to elicit a response, or vice versa, fail to cause tolerization of T cells. Cryptic epitopes presumably remain immunologically silent at physiological expression levels because their affinity to the MHC binding sites is below a threshold that is needed for efficacious T cell activation/tolerization. Overexpression of the antigen can counterbalance the low affinity, and thus result in a T cell response that could potentially react with self determinants.

DNA vaccines were shown to induce responses to epitopes that are not recognized upon immunization with a protein-based immunogen [17, 22, 41]. They were also shown to induce T cell responses in non-responder haplotypes [17], indicating that antigen as expressed by a DNA vaccine might cause exposure of hidden (cryptic) epitopes. This is most likely not caused by overexpression of the antigen, but might be a side effect of the persistent expression of the antigen. Lack of recognition of immunodominant epitopes, as was described in one system [41], might reflect a form of immunological tolerance – a highly speculative interpretation that remains to be addressed experimentally. In addition, exposure of cryptic epitopes that fail to eliminate/tolerize T cells during their maturation, could pose an increased risk for cross-reactive autoimmune responses. Again, this remains to be tested in a number of well-defined systems. In spite of these caveats, the apparent ability of DNA vaccines to overcome immunological non-responsiveness caused by Ir gene control could be exceedingly valuable for infectious diseases such as hepatitis B virus infections where current vaccines fail to induce an immune response in a significant percentage of humans. This might also be useful for immunotherapy of cancer where the patient's immune system might be rendered unresponsive to the immunodominant epitopes of tumor-associated antigens. Such antigens are expressed on cancer cells in absence of co-stimulatory molecules, and cause potentially immunological anergy.

The immune response of neonates to genetic vaccination

Neonates are generally not vaccinated (except to hepatitis B virus infections), for their immune system is partially immature. For example, neonates are incapable of responding to polysaccharide antigens due to a developmental delay in maturation of a subset of B cells [15]. Newborns can readily be tolerized to some antigens, such as alloantigens expressing lymphoid cells which can induce tolerance allowing subsequent transplantation of skin grafts syngeneic to the donor lymphocytes [6, 42, 58].

Three recent reports [21, 48, 51] have shown that neonatal mice can respond to either low doses of virus, protein antigen, or allogeneic cells provided the antigen was presented by APCs, suggesting that neonatal immunological immaturity is linked to antigen presentation rather than to T cell development.

We tested the effects of genetic immunization with a plasmid vector expressing the rabies virus G protein in neonatal mice. Mice of the C3H/He strain inoculated within 24–48 h after birth with a plasmid vector given subcutaneously developed both antibodies and T helper cells to rabies virus [62]. Some of the mouse pups failed to seroconvert, which was most likely due to variability in the delivery method rather than to the induction of tolerance. Qualitatively, the response was identical to that seen upon genetic immunization of adult mice, i.e., neonatal immunization resulted in T helper cells secreting IL-2 but not IL-4, and mixed antibody isotypes with IgG2a being predominant [62]. Two other groups reported successful immunization of neonatal mice [50] or non-human primates [46] with genetic vaccines, while one group described induction of tolerance upon inoculation of BALB/c mice with a vector encoding the circumsporoite antigen of *P. yoelii* [41]. The pathway(s) that determine if neonatal genetic immunization with a vector results in activation or tolerization of an immune response remain(s) to be elucidated. We used a vector expressing a cell surface protein in C3H/He mice. The group that reported induction of tolerance used a secreted protein in BALB/c mice that, unlike all other mouse strains, have a genetic defect in IL-12 receptor expression and are thus more prone to develop Th2-like responses. Both secretion of the antigen and the inability of BALB/c mice to respond appropriately to IL-12 might affect the outcome upon neonatal immunization. Nevertheles, although there is some concern that neonatal immunization might under exceptional circumstances result in tolerance, in general neonates seem to respond quite readily to genetic vaccines.

Advantages and disadvantages of genetic vaccines

One of the main advantages of vector vaccines, at least for experimentors, is the ease with which they can be constructed. Attenuating a pathogen in tissue culture often takes years, generating a recombinant vaccine takes months and producing a new genetic vaccine can be achieved in less than a week. Generation and purification of DNA is also quite simple and inexpensive. Unlike most other types of vaccines, DNA is remarkably heat stable, which is especially of benefit for vaccines in developing countries where cold chains are often difficult to maintain. Immunologically, genetic vaccines seem to provide their own adjuvant in form of CpG sequences and can be delivered in saline solutions. Unlike inactivated vaccines, genetic vaccines cause de novo synthesis of proteins in transfected cells, leading to association of antigenic peptides with MHC class I determinants and, hence, activation of cytolytic T cells. In mice inoculation of plasmid vectors causes, at least in some systems, life-long immunity, which would provide genetic vaccines with a tremendous advantage over traditional vaccines. Further studies in long-lived species are needed to confirm that life-long immunity upon genetic immunization is not just achieved in short-lived rodents. Genetic vaccines result in slowly rising antibody titers; this is of little concern for prophylactic vaccines, unless they are given after the onset of an epidemic. For post-exposure treatment of infections, such as to rabies virus, that is generally initiated in humans after contact with a rabid animal, a vaccine that requires weeks to elicit measurable antibody titers can not be recommended.

Genetic vaccines are subunit vaccines. The immune response to individual proteins is commonly under Ir gene control, resulting in immunological unresponsiveness in a significant percentage of an outbred population; genetic vaccines are apparently able to overcome this genetic unresponsiveness. To design a subunit vaccine intelligently, the primary and secondary structure of the pathogen's antigens that result in stimulation of a protective immune response have to be known. Although this has been achieved for many viruses, especially those that encode a limited number of proteins such as rabies virus, this often formidable task remains to be tackled for many of the more complex or newly emerging pathogens. For the latter, the development of genetic vaccines will remain a hit or miss approach. Using the recently described ELI (expression library immunization) approach might not be feasible for actual vaccination, but might be exceedingly useful to identify protective antigens.

Conclusions

Genetic vaccines have been tested in a number of different species against more than 25 pathogens and, generally, have been shown to result in an immune response that is protective to challenge with the pathogen. Two clinical trials in healthy human adults were already initiated in 1996. Only time will show if this vaccination approach that evolved from gene therapy and was initially developed mainly by molecular biologists will indeed fulfill our current high hopes. In addition, this rather application-oriented vaccine approach will provide basic immunologists with a simple tool to study the rules that govern induction of primary immune responses.

Acknowledgements. This work was funded by grants from NIH/NIAID. We wish to thank Ms. W. Giles-Davis and S. Shane for superb technical assistance, Mr. A. Assalian for help in preparation of the manuscript and Dr. L. Otvos for the critical review of this manuscript. We also would like to thank all of our colleagues who collaborated with us or provided us with advice or reagents.

References

1. Aldovini A, Young RA (1991) Humoral and cell-mediated immune responses to live recombinant BCG-HIV vaccines. Nature 351 : 479
2. Angus CW, Klivington D, Wyman J, Kovacs JA (1996) Nucleic acid vaccination against *Toxoplasma gondii* in mice. J Eukaryot Microbiol 43 : 117 S
3. Asakura Y, Hamajima K, Fukshima J, Mohri H, Okubo T, Okudo K (1996) Induction of HIV Nef-specific cytotoxic T lymphocytes by Nef-expressing DNA vaccine. Am J Hematol 53 : 116
4. Barry MA, Johnston SA (1997) Biological features of genetic immunization. Vaccine 15 : (in press)
5. Benacerraf B, McDevitt HO (1972) Histocompatibility-linked immune response genes. Science 175 : 273
6. Billingham RE, Brent L, Medawar PB (1953) Activity acquired tolerance of foreign cells. Nature 172 : 603
7. Boyer JD, Wang B, Ugen KE, Agadjanyan M, Javadian A, Frost P, Dang K, Carrano RA, Ciccarelli R, Coney L, Williams WV, Weiner DB (1996) In vivo protective anti-HIV immune responses in non-human primates through DNA vaccination. J Med Primatol 25 : 242
8. Ciernik IF, Berzofsky J, Carbone DP (1996) Induction of cytotoxic T lymphocytes and antitumor immunity with DNA vaccines expressing single T cell epitopes. J Immunol 156 : 2369
9. Cowdery JS, Chace JH, Yi A-K, Krieg AM (1996) Bacterial DNA induces NK cells to produce interferon-gamma in vivo and increases the toxicity of lipopolysaccharide. J Immunol 156 : 4570
10. Cox GJM, Zamb TJ, Babiuk LA (1993) Bovine herpes virus type I: immune responses in mice and cattle injected with plasmid DNA. J Virol 67 : 5664

11. Davis HL, Michel M, Whalen RG (1993) DNA based immunization for hepatitis B induces continuous secretion of antigen and high levels of circulating antibody. Hum Mol Genet 2 : 1847
12. Davis HL, Whalen RG, Demeneix BA (1994) Direct gene transfer into skeletal muscle in vivo: factors affecting efficiency of transfer and stability of expression. Hum Gene Ther 4 : 151
13. Davis HL, Michel M, Mancini M, Schleef M, Whalen RG (1994) Direct gene transfer in skeletal muscle: plasmid DNA-based immunization against the hepatitis B virus surface antigen. Vaccine 12 : 1503
14. Davis HL, McCluskie MJ, Gerin JL, Purcell RH (1996) DNA vaccine for hepatitis B: evidence for immunogenicity in chimpanzees and comparison with other vaccines. Proc Natl Acad Sci USA 93 : 7213
15. Doe B, Selby M, Barnett S, Baenziger J, Walker CM (1996) Induction of cytotoxic T lymphocytes by intramuscular immunization with plasmid DNA is facilitated by bone marrow-derived cells. Proc Natl Acad Sci USA 93 : 8578
16. Donnelly JJ, Friedman A, Montgomery D, Shiver JW, Leander KR, Perry H, Martinez D, Ulmer JB, Liu MA (1994) Polynucleotide vaccination against influenza p55. Vaccines 94. Cold Spring Harbor Laboratory Press, Cold Spring Harbor
17. Doolan DL, Sedegah M, Hedstrom RC, Hobart P, Charoenvit Y, Hoffman SL (1996) Circumventing genetic restriction of protection against malaria with multigene DNA immunization: $CD8^+$ cell-, interferon gamma-, and nitric oxide-dependent immunity. J Exp Med 183 : 1739
18. Eloit M, Gilardi-Hebenstrei P, Pericaudet M (1990) Construction of a defective adenovirus vector expressing the pseudorabies virus glycoprotein gp50 and its use as a live vaccine. J Gen Virol 71 : 2425
19. Ertl HCJ, Dietzschold B, Gore M, Otvos JRL, Larson JK, Wunner WH, Koprowski H (1989) Induction of rabies virus-specific T helper cells by synthetic peptides that carry dominant T helper cell epitopes of the viral ribonucleoprotein. J Viol 63 : 2885
20. Fooks AR, Jeevarajah B, Warnes A, Wilkinson GW, Clegg JC (1996) Immunization of mice with plasmid DNA expressing the measles virus nucleoprotein gene. Viral Immunol 9 : 65
21. Frosthuber T, Yip HC, Lehmann PV (1996) Induction of TH1 and TH2 immunity in neonatal mice. Science 271 : 1728
22. Fu TM, Friedman A, Ulmer JB, Liu MA, Donnelly JJ (1997) Protective cellular immunity: CTL responses against dominant and recessive epitopes of influenza virus nucleoprotein induced by DNA immunization. J Virol (in press)
23. Fuller DH, Haynes JR (1996) A qualitative progression in HIV type 1 glycoprotein 120-specific cytotoxic cellular and humoral immune responses in mice receiving a DNA-based glycoprotein 120 vaccine. AIDS Res Hum Retroviruses 10 : 1433
24. Fynan EF, Webster RG, Fuller DH, Haynes JR, Santoro JC, Robinson HL (1993) DNA vaccines: protective immunizations by parenteral, mucosal and gene-gun inoculations. Proc Natl Acad Sci USA 90 : 11478
25. Gonzales Armas JC, Morello CS, Cranmer LD, Spector DH (1996) DNA immunization confers protection against murine cytomegalovirus infection. J Virol 70 : 7921
26. Grey D (1993) Immunological memory. Annu Rev Immunol 11 : 49
27. Herrmann GE, Chen SC, Fynan EF, Santoro JC, Greenberg HB, Wang S, Robinson HL (1996) Protection against rotavirus infections by DNA vaccination. J Infect Dis 174 [Suppl 1] : S 93
28. Jacobs WR Jr, Tuckman M, Bloom RB (1987) Introduction of foreign DNA into mycobacteria using a shuttle plasmid. Nature 327 : 532
29. Johnston SA, Sykes KF, Barry MA (1997) DNA-based vaccines: extending the technology. In: Levine et al (ed) New generation vaccines, chapter 23. Marcel Dekker Inc, pp 279–286
30. Klinman DM, Yi AK, Beaucage SL, Conover J, Krieg AM (1996) CpG motifs present in bacterial DNA rapidly induce lymphocytes to secrete interleukin 6, interleukin 12 and interferon-γ. Proc Natl Acad Sci USA 93 : 2879
31. Krieg AM, Yi A-K, Matson S, Waldschmidt TJ, Bishop GA, Teasdale R, Koretsky GA, Klinman DM (1995) CpG motifs in bacterial DNA trigger direct B-cell activation. Nature 374 : 546
32. Laaging LM, Meyer K, Hoft D, Houghton M, Belshe RB, Ray R (1995) Immune responses to plasmid DNA encoding the hepatitis C virus core protein. J Virol 69 : 25859
33. Lanzavecchia A (1995) How cryptic epitopes trigger autoimmunity. J Exp Med 181 : 1945
34. Larson JK, Wunner WH, Ertl HCJ (1992) Immune response to the nominal phosphoprotein of rabies virus. Virus Res 23 : 73
35. Lowrie DB, Tascon RE, Colston MJ, Silva CL (1994) Towards a DNA vaccine against tuberculosis. Vaccine 12 : 1529
36. Lu S, Santoro SC, Fuller DH, Haynes JR, Robinson HL (1995) Use of DNAs expressing HIV-1 env and non infectious HIV-1 particles to raise antibody responses in mice. Virology 209 : 147

37. Luke CJ, Carnes K, Liang X, Barbour AG (1997) An OspA-based DNA vaccine protects mice against infection with *Borrelia burgdorferi*. J Infect Dis 175 : 91
38. Manickan E, Rouse RJD, Yu Z, Wire WS, Rouse BT (1995) Genetic immunization against herpes simplex virus: protection is mediated by CD4+ T lymphocytes. J Immunol 155 : 259
39. McAlleer WJ, Buynak EB, Maigetter RZ, Wampler DE, Miller JM, Hilleman MR (1984) Human hepatitis B vaccine from recombinant yeast. Nature 307 : 178
40. McClements WL, Armstrong ME, Keys RD, Liu M (1996) Immunization with DNA vaccines encoding glycoprotein D or glycoprotein B alone or in combination induces protective immunity in animal models of herpes simplex virus-2 disease. Proc Natl Acad Sci USA 93 : 11414
41. Mor G, Yamshchikov G, Sedegah M, Takeno M, Wang R, Houghten RA, Hoffman S, Klinman DM (1996) Induction of neonatal tolerance by plasmid DNA vaccination of mice. J Clin Invest 98 : 2700
42. Mosier DE, Zaldivar NM, Goldings E, Mond J, Scher I, Paul WE (1977) Formation of antibody in the newborn mouse: study of T-cell-independent antibody response. J Infect Dis 130 : S 14
43. Nossal GJV (1994) Negative selection of lymphocytes. Cell 76 : 229
44. Pertmer TM, Eisenbraun MD, McCabe D, Prayaga SK, Fuller DH, Haynes JR (1995) Gene gun-based nucleic acid immunization: elicitation of humoral and cytotoxic T lymphocyte responses following intradermal delivery of nanogram quantities of DNA. Vaccine 13 : 1427
45. Poirer JP, Kehoe M, Beachey EH (1988) Protective immunity provoked by oral administration of attenuated aroA *Salmonella typhimurium* expressing cloned streptococcal M protein. J Exp Med 168 : 25
46. Prince AM, Whalen R, Brotman B (1997) Successful nucleic acid based immunization of newborn chimpanzees against hepatitis B virus. Vaccine 15 : 916
47. Raz E, Carson DA, Parker SE, Barr TB, Abai AM, Achinger G, Gromkowski SH, Shing M, Lew D, Yankaukas MA, Bard SM, Rhodes GH (1994) Intradermal gene immunizations: the possible role of DNA uptake on the induction of cellular immunity to viruses. Proc Natl Acad Sci USA 91 : 9519
48. Ridge JB, Fuchs EG, Matzinger P (1996) Neonatal tolerance revisited: turning on newborn T cells with dendritic cells. Science 217 : 1723
49. Sakaguchi M, Nakamura H, Sonoda K, Hamada F, Hirai K (1996) Protection of chickens from Newcastle disease by vaccination with a linear plasmid expressing the F protein of Newcastle disease virus. Vaccine 14 : 747
50. Sarzotti M, Dean TA, Remington MP, Ly CD, Furth PA, Robbins DS (1997) Induction of CTL responses in newborn mice by DNA immunization. Vaccine 15 : 795
51. Sarotti M, Robbins DS, Hoffman PM (1996) Induction of CTL responses in newborn mice by a murine retrovirus. Science 271 : 1726
52. Sato Y, Roman M, Tighe H, Lee D, Corr M, Nguyen MD, Silverman GL, Lotz M, Carson DA, Raz E (1996) Immunostimulatory DNA sequences necessary for effective intradermal gene immunization. Science 273 : 352
53. Schirmbeck R, Bohm W, Reimann J (1996) DNA vaccination primes MHC class I-restricted, simian virus 40 large tumor antigen-specific CTL in H-2^d mice that reject syngeneic tumors. J Immunol 157 : 3550
54. Sedegah M, Hedstrom R, Hobart P, Hoffman SL (1994) Protection against malaria by immunization with plasmid DNA encoding circumsporozoite protein. Proc Natl Acad Sci USA 91 : 9866
55. Sercarz EE, Lehmann PV, Ametani A, Benichou G, Miller A, Moudgli K (1993) Dominance and cryptivity of T cell antigenic determinants. Annu Rev Immunol 11 : 729
56. Sprent J (1994) T and B cell memory. Cell 76 : 315
57. Stevenson FK, Zhu D, King CA, Ashworth LJ, Kumar S, Thompsett A, Hawkins RE (1995) A genetic approach to idiotypic vaccination for B cell lymphoma. Ann NY Acad Sci 772 : 209
58. Streilein JW (1991) Neonatal tolerance of H-2 allantigens. Transplantation 52 : 1
59. Tang D, DeVit M, Johnston SA (1992) Genetic immunization is a simple method for eliciting an immune response. Nature 356 : 152
60. Ulmer JB, Donnelly JJ, Parker SE, Rhodes GH, Felgner PL, Dwarki VJ, Gromkowski SH, Deck RR, DeWitt CM, Friedman A, Hawe LA, Leander KR, Martinez D, Perry HC, Shiver JW, Montgomery DL, Liu MA (1993) Heterologous protection against influenza by injection of DNA encoding a viral protein. Science 259 : 1745
61. Wang B, Ugen KI, Srikantan V, Agadjanyan MG, Dang K, Refaeli Y, Sato AI, Boyer J, Williams WV, Weiner DB (1993) Gene inoculation generates immune responses against immunodeficiency virus type I. Proc Natl Acad Sci USA 90 : 4156
62. Wang Y, Zhiquan X, Pasquini S, Ertl HCJ (1996) Immune responses to neonatal genetic immunization. Virology 228 : 278

63. Webster RG, Fynan EF, Santoro JC, Robinson H (1994) Protection of ferrets against influenza challenge with a DNA vacine to the hemagglutinin. Vaccine 16 : 1495
64. Wiktor TJ, MacFarlan RT, Reagan K, Dietzschold B, Curtis PJ, Wunner WH, Kieny MP, Lathe R, Lecoq JP, Mackett M, Moss B, Koprowski H (1984) Protection from rabies by a vaccinia rabies recombinant containing the rabies virus glycoprotein gene. Proc Natl Acad Sci USA 81 : 7194
65. Wolff JA, Malone RW, Williams P, Chong W, Acsadi G, Jani A, Felgner PL (1990) Direct gene transfer into mouse muscle in vivo. Science 247 : 1465
66. Wolff JA, Ludtke JJ, Ascadi G, Williams P, Jani A (1992) Long-term persistence of plasmid DNA and foreign gene expression in mouse muscle. Hum Mol Genet 1 : 363
67. Xiang ZQ, Spitalnik S, Tran M, Wunner WH, Cheng J, Ertl HCJ (1994) Vaccination with a plasmid vector carrying the rabies virus glycoprotein gene induces protective immunity against rabies virus. Virology 199 : 132
68. Xiang ZQ, Spitalnik L, Cheng J, Erikson J, Wojczyk B, Ertl HCJ (1995) Immune responses to nucleic acid vaccines to rabies virus. Virology 209 : 569
69. Xiang ZQ, Yang Y, Wilson JM, Ertl HCJ (1996) A replication-defective human adenovirus recombinant serves as a highly efficacious vaccine carrier. Virology 219 : 220
70. Xy D, Liew FY (1994) Genetic vaccination against leishmaniasis. Vaccine 12 : 1534
71. Yamamoto S, Yamamoto T, Kataoka T, Kuramoto E, Yano O, Tokinaga T (1992) Unique palindromic sequences in synthetic oligonucleotides are required to induce IFN and augment IFN-mediated natural killer cell activity. J Immunol 148 : 4072
72. Yakaukas MA, Marrow JE, Parker SE, Abai A, Rhoes GH, Dwarki VJ, Gromkowski SH (1993) Long-term anti-nucleoprotein cellular and humoral immunity is induced by intramuscular injection of plasmid DNA containing NP gene. DNA Cell Biol 12 : 771
73. Yang Y, Li Q, Ertl HCJ, Wilson JW (1995) Cellular and humoral immune responses to viral antigens create barriers to lung-directed gene therapy with recombinant adenoviruses. J Virol 69 : 2004
74. Yokoyama M, Zhang J, Whitton JL, (1995) DNA immunization confers protection against lethal lymphocytic choriomeningitis infection. J Virol 69 : 2684

MIX
Papier aus verantwortungsvollen Quellen
Paper from responsible sources
FSC® C105338

FSC
www.fsc.org

If you have any concerns about our products,
you can contact us on
ProductSafety@springernature.com

In case Publisher is established outside the EU,
the EU authorized representative is:
Springer Nature Customer Service Center GmbH
Europaplatz 3, 69115 Heidelberg, Germany

Printed by Libri Plureos GmbH
in Hamburg, Germany